# Brain Insults in Infants and Childr
# Pathophysiology and Managem

# Brain Insults in Infants and Children: Pathophysiology and Management

Edited by

Hector E. James, M.D.

*Associate Professor of Neurosurgery and Pediatrics*
*School of Medicine*
*University of California*
*San Diego, California*

Nick G. Anas, M.D.

*Assistant Professor of Pediatrics*
*Division Critical Care Medicine*
*University of California, Irvine*
*Irvine, California*

Ronald M. Perkin, M.D.

*Assistant Professor of Pediatrics*
*University of California, Irvine;*
*Director of Pediatric Intensive Care*
*Children's Hospital of Orange County*
*Irvine, California*

G&S

GRUNE & STRATTON, INC.

(Harcourt Brace Jovanovich, Publishers)

Orlando San Diego New York
London Toronto Montreal Sydney Tokyo

**Library of Congress Cataloging in Publication Data**
Main entry under title:

Brain insults in infants and children.

Includes index.
1. Brain—Wounds and injuries—Complications and sequelae. 2. Pediatric neurology. I. James, H. E. II. Anas, Nicholas G. III. Perkin, Ronald M. [DNLM: 1. Brain Injuries—in infancy & childhood. 2. Brain Injuries—therapy. WS 340 B814]
RD594.B73 1985 617'.481044 85-939
ISBN 0-8089-1723-4



*Grune & Stratton, Inc.*
*Orlando, FL 32887*

Distributed in the United Kingdom by
*Grune & Stratton, Ltd.*
*24/28 Oval Road, London NW 1*

Library of Congress Catalog Number 85-939
International Standard Book Number 0-8089-1723-4

Printed in the United States of America
85 86 87 88 10 9 8 7 6 5 4 3 2 1

# Contents

# Preface

The management of brain insults from its onset is one of the most complex and difficult health care problems in existence today. There have been tremendous strides in research—both from the experimental and clinical standpoint. Diagnosis and various therapeutic modalities have grown dramatically over the past decade.

An even greater challenge in the health care of acute brain insults in infants, children, and adolescents is that the primary physician, nurse, and allied health care personnel caring for the child have had limited training in the neurosciences. Pediatricians, family practice physicians, nurses, and nurse practitioners are not significantly trained in any neuroscience specialties. Consequently, there is a dichotomy in the health care delivery of children. There is no question that the first person coming into contact with the brain dysfunctional child is a pediatrician. The assessment, decision-making, and initial therapy will be performed according to his or her level of expertise. In acute brain insults, the initial therapy is the one that determines the outcome.

It is the aim of *Brain Insults in Infants and Children: Pathophysiology and Management* to enhance the neuroscientific knowledge of the primary caretakers of infants, children, and adolescents with brain injury. Although this book does not present a complete analysis of neuroscience, neuroimaging, and the therapeutic facets of brain insults, we hope it may help the reader to better understand underlying physiopathology in acute therapy decisions.

# Contributors

**Nick G. Anas, M.D.** Assistant Professor of Pediatrics, Division Critical Care Medicine, University of California, Irvine, California

**Alex Baethmann, M.D.** Professor, Institute for Surgical Research, Ludwig-Maximilians University, Munich, West Germany

**Raul Bejar, M.D.** Associated Physician, Division of Perinatal/Neonatal Medicine, Department of Pediatrics, School of Medicine, University of California, San Diego, California

**Derek A. Bruce, M.D., Ch.B.** Associate Professor of Neurosurgery and Pediatrics, School of Medicine, University of Pennsylvania, Philadelphia, Pennsylvania

**Ronald Coen, M.D.** Associate Professor, Division of Perinatal/Neonatal Medicine, Department of Pediatrics, School of Medicine, University of California, San Diego, California

**Hector E. James, M.D.** Associate Professor of Neurosurgery and Pediatrics, Division of Neurosurgery, School of Medicine, University of California, San Diego, California

**Martin Jansen, M.D.** Institute of Surgical Research, Ludwig-Maximilians University, Munich, West Germany

**Oliver Kempski, M.D.** Institute of Surgical Research, Ludwig-Maximilians University, Munich, West Germany

**Thomas G. Luerssen, M.D.** Assistant Professor, Neurosurgery and Pediatrics, Division of Neurosurgery, University of California Medical Center, San Diego, California

**J. Gordon McComb, M.D.** Associate Professor of Neurological Surgery, School of Medicine, University of Southern California, Los Angeles, California

**Arno Neu, M.D.** Institute of Surgical Research, Ludwig-Maximilians University, Munich, West Germany

**Robert C. Pascucci, M.D.** Instructor in Anesthesia (Pediatrics), Harvard Medical School, Boston, Massachusetts

**Ronald M. Perkin, M.D.** Assistant Professor of Pediatrics, University of California, Irvine; Director of Pediatric Intensive Care Unit, Children's Hospital of Orange County, Irvine, California

**Mark A. Rockoff, M.D.** Assistant Professor of Anesthesiology and Pediatrics, Associate Director, Multidisciplinary Intensive Care Unit, Children's Hospital, Boston, Massachusetts

**Sylvia Schneider** Institute of Surgical Research, Ludwig-Maximilians University, Munich, West Germany

**Doris A. Trauner, M.D.** Associate Professor, Neurosciences and Pediatrics, Department of Neurosciences, School of Medicine, University of California, San Diego, California

**Andreas Unterberg, M.D.** Institute of Surgical Research, Ludwig-Maximilians University, Munich, West Germany

**Friedirich F. von Rosen, M.D.** Candidate, Institute of Surgical Research, Ludwig-Maximilians University, Munich, West Germany

**Markus Zimmer, M.D.** Institute of Surgical Research, Ludwig-Maximilians University, Munich, West Germany

**Robert A. Zimmerman, M.D.** Professor of Radiology, School of Medicine, University of Pennsylvania, Philadelphia, Pennsylvania

# PART I

# Functional Basics

*Alexander Baethmann*

# 1

# Steroids and Brain Function

Corticosteroid treatment has been attempted in most of the acute or chronic diseases of the central nervous system (CNS), particularly in disorders associated with cerebral edema; however, it is a common clinical experience that the therapeutic efficiency of corticosteroids varies. Brain edema developing slowly as in a chronic process, such as a cerebral tumor or an abscess is more susceptible to treatment with steroids than is acute edema resulting from head injury or cerebral infarction, where the administration of these compounds appears to be less satisfying.[8,33,41]

Figure 1-1 summarizes schematically the efficiency of corticosteroids in various cerebral processes, such as metastases, cerebral tumors, and head injury. Few clinical studies of head injury or cerebral ischemia have demonstrated a clear benefit of steroids. Nevertheless, clinicians continue to employ these compounds for treatment, although they maintain a certain skepticism about its rationale. Corticosteroids are also considered an attractive form of treatment for acute cerebral disorders probably because their therapeutic potential has been more clearly established under respective experimental conditions than is possible in the clinical situation. Certainly, the therapeutic efficiency of these drugs is far more difficult to evaluate in the complex clinical situation, where many factors influence outcome, such as onset and quality of first aid on the scene, the time interval between the acute (ischemic, or traumatic) insult and its diagnosis and finite treatment, and the efficiency of intensive care. A purpose of this chapter is to provide insight into the different physiological functions of this interesting group of drugs in the normal brain, which may help to understand steroid mechanisms in the diseased brain.

BRAIN INSULTS IN INFANTS AND CHILDREN
0-8089-1723-4

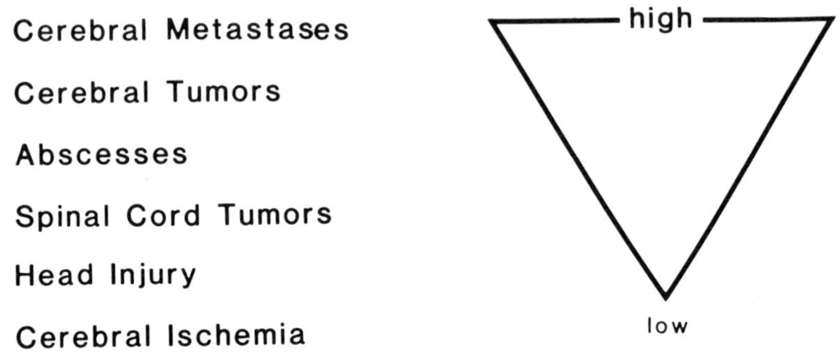


**Fig. 1-1.** Schematic representation of the efficiency of corticosteroids in the treatment of different, acute, and chronic cerebral processes associated with cerebral edema. From Reulen HJ, Hadjidimos A, Hase U: Steroids in the treatment of brain edema. Adv Neurosurg 1:105, 1973. With permission.

## BIOCHEMICAL PATHWAYS MEDIATING STEROID MECHANISMS IN THE CNS

First, let us consider why steroid molecules are also suitable messengers of biological signals for the brain. The CNS is a particularly appropriate target[27] because of the richness of lipids, making it easy for steroid compounds to cross the blood–brain barrier and reach the receptor sites. Steroid receptors are *intracellular* binding proteins, in contrast to the extracellular structural receptors of peptide hormones, for example, or transmitter compounds localized on the external surface of cell membranes.[16,27] Cerebral tissue, like other organs, has highly specific, intracellular receptors for glucocorticosteroids and mineralocorticosteroids and for other steroids, such as the sexual hormones.[2,35] Binding of steroids in cerebral tissue may result in an accumulation of these substances 20–30 times the concentration present in plasma.[51] The high-affinity binding proteins for the different steroids provide the steroid action with the required degree of specificity. There is, in fact, a close correlation between the affinity of different steroids for their intracellular receptor and the physiological efficiency.[16]

It is generally accepted now that steroid hormones exert biological effects by entertaining distinct biochemical pathways. The receptor–steroid complex is attached to the chromatin of the cell nucleus, leading to de novo synthesis of RNA and, subsequently, of proteins, finally resulting in the physiological expression of the steroid-specific effect in the cell or organ (Fig. 1-2). Many observations, including those of the brain, suggest that steroid mechanisms in a tissue are mediated through the synthesis of enzymes.[4,14,20]

The sequence of molecular-biological reactions initiated by steroids has

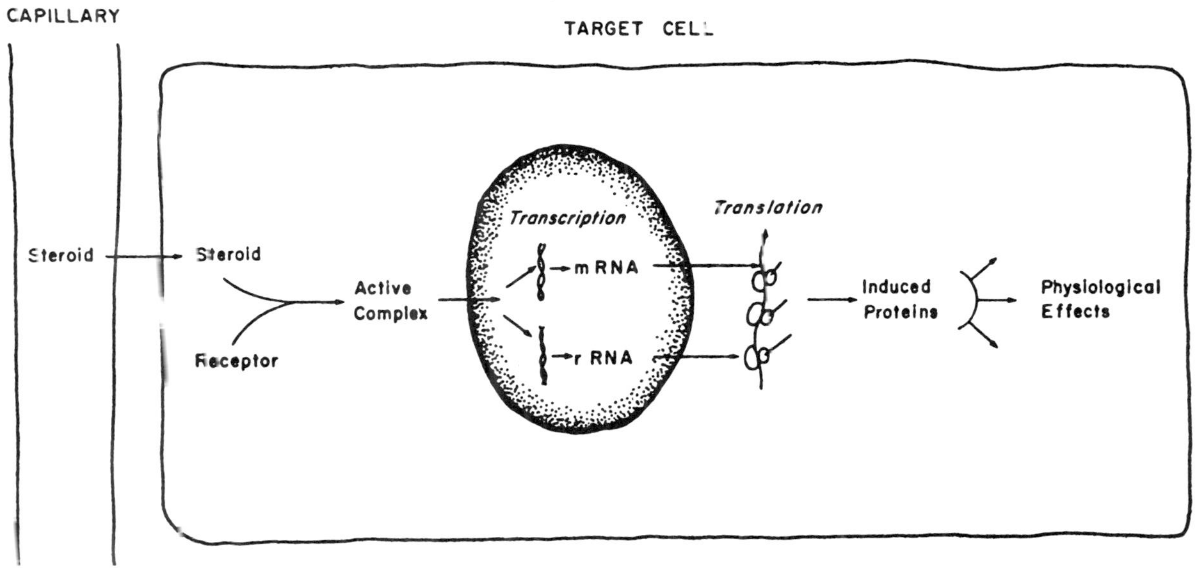


**Fig. 1-2.** Molecular-biological pathway of de novo synthesis of enzymes via intracellular penetration of the steroid compound, formation of the activated steroid–receptor complex in the cytosol, attachment to the nuclear chromatin, and activation of de novo RNA synthesis and translation into proteins. The proteins induced are enzymes of the intermediary and transmitter metabolism or are involved in membrane transport and provide the biochemical basis for the physiological expression of steroids in the cell, organ, and organism. From Edelman IS, Mechanism of action of steroid hormones. J Steroid Biochem 6:148, 1975. With permission.

been fairly well understood. Information is missing, however, on how the final physiological and biochemical effects in cells, organs, and the total oganism are mediated. There is also insufficient information on the effects of steroid mechanisms on electrical activity of nerve cells or the entire brain and on behavioral aspects and mental function.[13,18] Moreover, our ignorance of steroid mechanisms also includes the therapeutic efficiency of these drugs in pathophysiological conditions ranging from epilepsy to cerebral edema. It is also not clear why steroids of the same species, which differ in only minor chemical details, such as methylprednisolone and dexamethasone, have different effects on behavior, electroencephalogram (EEG) activity, and so on.[24]

## STEROIDS AND CEREBRAL DEVELOPMENT

Steroids have been shown to affect CNS development. Vernadakis and Woodbury[47] have shown that cortisol, the physiologically occurring glucocorticosteroid in humans, accelerates brain maturation, as studied by the CNS response to electrical stimulation. Control of cerebral development by steroids is not homogeneously exerted, however, but varies with the phase of brain growth. A parameter for analysis of this effect is the induction of enzymes, such as tyrosine hydroxylase, or dopamine $\beta$-hydroxylase by nerve growth factor (NGF), which in rat sympathetic ganglia is enhanced by glucocorticosteroids.[38] These findings may relate with the observation that a steroid compound (i.e. $\beta$-estradiol, but not testosterone, hydrocortisone or aldosterone) stimulates the formation of nerve growth factor by glial cells.[39]

Puro[40] studied the effect of glucorticosteroids on the control of synaptic development in a retina-muscle cell culture system. In this model the author found that the hormone accelerated the maturation of the stimulus-evoked transmitter release, suggesting steroids tune the coupling of nerve cell depolarization with transmitter release.

It is important to distinguish between physiological and pharmacological effects of steroids on CNS development. Glucocorticosteroids may suppress somatic growth by inhibition of cell proliferation. Administration of corticosteroids in a dose only 2–3 times that normally produced by endogenous secretion may suffice to suppress somatic growth in children.[29] Growth retardation by steroids may also affect the CNS.[48] Oda and Huttenlocher[36] cite observations that neurological deficits have resulted from steroid administration directly to infants, children, and pregnant women. Treatment of neonatal animals with corticosteroids was found to result in irreversible decrease in weight of the cerebrum. Disturbances of brain growth may be associated with long-term functional deficits, such as spontaneous locomotor activity, which may occur after even relatively small doses of cortisol. The authors conducted experimental studies in rats 6–12 days after birth. Treatment with excessive doses of methylprednisolone (i.e., 60–80 mg/kg body weight) resulted in a decrease of the number of dendritic branches in layers 3 and 5 of the cerebral cortex a few weeks later. The number of intersections and terminations of the dendritic processes decreased as well.[36] Shapiro et al[44] found retardation of growth of visual cortex dendritic spines in neonatal rats receiving cortisol.

## INDUCTION OF ENZYMES IN CEREBRAL TISSUE BY CORTICOSTEROIDS

De novo synthesis of enzymes involved in the intermediary metabolism of the cell probably is an essential step for the physiological expression of steroids in an organ.[20] This is also valid for CNS tissue. Metabolic effects through induction of enzymes may explain earlier observations on cerebral blood flow and metabolism following adrenalectomy. Glycerolphosphate dehydrogenase is a classical example. The enzyme is regulated by corticosteroids in almost all cerebral areas of the hemispheres, cerebellum, and brainstem, whereas it is not responsive in peripheral tissues, such as liver or muscle.[12] Control of brain tissue metabolism by steroids is not restricted to this enzyme, but involves a spectrum of cystolic, mitochondrial, and membrane-bound enzymes, including glutamate oxaloacetate transaminase (GOT), glutamate dehydrogenase, glutamate synthetase—an enzyme probably involved in the control of normal extracellular glutamate levels, sodium-potassium adenosinetriphosphatase ($Na^+$-$K^+$-ATPase), and other enzymes.[4,11,34,45]

Baethmann and Van Harreveld[4] have reported that corticosteroid deprivation by adrenalectomy in experimental animals (rats) causes a significant decrease in activity of NADP-dependent isocitric dehydrogenase, glutamate dehydrogenase, and GOT in the brain. If the adrenalectomized animals were substituted with either aldosterone (100 $\mu$g/kg body weight), or dexamethasone (400 $\mu$g/kg body weight), respectively, the activity of these enzymes increased significantly in the cerebral cortex (Fig. 1-3). These finding may have a bearing on the therapeutical function of steroids in cerebral edema. Concurrent studies have demonstrated that adrenalectomy of animals without substitution causes a significant increase of the cerebral water and $Na^+$ content, which could be prevented by corticosteroid administration. (Fig. 1-4).[4] It is noteworthy in this context that not only glucocorticosteroids but also mineralocorticosteroids were effective in preventing disturbances of the cerebral electrolyte- and water content, as well as the decrease of the specific enzyme activities of the citric acid cycle (Figs. 1-3 and 1-4).

Sodium potassium ATPase is an important enzyme of the cellular plasma membrane because it is involved in the control of the intra- and extracellular electrolyte- and fluid distribution. Corticosteroids, such as cortisol, or methyl-

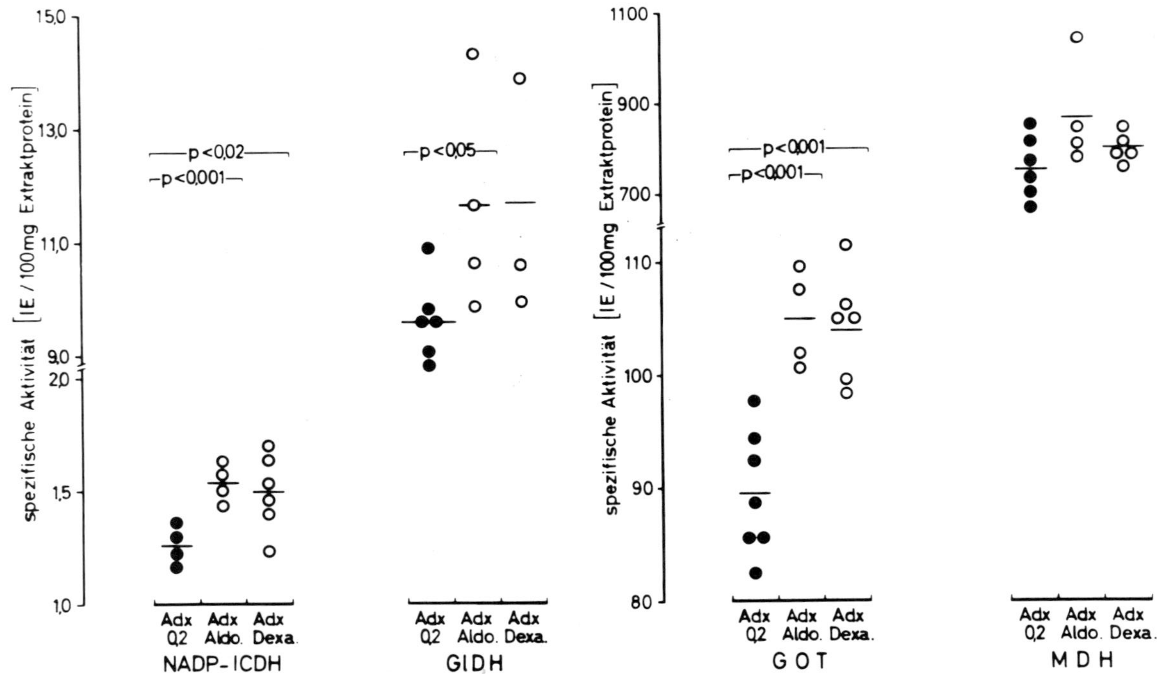


**Fig. 1-3.** Activity of different Krebs cycle enzymes studied in the gray matter of adrenalectomized rats with and without daily administration of aldosterone (100 $\mu$g/kg) or dexamethasone (400 $\mu$g/kg). Adrenalectomized animals received 0.2 percent NaCl as drinking fluid to replace losses of $Na^+$ through urinary excretion. Both aldosterone and dexamethasone substitution led to a significant increase of the specific activity of NADP-dependent isocitric dehydrogenase, glutamate dehydrogenase, and GOT. Malate dehydrogenase (MDH) was not affected. From Baethmann A, Van Harreveld A: Physiological and biochemical findings in the central nervous system of adrenalectomized rats and mice, in Reulen HJ, Schurmann K (Eds): Steroids and Brain Edema. Berlin, Springer, 1972, p 201. With permission.

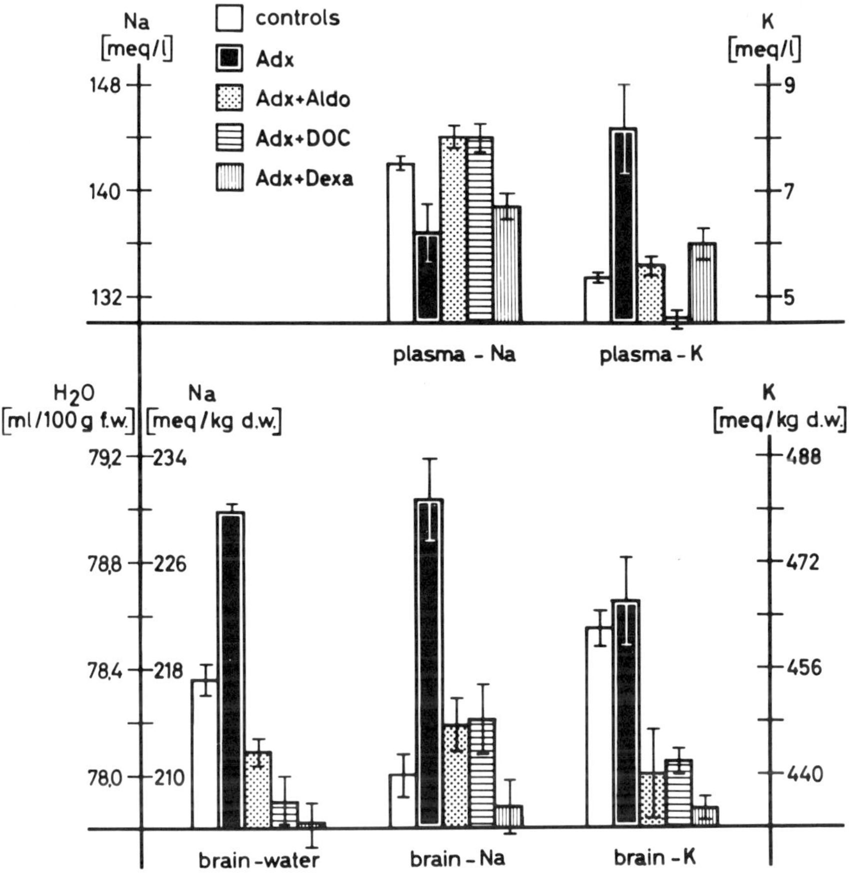


**Fig. 1-4.** Cerebral water and electrolytes (ml/100 g fresh weight, mEq/kg dry weight, respectively) of adrenalectomized animals with and without steroid substitution. The corresponding $Na^+$ and $K^+$ concentrations of plasma are also given, demonstrating the inverse change of plasma $Na^+$ and $K^+$ in adrenal insufficiency and normalization by steroid substitution. Intact controls are shown for comparison. Adrenalectomized animals without steroid substitution had a significant increase of the cerebral water and sodium content (black bars), which was completely prevented by simultaneous administration of the different corticosteroids. Completeness of adrenalectomy was tested prior to substitution by a water retention test. From Baethmann A, Van Harreveld A: Physiological and biochemical findings in the central nervous system of adrenalectomized rats and mice, in Reulen HJ, Schurmann K (Eds): Steroids and Brain Edema. Berlin, Springer, 1972, p 201. With permission.

prednisolone induce the enzyme in cerebral tissue. Stastny[45] has considered the control of ATPase activity by steroids through the classical pathways involving de novo synthesis, whereas Braughler and Hall[11] suggest alternative mechanisms in addition. Within 5 minutes, intravenous (IV) methylprednisolone led to a twofold rise of activity of synaptosomal $Na^+$-$K^+$-ATPase, which might be too short a time period for enzyme induction. The authors suggest a direct effect on the enzyme activity in situ. This conclusion is supported by the observation that the time course of activation and deactivation of $Na^+$-$K^+$-ATPase closely followed the accumulation and subsequent disappearance of methylprednisolone in the tissue. Steroids are considered to interfere with a functional inhibition of ATPase by lipid peroxides.[11] Cerebral glutamine synthetase is exclusively localized in astrocytes[31] and is also regulated by corticosteroids.[23,34] Induction of the enzyme by corticosteroids has been studied in chick retina, cerebral hemispheres, and cultures of glial cells.[23,26] Glutamine synthetase catalyzes formation of glutamine from glutamate. This is an important step for the inactivation of glutamic acid following its extracellular release during synaptic excitation and uptake into perisynaptic glial elements. Inactivation of extracellular glutamate obviously has a high biological priority, as inferred from the energy expenditure involved in its uphill transport into glial cells, taking along sodium ions, and subsequent metabolization requiring 1 mole of ATP per mole of glutamine formed.[10] Release of glutamate leading to excessive extracellular accumulation occurs under pathophysiological conditions, such as cerebral ischemia and traumatic insults and is considered as a mechanism of secondary cytotoxic cell swelling.[7,28,30] High concentrations of glutamate in the extracellular space increase membrane permeability for $Na^+$ ions.[1,37] This, in turn, causes an intracellular influx of $Na^+$ ions together with $Cl^-$ and water. Treatment of cerebral edema with steroid compounds, among others, may result in an enhanced inactivation of glutamate by induction of glutamine synthetase.

Global aspects of cerebral metabolism influenced by steroids pertain to the cerebral oxygen uptake and glucose consumption.[51] Baethmann et al[6] observed acute adrenalectomy in dogs without steroid substitution to significantly decrease cerebral blood flow and metabolism, which was reversed by substitution with either aldosterone, or dexamethasone, respectively (Fig. 1-5). Activation of the cerebral energy metabolism by steroids may support resolution of cerebral edema from the cerebral tissue by enhancing clearance of both extra- and intracellular fluid accumulation.

## EFFECTS OF STEROIDS ON ELECTROPHYSIOLOGICAL FUNCTION IN CNS TISSUE

Since disorders of the adrenal cortex have been recognized as pathological entites, either hyper- or hypofunction of the organ is known to influence

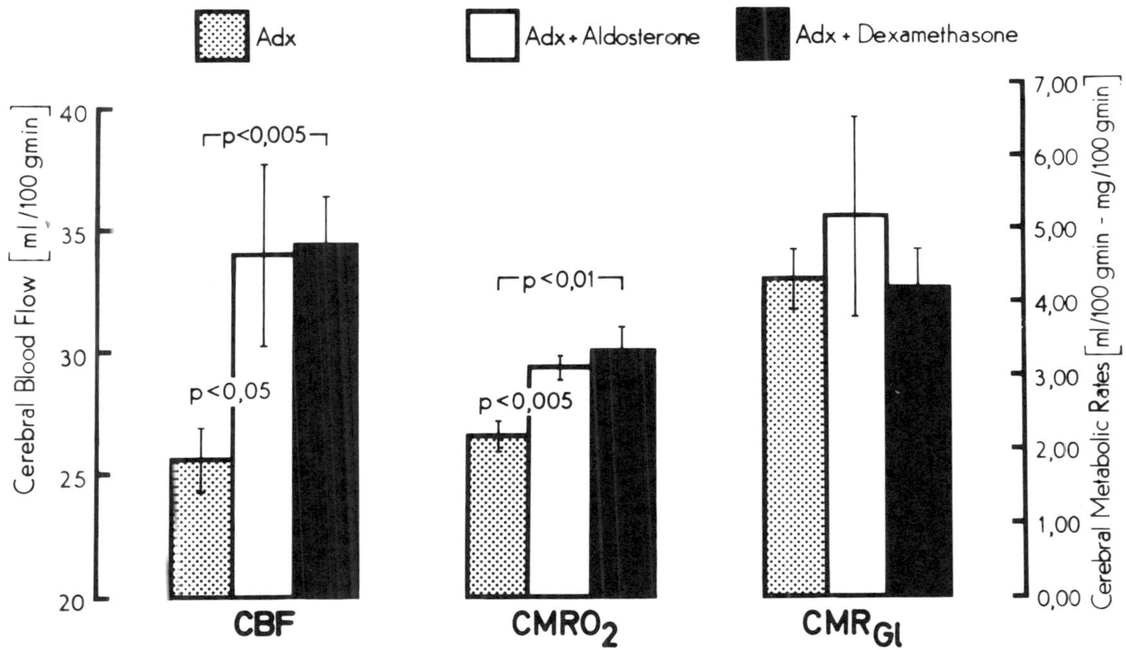


**Fig. 1-5.** Cerebral blood flow, cerebral oxygen, and glucose consumption of adrenalectomized dogs without steroid substitution, and acutely (3 hours) after intra-arterial administration of aldosterone or dexamethasone (0.2 mg/kg body weight), respectively. Adrenalectomy led to a significant decrease of cerebral blood flow which was markedly improved within hours after administration of either aldosterone or dexamethasone. From Baethmann A, Oettinger W, Chaussy L, et al: Corticosteroid effects on cerebral blood flow and metabolism; a potential mechanism in brain edema. Acta Neural Scand 60, Suppl 72:371, 1979. With permission.

CNS function and mental behavior. Addison's disease may be associated with depression, anxiety, apathy, and other symptoms, whereas adrenocortical hyperfunction in Cushing's syndrome may induce psychotic behavior or mania, but also depression, mental irritability, agitation, anxiety, and noncooperative behavior.[9,51] Apathy and mental depression, found in adrenocortical insufficiency, might reflect underlying metabolic and blood flow conditions of the brain, whereas states of mental irritability and excitation evolving in hyperfunction or following excessive steroid administration would agree with an experimently assessed enhancement of susceptibility of the brain to seizures following electrical or chemical stimulation.[50]

The situation is more complex, however, since adrenal insufficiency is also associated with enhanced seizure susceptibility either electrically or audiogenically induced, or by insulin or water intoxication. Steroid deprivation results in a slow-wave activity (2–6 Hz) and high voltage EEG and a decrease of the dominant frequency. Conversely, ACTH and corticosteroids may also induce slow-wave activity (4–7 Hz) and high-voltage amplitudes in humans and experimental animals and increases hyperventilation.[51] Electroencephalographic abnormalities in epileptic patients can be enhanced by ACTH or cortisone.[21] On the other hand, IV dexamethasone was reported by Matsuoka et al.[32] to reduce delta activity in patients with malignant or metastatic brain tumors, which was attributed to an amelioration of cerebral edema.

In general, studies on cerebral administration of steroids by intraventricular injection suggest enhancement, rather than depression, of excitability. After infusion of 1.5 mg of cortisol into different cerebral tissue areas, Feldman observed the hippocampus to be mostly susceptible as seen from high-voltage spikes and epileptic discharges.[19] The hypothalamus and the midbrain reticular formation were less sensitive. Studies of evoked potentials secondary to stimulation of the sciatic nerve demonstrated a marked increase of the amplitude in the medial lemniscus, midbrain reticular formation, and thalamic nuclei. Furthermore, nerve cells of the posterior hypothalamus and other areas markedly enhanced spontaneous firing after steroid administration.[18] Similar effects, however, such as an increase of single cell discharge, were also provoked by steroid deprivation, making the function of steroids in electrophysiological processes difficult to evaluate.[18]

Modification of the cerebral excitability by steroids or, conversely, by steroid deprivation (adrenalectomy) has also been observed.[46] The authors studied normal and adrenalectomized animals during exposure to an ambient oxygen pressure of 6 ata [1 technical atmosphere (of absolute pressure)]. The latency until appearance of electrical discharges was taken as a measure of excitability. Surprisingly, high oxygen pressure was better tolerated in adrenalectomized animals than in controls early after steroid deprivation, whereas increased duration of adrenal insufficiency resulted in enhanced excitability of the brain.[46] Taken together, complex and differentiated modifications of the nerve cell function by steroids must be assumed, rather than gross increase in CNS excitability or decrease by steroid deprivation, respectively. This is also supported by the more recent studies of Avanzino et al.,[3] who administered cortisol or corticosterone per microelectrophoresis to single neurons of the reticular formation in the brainstem. An excitatory nerve cell activity was found in 26 percent, inhibition was observed in 15 percent, whereas no effect was observed in 60 percent of the nerve cell population. Caudal areas of the reticular formation had a predominantly excitatory response, whereas inhibition prevailed in rostral areas.[3]

## STEROID EFFECTS ON SPINAL CORD AND NEUROMUSCULAR JUNCTION

Respective observations have been made concerning spinal cord injury and miniature endplate potential (MEPPs) at the neuromuscular synapse. The administration of steroids was reported to preserve function of the nerve fibers following cross section of the spinal cord.[22] Respective studies were based on earlier observations that glucocorticosteroids have a potency to enhance excitability and facilitatory functions of motor axons.[42] In studies by Hall et al.,[22] adult cats received triamcinolone [8 mg/kg body weight intramuscularly (IM) per day] for 1 week to analyze segmental spinal reflexes after cord section at C1. The function of the segmental reflex pathways was studied at the ventral root of L7. Animals receiving triamcinolone for 7 days had markedly improved monosynaptic responses after stimulation of a peripheral nerve, as compared to the controls. Hall et al.[22] suggest that steroids act on the primary afferent terminals by increasing the responsiveness and the release of transmitter compounds upon stimulation.

The preservation of nerve fibers after sectioning is also supported by the morphological studies by Drakontides,[15] who observed the degenerative changes of the motor nerve terminals of rat diaphragm to be less severe and to develop more slowly in animals receiving triamcinolone. Degeneration of nerve terminals following cord sectioning without treatment is associated with swelling and disruption of mitochondria, loss of synaptic vesicles, and formation of vacuoles and dense bodies.[15] The nerve terminals later become fragmented, disappear, and are replaced by Schwann cells. Although steroids cannot prevent this process, they markedly reduce its severity and increase the time interval until degeneration is complete.[15]

Beneficial effects of corticosteroids in neuromuscular diseases, such as myasthenia gravis, are usually attributed to an influence of the underlying immunological process, but rarely to direct effects on the neuromuscular junction. Experimental studies support the latter, nevertheless. Wilson et al.[49] analyzed MEPP frequency as a measure of random liberation of acetylcholine at the neuromuscular synapse (i.e., motor endplate). Prednisolone (0.5 mM or higher) led to MEPP increase of up to 2 times what was found under control conditions, together with a simultaneous decrease of MEPP amplitude. Removal of prednisolone was found to result in normalization of the MEPPs.[49] The authors consider such an effect on the neuromuscular junction instrumental in the therapeutic efficiency of steroids in myasthenia gravis.

The effect of steroids on transmitter metabolism in cerebral tissue may contribute to the enhancement of excitability and preservation of function in degenerating nerve terminals. Cortisol given acutely or chronically raises concentrations of excitatory aminoacids in the brain but decreases $\gamma$-aminobutyric acid (GABA) and glutamine. Desoxycorticosterone acetate (DOC), a predominantly mineral active steroid, has the opposite effect.[51] Woodbury[51] considers the glutamate:glutamine concentration ratio to reflect the state of excitability. The ratio is increased following cortisol treatment. The increased excitability by glucocorticosteroids may also be attributed to the increased availability of excitatory transmitters, such as glutamate and a decrease of inhibitory transmitters, such as GABA. Subsequent steps, finally leading to the electrophysiological, or even more complex behavioral phenomenal expression of steroid mechanisms (excitation, increased responsiveness of the neuromuscular junction, psychoses, depression, etc.), are not yet understood on a cell physiological basis. Quantitative aspects of the actual steroid doses and concentrations at different cerebral targets are undoubtedly of importance and require the differentiation of physiological steroid functions from pharmacological, or even toxicological, side effects. Table 1-1

**Table 1-1** *Physiological and Biochemical Mechanisms of Corticosteroids in the Central Nervous System**

- Influence of nerve cell activity in distinct cerebral areas; lowering of the seizure threshold to electrical or chemical stimulation
- Increase of excitatory transmitter concentrations and release
- Enhanced sensitivity to barbiturates by steroid deprivation
- De novo synthesis of enzymes, e.g., $Na^+ - K^+$ –ATPase, glycerol phosphate dehydrogenase, glutamine synthetase, citric acid cycle enzymes
- Influence of intermediary and transmitter metabolism
- Stimulation of $O_2$ and glucose consumption
- Modification of CSF formation and absorption
- Normalization of blood–brain barrier permeability in pathophysiological conditions

*From Baethman A, Grossman R, Terapie dis ischämischen Hirnödems, in Paal G. (Ed.): Treatment of Cerebral Ischemia. Edition Medizin, Verlag Chemie GmbH, 1984, pp. 370–427. With permission.

contains additional mechanisms suggested to be modified by steroids, such as permeability of the blood–brain barrier, cerebral spinal fluid (CSF) formation and absorption, and sensitivity to barbiturates. The reader is referred to the respective literature.[5,17,25,43]

### Acknowledgments

This work was supported by Deutsche Forschungsgemeinschaft: Ba 452/6-5. Invaluable assistance for the preparation of the manuscript was provided by Ruth Demmer, Friederike Helmes, and Ulrike Goerke.

### REFERENCES

1. Ames A, Tsukada Y, Nesbett FB: Intracellular $Cl^-$, $Na^+$, $K^+$, $Ca^{++}$, $Mg^{++}$ and P in nervous tissue; response to glutamate and to changes in extracellular calcium. J Neurochem 14:145–159, 1967
2. Anderson NS, Fanestil DD: Corticoid receptors in rat brain: Evidence for an aldosterone receptor. Endocrinology 98:676–684, 1976
3. Avanzino GL, Celasco G, Cogo CE, et al: Actions of microelectrophoretically applied glucocorticoid hormones on reticular formation neurones in the rat. Neurosci Lett 38:45–49, 1983
4. Baethmann A, Van Harreveld A: Physiological and biochemical findings in the central nervous system of adrenalectomized rats and mice, in Reulen HJ, Schurmann K (Eds): Steroids and Brain Edema. Berlin, Springer, 1972, pp 195–202
5. Baethmann A: Treatment of cerebral edema with steroid compounds, in Addison GM, et al., (Eds): Aldosterone Antagonists in Clinical Medicine. Amsterdam Oxford, Excerpta Medica, 1978, pp 386–392
6. Baethmann A, Oettinger W, Chaussy L, et al.: Corticosteroid effects on cerebral blood flow and metabolism; a potential mechanism in brain edema. Acta Neurol Scand 60, Suppl 72:370–371, 1979
7. Baethmann A, Oettinger W, Rothenfusser W, et al.: Brain edema factors: Current state with particular reference to plasma constituents and glutamate. Adv Neurol 28:171–195, 1980.
8. Baethmann A, Grossmann R: Terapie des ischämischen Hirnödems, in Paal G (Hrsg): Die Therapie der zerebralen Durchblutungsstorungen, Weinheim, Verlag Chemie GmbH, Edition Medizin, 1984, pp 370–427.
9. Baxter JD, Forsham PH: Tissue effects of glucocorticoids. Am J Med 53:573–589, 1972
10. Benjamin AM, Quastel JH: Fate of glutamate in the brain. J Neurochem 23:457–464, 1974
11. Braughler JM, Hall ED: Acute enhancement of spinal cord synaptosomal $(Na^+ + K^+)$-ATPase activity in cats following intravenous methylprednisolone. Brain Res 219:464–469, 1981
12. Breen GAM, De Vellis J: Regulation of glycerol phosphate dehydrogenase by hydrocortisone in rat brain explants. Exp Cell Res 91:159–169, 1975
13. Carpenter WT, Gruen PH: Cortisol's effects on human mental functioning. J Clin Psychopharmacol 2:91–101, 1982
14. De Vellis J, Inglish D: Hormonal control of glycerol phosphate dehydrogenase in the rat brain. J Neurochem 15:1061–1070, 1968
15. Drakontides AB: The effect of glucocorticoid treatment on denervated rat hemidiaphragm. Brain Res 239:175–189, 1982
16. Edelman IS: Mechanism of action of steroid hormones. J Steroid Biochem 6:147–159, 1975

17. Eisenberg HM, Barlow CF, Lorenzo AV: Effect of dexamethasone on altered brain vascular permeability. Arch Neurol 23:18–22, 1970
18. Feldman S, Dafny N: Effects of adrenocortical hormones on the electrical activity of the brain. Progr Brain Res 32:90–100, 1970
19. Feldman S: Electrical activity of the brain following cerebral microinfusion of cortisol. Epilepsia 12:249–262, 1971
20. Fimognari GM, Porter GA, Edelman IS: The role of the tricarboxylic acid cycle in the action of aldosterone on sodium transport. Biochem Biophys Acta 135:89–99, 1967
21. Glaser GH, Merritt HH: Effects of corticotropin (ACTH) and cortisone on disorders of the nervous system. JAMA 148:898–904, 1952
22. Hall ED, Baker T, Riker WF: Glucocorticoid effects on spinal cord function. J Pharmacol Exp Ther 206:361–370, 1978
23. Hallermayer K, Harmening CH, Hamprecht B: Cellular localization and regulation of glutamine synthetase in primary cultures of brain cells from newborn mice. J Neurochem 37:43–52, 1981.
24. James HE: Effects of steroids on behavior, electrophysiology, water content and intracranial pressure in cerebral cytotoxic edema. Pharmacol Biochem Behav 9:653–657, 1978
25. Johnston I, Gilay DL, Hendrick EB: Experimental effects of steroids and steroid withdrawal on cerebrospinal fluid absorption. J Neurosurg 42:690–695, 1975
26. Juurlink B, Schousboe A, Jorgensen O, et al: Induction by hydrocortisone of glutamine synthetase in mouse primary astrocyte cultures. J Neurochem 36:136–142, 1981
27. Karlson P: Why are so many hormones steroids? Hoppe-Seyler's Z Physiol Chem 364:1067–1087, 1983
28. Kempski O, Gross U. Baethmann A: An in vitro model of cytotoxic brain edema: Cell volume and metabolism of cultivated glial- and nerve-cells. Adv Neurosurg 10:254–258, 1982
29. Loeb JN: Corticosteroids and growth. New Engl J Med 295:547–552, 1976
30. Maier-Hauff K, Lange M, Schurer L, et al: Glutamate and free fatty acid concentrations in extracellular vasogenic edema fluid, in Go KG, Baethmann A (Eds): Recent Progress in the Study and Therapy of Brain Edema. New York, Plenum Press, 1984, pp 183–192
31. Martinez-Hernandez A, Bell KP, Norenberg MD: Glutamine synthetase: Glial localization in brain. Science 195:1356–1358, 1977
32. Matsuoka S, Arakaki Y, Numaguchi K, et al: The effect of dexamethasone on electroencephalograms in patients with brain tumors. J Neurosurg 48:601–608, 1978
33. Maxwell RE, Long DM, French LA: The clinical effects of a synthetic glucocorticoid used for brain edema in the practice of neurosurgery, in Reulen HJ, Schurmann K (Eds): Steroids and Brain Edema. Berlin, Springer, 1972, pp 219–232
34. Moscona AA, Piddington R: Stimulation by hydrocortisone of premature changes in the developmental pattern of glutamine synthetase in embryonic retina. Biochim Biophys Acta 121:409–411, 1966
35. McEwen BS, Weiss JM, Schwartz LS: Uptake of corticosterone by rat brain and its concentration by certain limbic structures. Brain Res 16:227–241, 1969
36. Oda MAS, Huttenlocher PR: The effect of corticosteroids on dendritic development in the rat brain. Yale J Biol Med 3:155–156, 1974
37. Onodera K, Takeuchi A: Permeability changes produced by L-glutamate at the excitatory post-synaptic membrane of the crayfish muscle. J Physiol 255:669–685, 1976
38. Otten U, Thoenen H: Effect of glucocorticoids on nerve growth factor-mediated enzyme induction in organ cultures of rat sympathetic ganglia: Enhanced response and reduced time requirement to initiate enzyme induction. J Neurochem 29:69–75, 1977

39. Perez-Polo JR, Hall K, Livingston K, et al: Steroid induction of nerve growth factor synthesis in cell culture. Life Sci 21:1535–1544, 1977
40. Puro DG: Glucocorticoid regulation of synaptic development. Develop Brain Res 8:283–290, 1983
41. Reulen HJ, Hadjidimos A, Hase U: Steroids in the treatment of brain edema. Adv Neurosurg 1:92–105, 1973
42. Riker WF, Baker T, Okamoto M: Glucocorticoids and mammalian motor nerve excitability. Arch Neurol 32:688–694, 1975
43. Sato O, Hara M, Asai T, et al: The effect of dexamethasone phosphate on the production rate of cerebrospinal fluid in the spinal subarachnoid space of dogs. J Neurosurg 39:480–484, 1973
44. Schapiro S, Vukovich K, Globus A. Effects of neonatal thyroxine and hydrocortisone administration on the development of dendritic spines in the visual cortex of rats. Exp Neurol 40:286–296, 1973
45. Stastny F: Hydrocortisone as a possible inductor of $Na^+$-$K^+$-ATPase in the chick embryo cerebral hemispheres. Brain Res 25:397–410, 1971
46. Torbati ID, Harel D, Lavy S: Excitability of the cortex in normal and adrenalectomized rats during repeated exposures to high oxygen pressure. Aviat Space Environ Med 46:241–243, 1975
47. Vernadakis A, Woodbury DM: Effect of cortisol on the electroshock seizure thresholds in developing rats. J Pharmacol Exp Ther 139:110–113, 1963
48. Weichsel ME: The therapeutic use of glucocorticoid hormones in the perinatal period: Potential neurological hazards. Ann Neurol 2:364–366, 1977
49. Wilson RW, Ward MD, Johns TR: Corticosteroids: A direct effect at the neuromuscular junction. Neurology 24:1091–1095, 1974
50. Woodbury DM, Vernadakis A: Effects of steroids on the central nervous system. Methods Hormone Res 5:1–57, 1966
51. Woodbury DM: Biochemical effects of adrenocortical steroids on the central nervous system, in Lajtha A (Ed): Handbook of Neurochemistry, Vol 7. New York, Plenum, 1972, pp 255–287

*Derek A. Bruce*

# 2

# Concepts of Intracranial Volume and Pressure

The intracranial space, even in the child with an open fontanel and nonfused sutures, can be considered to be fixed to acute changes in volume. It is erroneous to presume that the presence of an open fontanel protects the child against elevated intracranial pressure (ICP). It may add some small extra compensatory volume, but the presence of split sutures and a bulging fontanel denotes elevated ICP, and that compensatory mechanisms have become exhausted.[2]

## THE INTRACRANIAL COMPARTMENTS

Inside the cranium are brain, blood, and cerebrospinal fluid (CSF). Any change in volume of one of these components is compensated for by a reciprocal change in volume in one of the other components. The intracranial volume does not change; it is the balance between the contents that alters. As long as a change in volume is not too great or occurs too quickly, no overall change in pressure takes place. Rapid changes of volume of one intracranial component will produce a rise in pressure that is then partially compensated for by a decrease in one of the other components, and also by the short-lived nature of the change (e.g., coughing). Coughing increases venous volume intracranially. This is compensated for by displacement of CSF into the spinal subarachnoid space, but the ICP still rises. If the venous congestion does not resolve as in a coughing fit, fixed increase in ICP may occur. Cough syncope, for example, is probably the result of the ICP and systemic arterial pressure (SAP) becoming equal and producing a marked decrease in cerebral blood

BRAIN INSULTS IN INFANTS AND CHILDREN
0-8089-1723-4

flow (CBF). Even under normal physiological conditions, therefore, the compensatory mechanisims are not perfect.[1,5,6]

### Cerebrospinal Fluid

The major compensatory mechanism is CSF. This accounts for approximately 10 percent of intracranial volume, which in an adult is approximately 1800–2000 ml. The majority of the CSF is in the subarachnoid spaces of the brain and spinal dural sac, and only 10 percent is in the ventricular system. The ability of the CSF to compensate for the volume changes in other intracranial compartments is dependent on an open subarachnoid space. Once the subarachnoid passages are obstructed (e.g., as in temporal lobe parahippocampal gyrus herniation), an acute decrease in the ability of the CSF to compensate for volume changes will occur. In a clinical setting, this observation implies that even though one ICP wave was well tolerated the next one might not be, and if a change in the degree of herniation occurs with the next similar increase in intracranial volume, much higher elevations of ICP may occur because the CSF can no longer be displaced as a result of a subarachnoid occlusion.[5] The CSF is displaced into the venous sinuses and also through the foramen magnum into the spinal sac. Cerebrospinal fluid production is minimally affected by elevated ICP until CBF begins to fall, at which time CSF production decreases. Cerebrospinal fluid clearance, however, is increased by elevated ICP.[5]

### The Vascular Compartment

The exact role of changes in blood volume in the cranium to compensate for changes in other components is not clear. With elevated ICP produced by an increase in CSF volume, an increase in intraparenchmyal blood volume occurs as a result of cerebrovascular dilatation in an effort to maintain CBF. In this case, the cerebral blood volume (CBV) does not act as a compensatory mechanism, but compounds the problem. It is likely that some decrease in cerebral arachnoid venous volume occurs, however, which more than offsets the increase in intraparenchymal blood volume. Blood volume has been suggested to account for 10 percent of the intracranial space. This would mean the total blood volume in an adult would be 150 ml. The actual intraparenchymal blood volume is approximately 3 ml/100 g of brain, giving a total of approximately 60 ml; thus 67 percent of the cerebral blood volume is in the dural sinuses and the subarachnoid veins. It has been suggested that as ICP continues to rise, a pressure is reached at which the veins are compressed as they enter the sagittal sinus; hence an increase in intracranial venous volume occurs, adding to the increasingly rapid decompensation.[3] Although this mechanism has been repeatedly suggested over the years, it remains unproven.

It does appear, however, that in the late stages of cerebral decompensation there are increases in venous volume that are detrimental and act against cerebral spatial compensation.[4]

### The Brain Parenchyma

The brain itself, although generally stated to be incompressible, clearly can be both displaced and compressed (e.g., by hydrocephalus or an expanding epidural hematoma). This displacement is potentially deleterious as herniation of cerebral tissue can be produced. The sites of herniation are below the falx cerebri from one side of the brain to the other, retrograde over the sphenoid wing, from the supratentorial to the infratentorial space (tentorial herniation), or through the foramen magnum. The brain displacement is accompanied by cerebrovascular compression and tissue ischemia and obstruction of the CSF spaces. The fact that displacement can occur suggests that some pressure gradients must exist within the cranial cavity during the expanding phase of any intracranial mass lesion.[3]

### The Volume–Pressure Curve

The simple equation describing the volume and pressure relationships can be expressed as follows:

$$V_{\text{tissue}} + V_{\text{blood}} + V_{\text{CSF}} + V_{\text{other}} = V_{\text{total}} = V_{\text{eq}} + V_{\text{elastic}}$$

where, $V_{\text{eq}}$ represents the equilibrium volume of the craniospinal axis where the ICP is within the normal range (i.e., compensation is taking place) and $V_{\text{elastic}}$ represents elastic volume, which is a measure of the elastic properties of the cerebral tissue and is important when the ICP is elevated. The volume–pressure curve can be depicted graphically (Fig. 2-1).

Currently, we believe that the flat portion of the volume–pressure curve is that portion during which spatial compensation is occurring while one compartment is expanding, the other compartments are contracting, and thus little increase in pressure occurs. The steep portion of the curve is the area of exhausted spatial compensation and essentially represents brain elasticity. Graphic representation is important because it demonstrates that a normal ICP does not by itself define whether that patient is near the point of compensation exhaustion and, therefore, able to tolerate a further increase in volume of one of the intracranial components without developing raised ICP. Clinically, other clues (e.g., papilledema, episodic headaches, intermittent blindness) and computed tomography (CT) scan findings of the presence of midline displacement or absence of CSF spaces are helpful in suggesting that this patient may have little residual compensatory ability and hence is at risk for acute herniation.[1]

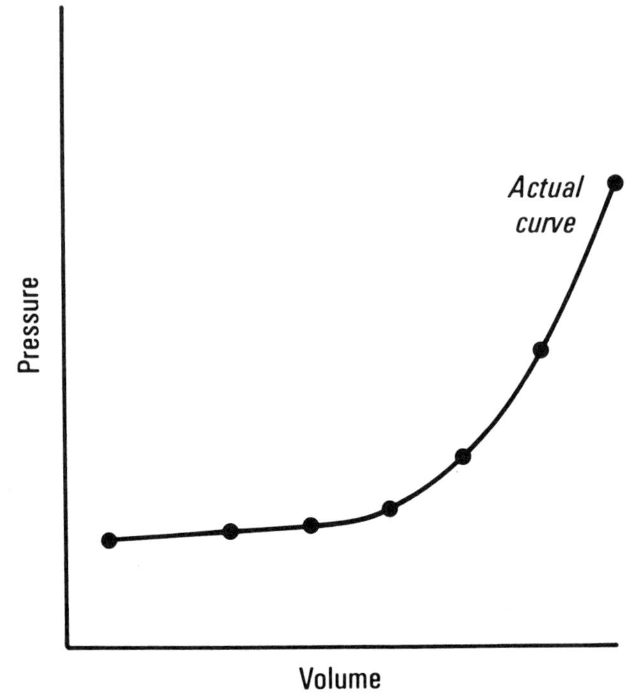


**Fig. 2-1.** Intracranial volume-pressure curve obtained in animals with an expanding epidural balloon.

## CLINICAL ASPECTS

Clinical episodes that can easily produce deterioration are seizures or an acute elevation in $CO^2$ both of which acutely increase cerebral blood volume or further mass expansion with occlusion of CSF spaces.[1] Increase in systemic arterial pressure will render the brain less resilient and decrease the elastic volume, making the steep portion of the curve even steeper.[3] Stressing the intracranial space by adding a small volume of CSF to the ventricles has been suggested as a method to check the patient's position on the volume pressure curve.[5] This is the volume–pressure response (VPR). Unfortunately, this test does not indicate how the intracranial space in this patient will respond to an increase in volume produced by either increase in brain mass or increase in blood volume. The test gives information only about what will occur if the situation remains the same and CSF is added. From a clinical point of view, therefore, misleading information can be generated by use of the VPR.[5] It seems safer in each individual patient to consider the potential spatial decompensation, the patient's clinical symptomatology, and the CT scan. It is also safer to assume that any patient who manifests some V/P disturbance is potentially close to the decompensation point and should be treated aggressively in an effort to restore adequate spatial compensation. In patients manifesting disturbances in intracranial volume and pressure relationships, the various therapies discussed later in this book are designed to differentially affect either CSF volume, brain volume, or blood volume.

## REFERENCES

1. Bruce DA, Berman WA, Schut L: Cerebrospinal fluid pressure monitoring in children. Pathophysiology, pathology and clinical usefulness, in Advances in Pediatrics, vol 24, New York, Yearbook Medical Publishers, 1977, pp 223–290
2. Bruce, A: The pathophysiology of increased intracranial pressure. Current Concepts, Upjohn Company Publication, 1978
3. Langfitt, TW: Increased intracranial pressure. Clin Neurosurg. 16:436–471, 1969
4. Lofgren J, Van Essen C, Swetnow, NN: The pressure–volume curve of cerebrospinal fluid space in dogs. Acta Neurol Scand 49:551–574, 1973
5. Marmarou A, Schulman K: Pressure–volume relationships—basic aspects, in McLaurin RL (Ed): Head Injuries. New York, Grune & Stratton, 1976, pp 233–236
6. Shapiro K, Marmarou A: Mechanisms of intracranial hypertension in children, in Pediatric Neurosurgery. New York, Grune & Stratton, 1982, pp 255–264

*Alexander Baethmann*
*Oliver Kempski*
*Sylvia Schneider*
*Markus Zimmer*
*Arno Neu*
*Friedirich F. von Rosen*
*Martin Jansen*

# 3

# Normal and Abnormal Neuronal and Glial Volume

Swelling of nerve and glial cells—that is, cytotoxic brain edema—may occur in various forms of cerebral disorders independently from a failure of the blood–brain barrier. The significance of cytotoxic brain edema is underestimated as compared to the vasogenic type, which develops in many common neurological disorders, such as trauma, tumor, and inflammation secondary to ischemia and so on.[5,46] Even with the use of computed tomography, (CT) or other imaging techniques of the brain, diagnosis of cytotoxic brain edema is difficult to establish under clinical circumstances. Nevertheless, swelling of nerve and glial cells is an important component of acute, or chronic forms of cerebral damage or disorders, since it evolves almost always concomitantly with vasogenic brain edema and is a predominant feature early after onset of cerebral ischemia.[5,23,29,53] Primary forms of cytotoxic edema are associated with metabolic disorders, such as in Reye's syndrome and following intoxication.[3,39,44,45] Vacuolization of myelin lamellae in the white matter evolving

BRAIN INSULTS IN INFANTS AND CHILDREN
0-8089-1723-4

after intoxication, for example, by hexachlorophene, or secondarily in traumatic or other lesions of the brain is another pertinent form of cytotoxic brain edema.[45] Splitting of myelin lamellae is the ultrastructural equivalent of the spongy state seen under the light microscope. Although the mechanisms causing cytotoxic brain edema remain elusive so far, three major processes might be considered alone or in combination:[5]

1. Increase of membrane permeability to $Na^+$ ions of affected cells. This would allow for a downhill influx of $Na^+$ into cells together with chloride and water. The mechanism might operate, if compounds raising membrane permeability accumulate in the extracellular compartment. Excitatory transmitters such as acetylcholine or glutamic acid may serve as examples.[25] Abnormal concentrations of glutamate in the cerebral extracellular space have been observed indeed under pathological conditions.[35]
2. Inhibition, or disturbances of active pumping mechanisms, that is, $Na^+$-$K^+$-ATPase responsible for the normal concentration gradients of ions between the intra- and extracellular compartment. A failure to pump back $Na^+$ ions constantly leaking into cells, particularly during excitation, would suffice to cause eventual swelling of nerve and glial cells. Cerebral administration of ouabain, to inhibit $Na^+$-$K^+$-ATPase was found to induce cytotoxic brain edema.[20,37] Cerebral tissue contains endogenous ATPase inhibitors[22] which may become activated under pathological circumstances
3. Finally, inhibition of energy metabolism fueling the active pumps might be proposed by either anoxia or other metabolic disturbances. Experimental examples abound to support this point.[3,4,53]

Understanding of swelling mechanisms on a molecular level in vivo is obscured because of a multitude of parameters that are liable to change simultaneously under conditions associated with and leading to cell swelling. This makes impossible an in depth analysis to provide a basis for an improvement of current forms of treatment by increasing specificity.

Advances in flow cytometry allowing for reliable and rapid analysis of pertinent parameters, such as the actual cell volume of living cells in vitro together with the availability of stable cell lines of central nervous system tissue (CNS) with glia- or neuron-specific properties, may provide novel approaches to the problem. The in vitro model, discussed in the following section, was established for the study of cytotoxic swelling mechanisms of defined cells under defined conditions.[17,31] Quantitative aspects of cell volume of nerve and glial cells in the normal state are first considered as investigated by morphometric techniques together with derangements observed largely in vivo.

## CELL VOLUME OF NERVE AND GLIAL CELLS IN VIVO

### Under Normal Conditions

Although absolute figures of nerve or glial cell volume are of limited significance, quantitative estimates are necessary for the evaluation of pathological changes, such as in brain edema. Moreover, comparison of respective findings from morphological studies with data obtained by flow cytometric sizing of suspended cells taken from culture as used for in vitro studies of cytotoxic brain edema may be of interest. Since cerebral tissue contains many types of nerve and glial cells, a discussion of the subject must be limited. One may remember that the nerve cell volume changes already under normal conditions, such as during CNS development. Nerve cells increase in volume to an almost fourfold level at maturation of the brain when compared to the neonatal state.[48] In addition, nerve cell processes (e.g., axons, dendrites) may undergo reversible volume changes during physiological events, such as electrical excitation,[50,57] and probably also during formation of memory traces through activation of specific nerve cell circuits.[56] Cell volume changes of clinical relevance under pathophysiological conditions occur in epileptic seizures, cerebral ischemia, and metabolic disturbances of the brain. Spreading depression may be also mentioned in this context, although its significance as a physiological or pathophysiological phenomenon is barely understood.[55]

In the following paragraphs, measures of quantitative cell volume estimates are given, either as diameter of cell body, occasionally as cell surface, or if available as volume proper in cubic micra. Attempts are not made to calculate cell volume from diameter of cell bodies or processes, because such a measure, when obtained from light microscopic or electron microscopic preparations, is influenced by the cutting plane and hence subjected to technical error and also because these structures are cellular components only and cannot be considered a reliable parameter of total cell volume, particularly in view of an extensive formation of processes forming the neuropil.

Valuable information on structure and morphology is found in electron microscopic studies conducted by the Palays[43] on the cerebellum. The authors published a highly comprehensive cytological atlas on the light and electron microscopic levels of the cerebellum of rats, also providing quantitative data concerning cell size. Still, morphological studies at this level in an organ as complex as the cerebellum demonstrate the limited significance of cell volume as such. As mentioned earlier, metric data given on cell components as the cell soma or cell processes underestimate real cell size. This is particularly obvious in the case of the Purkinje cells, where an enormous dendritic arborization probably comprises the overwhelming mass of the cell (Table 3-1). Nevertheless, cell bodies of Purkinje cells are among the largest in the brain. Cell bodies

**Table 3-1** *Size and Volume of Cells, or Cell Components of Nerve and Glial Cells In Vivo and In Vitro Under Normal Conditions*

| | Diameter ($\mu$) | Volume ($\mu^3$) | Method* | Reference |
|---|---|---|---|---|
| Nerve cells, third layer cerebral cortex (human) | | | | |
| Newborn | | 240 | | 48 |
| 6 months | | 610 | | 48 |
| 2 years | | 990 | | 48 |
| Adult | | 1040 | | 48 |
| Purkinje cells (human) | | | | |
| Cell body, transversal | 35–65 | | M | 43 |
| Cell body, longitudinal | 50–70 | | M | 43 |
| Dendritic surface area | 250,000 $\mu^2$ | | | 48 |
| Granule cell body | 5–8 | | M | 43 |
| Golgi cell body | 11–24 | | M | 43 |
| Nerve cells, cortex (rat) | | 3636 | † | 7 |
| Nerve cell body, isolation in vitro (rat) | 15–19 | | M | 40 |
| Fetal nerve cell body, primary culture (human) | 7–9 | | M | 18 |
| Nerve cell body, hippocampus (human) | | | | |
| <5 years | | 3800 | M | 51 |
| >10 years | | 5271 | M | 51 |
| F115 neuroblastoma, culture | | 1083 | ES | 17 |
| C1300 neuroblastoma, culture | | 3380 | ES | 17 |
| Protoplasmatic astrocyte body (rat) | 5–8 | | M | 43 |
| Oligodendrycyte body (rat) | 5–6 | | M | 43 |
| Astrocyte body (rabbit) | | 358 | M,FS | 19 |
| Oligodendrocyte body (rabbit) | | 105 | M,FS | 19 |
| Oligodendrocyte body (rat) | 7.0 | | M | 34 |
| Astrocyte body (rat) | 6.3 | | M | 34 |
| Astrocyte body (cat) | 6.2–10.4 | 190–320 | M | 58 |
| Astrocyte volume (cat; body + processes) | | 570 | M | 58 |
| Astrocyte body, primary culture of fetal brain (human) | 15–20 | | M | 18 |
| Astrocytes, primary culture (rat, newborn) | | 1200–1350 | ES | 42 |
| C6 glioma, culture | | 951 | M | 33 |
| | | 1320 | CyC | 33 |
| | | 869 | M | 33 |
| C6 glioma, culture | | 980–1033 | ES | 17 |

*Abbreviations: M, morphometry; ES, electrical sizing; FS, fixation by freeze substitution; CyC, volume measurement by cytocentrifugation.

†Cell volume was calculated from data given by the author and assuming a proportion of nerve cells of 60 and 20 percent extracellular fluid space.

in humans range from 35 to 65 $\mu$ in diameter and 50 to 70 $\mu$ in length.[43] Cell body diameters and length of Purkinje cells in rats are 21 or 25 $\mu$, respectively. Cerebellar granule cell are found at the opposite end of the spectrum of nerve cell size. Their cell bodies have diameters of only 5 to 8 $\mu$, which is close to that of red blood cells. Cell bodies of oligodendroglia and protoplasmic astroglia in cerebellum assume similar dimensions, whereas cell bodies of Golgi cells are somewhat larger, with diameters of 11–15 $\mu$.[43] Data on cell body diameter or volume are summarized in Table 3-1.

In studies on isolated nerve cell soma obtained from rat telencephalon following filtration of minced tissue blocks through nylon meshes and centrifugation on a discontinuous sucrose gradient, cell body diameters of 15–19 $\mu$ were found.[40] Direct estimates of nerve cell volumes are given by Schade and Ford.[48] Human nerve cells studied in layer III of cerebral cortex (middle frontal gyrus) have a cell volume of 250 $\mu^3$ in the newborn, 610 $\mu^3$ at 6 months, 990 $\mu^3$ at 2 years, and 1040 $\mu^3$ in the adult brain. An increase in cell size of this order is possible only by a simultaneous decrease in cell density found to decrease from 99 $\times$ $10^3/mm^3$ of fresh tissue in the newborn to 12.5 $\times$ $10^3/mm^3$ in the adult. Analysis of cell volume in vivo of nerve and glial cells thus requires consideration of the actual phase of cerebral development. A nerve cell volume of 1040 $\mu^3$ in adult cerebral cortex is in surprising agreement with the volume of cultured F115 neuroblastoma cells, that is, 1083 $\pm$ 23 $\mu^3$ of the mouse.[17] Yet, variability in volume of nerve cells is considerable, as reflected by a range of 500 $\mu^3$ (cerebellar granule cells) up to 70,000 $\mu^3$ (spinal cord motoneurons). The particularly developed dendritic system of Purkinje cells assumes a surface area per cell of no less than 250,000 $\mu^2$.[48]

Primary tissue cultures of the CNS are also employed for analysis of size of nerve and glial cells. Choi and Lapham[18] cultured specimen of fetal human brain and observed growth of two groups of cells having diameters of either 7–9 or 15–20 $\mu$. Further structural differentiation of the cells in culture let the authors identify small elements as neurons and large as astrocytes. This reemphasizes the influence of the actual state of cerebral development on cell volume.

Provided techniques are subtle and accurate quantitative studies on cerebral cytoarchitectonic, DNA content and similar factors may be also used to arrive at quantiative cell volume estimates. Investigations by Bass et al.[7] on the quantitative distribution and DNA content of nerve versus glial cells in the sensory cortex of rats may serve as an example. The mean cell volume of a given cell type can be calculated in a defined volume of tissue provided its ratio and number is known as well as the size of the extracellular fluid space. Taking a mean neuronal proportion of 60 percent per tissue volume unit, an extracellular space of 20 percent and a cell count of 132,000/$mm^3$ of fresh tissue as found by Bass et al.,[7] a cell volume of 3636.4 $\mu^3$ is obtained. Such an approach takes into account all structural components such as cell soma and processes provided they do not exceed the tissue unit under study.

**Under Pathophysiological Conditions**

Morphological techniques were also employed to study cell volume changes under different pathophysiological conditions, including spreading depression, hypothermia, and anoxia. An important improvement for morphometric cell sizing was the employment of freeze substitution as a fixation method, which was introduced for the CNS by Van Harreveld[52] to prevent distortion of cell dimensions. Morphometric studies by light microscopy of glial cells of freeze-substituted brain specimen of rabbits were made by Collewijn and Schade[19] using planimetric measurement of cell surfaces for volume calculation. Such an approach requires determination of many cells to obtain reliable data. This renders the method rather laborious, even if modern computerized image-analyzing systems are used. Collewijn subjected animals either to hypothermia at 28 or 20°C, to 10 minutes of global cerebral ischemia in normothermia or induced spreading depression by focal administration of glutamate crystals on the exposed cerebral cortex in vivo.

Oligodendroglia was found to increase cell volume during ischemia, whereas astroglia shrank. Normal astrocytes had a volume of 385 $\mu^3$, and oligodendroglia, 105 $\mu^3$. Volume of the latter increased to 140 $\mu^3$ during ischemia, that is, to 133 percent of normal. Hypothermia at 28°C led to an increase in astrocytic volume to 410 $\mu^3$ ($p < .02$) while further cooling to 20°C resulted in shrinking. On the other hand, oligodendrocytes increased cell volume to 118 percent at 20°C. Spreading depression elicited by glutamate did not increase, but rather reduced astrocytic volume.[19] The finding may be explained by a preferential fluid shift into dendrites rather than glia during spreading depression as demonstrated by Van Harreveld.[54]

Electron microscopic studies were conducted by Van Harreveld on molecular layers of cerebellar cortex of mice employing freeze substitution 8 minutes after circulatory arrest. Contrary to the above-cited observations of Collewijn, marked swelling of Bergmann fibers (glia) and their endfeet leading to an increase of electron transparency was found. Glial elements in the neuropil and the dendritic structures were also swollen. A normally visible extracellular space had almost disappeared as a result of the asphyxial shift of interstitial fluid into the cell elements.[54]

Van Harreveld[53] analyzed quantitative changes of dendritic diameters during spreading depression as shown in Figure 3-1. As seen, the phenomenon led to swelling of diameters of up to 122 percent (maximum) as compared to the nondepressed control hemisphere. The tissue was again freeze-substituted for fixation. Figure 3-2 is also taken from work of Van Harreveld,[53] giving a statistical analysis of ischemic swelling of Bergman fibers of rabbit or rat cerebellar cortex, respectively. The diameter histograms were obtained from experiments in 12 rabbits and 16 rats (controls, experimental) with measurements of 600 or 800 fibers per experiment. It demonstrates the enormous amount of measurements required to obtain reliable data. As shown in Figure

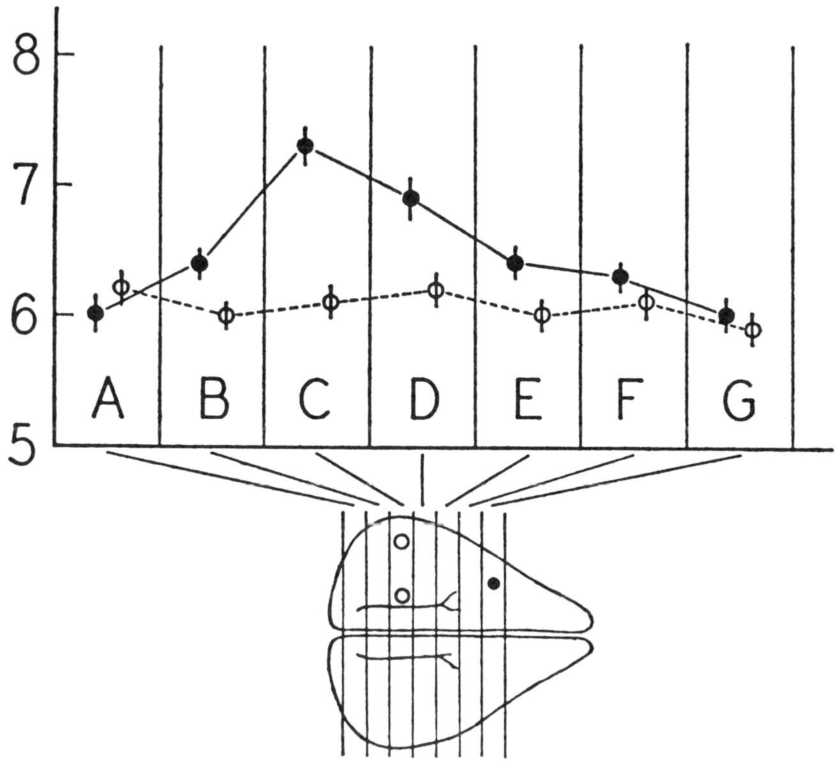


**Fig. 3-1.** Dendritic diameter given in arbitrary units (mean ± SE) of cerebral hemispheres with (filled circles) and without (open circles) spreading depression (SD). The diameters were morphometrically determined in slices A–G cut as shown in the inset. Spreading depression propagated from right (G) to left (A). From Van Harreveld A: Brain tissue electrolytes, in Bittar EE (Ed): Molecular Biology and Medicine Series. London, Butterworths, p 120. With permission.

3-2, interruption of the cerebral circulation for 6–8 minutes led to a clear shift of the histogram to larger diameters. The mean diameter increased by about 100 percent.[53] It was assumed then that it is not a lack of $O_2$ per se causing swelling of cell processes. Both spreading depression and asphyxiation elicit a release of glutamate from the cells into the extracellular space.[54] High extracellular concentrations of glutamate raise $Na^+$ permeability of the membranes, thus causing a downhill intracellular influx together with chloride and water, resulting in swelling. Instead of glutamate, discharge of $K^+$ ions is considered as a swelling-inducing factor. Incubation of cerebral tissue in medium containing high $K^+$ concentrations was found to cause intracellular swelling.[12,41] Extracellular release of $K^+$ is a regular phenomenon under these circumstances.[9,36,49]

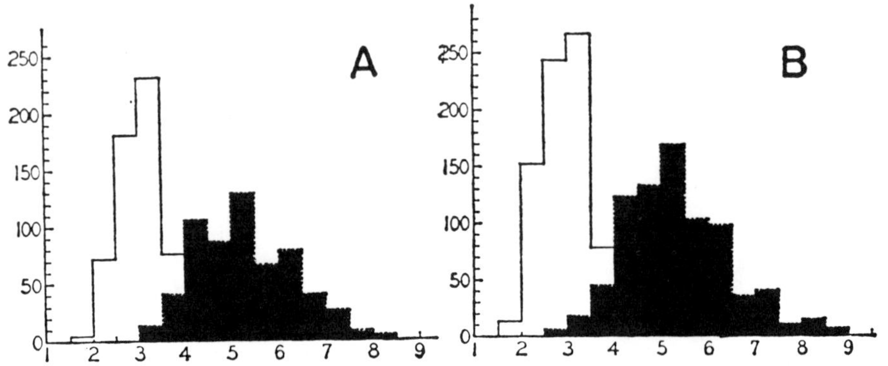


**Fig. 3-2.** Frequency distribution of diameters of Bergmann fibers obtained from rabbit (**A**) or rat (**B**) cerebellar cortex after 6–8 minutes of circulatory arrest (*black areas*). Morphometric determination of diameters involved freeze substitution as fixation method to maintain in vivo intracellular fluid distribution. Interruption of cerebral blood flow led to a marked shift of the histograms to larger diameters of approximately 100 percent. From Van Harreveld A: Brain tissue electrolytes, in Bittar EE (Ed): Molecular Biology and Medicine Series. London, Butterworths p 120. With permission.

The discussion of glutamate versus $K^+$ ions as mediators of ischemic cell swelling in nervous tissue demonstrates perfectly the problem encountered in studies of the living brain. Both are released in the extracellular space under these circumstances. Generally, analysis of cytotoxic swelling mechanisms in vivo is impeded by the complexity of changes occurring at the same time in a given pathophysiological situation. Progress might be expected from investigations of the phenomenon in a simple system allowing for control of as many as possible parameters. The development of an in vitro model using cultured nerve and glial cells and the availability of rapid and reliable cell sizing techniques provide the basis for such a venture.[17,30,31] The system currently available in our laboratory is discussed in the following paragraphs in greater detail.

## THE EXPERIMENTAL MODEL

The C6 glioma, or F115 neuroblastoma cell lines are used for experimentation. The C6 glial cell line, which is most frequently employed, is derived from a chemically induced glioma in rats.[8] The cells are available for many years and display remarkably stable properties. The glial origin can be tested by analysis of markers (e.g. S-100 protein), or specific enzymes.[21,26] Respective nerve cell lines were also derived from tumors induced in experimental animals. The cells are culture grown in Dulbeccos minimal essential medium (MEM) and 10 percent fetal calf serum (FCS) by standard procedures. On confluency, the cells are harvested for the experiment from the culture vessel, subsequently washed for removal of FCS, and then resuspended in medium. Trypsin used for detachment of cells from the dish and desaggregation is inactivated thereafter. Harvesting of nerve cells was usually conducted without trypsin. The suspended cells remain in steady-state conditions over long periods. Maintenance in culture medium at room temperature or 37°C in the incubation chamber (Fig. 3-3) did not change viability or the volume under normal conditions. The C6 glial cells had a constant volume and viability during observation periods of 7 hours or more.[17]

The majority of experiments are conducted in a plexiglas test chamber of 10 ml volume (Fig. 3-3). Suspension of cells after harvesting in the chamber allows for continuous control of pH, temperature, and $O_2$ tension by use of a thermocouple and respective electrodes. The medium was supplied with $O_2$ and $CO_2$ through a gas-permeable silicon rubber tube to avoid direct bubbling of the medium. The pH was adjusted by bicarbonate and control of the $CO_2$ supply. A magnetic stirrer prevents sedimentation and aggregation of the suspended cells. Stainless steel cannulas are inserted into the chamber for retrieval of cells or medium. Sizing of the suspended cells is conducted electrically by Metricell, a method based on the Coulter principle (Fig. 3-4). The suspended cell particles are aspirated for measurement by a vacuum pump through a small aperture with a diameter of 50, 100, or 150 $\mu$. Passage of a cell through the orifice imparts a sudden rise of electrical resistance to a constant current also flowing through the aperature. This induces a voltage pulse($\triangle u$) that is processed by the system. Increase in resistance during passage of the particle can be attributed to the electrical conductivity of the cell membrane being substantially lower than that of the suspension medium. The principle is used by the Coulter technique for counting of particles. The current model takes advantage of a quantitative relationship between cell size and resistance change during passage of the orifice, or the voltage pulse induced, respectively. The physical relationship is described by an equation used for volume determination as developed by Grover from the basic equations of Maxwell and Fricke:[30]

$$V = \frac{q^2 f_k}{\rho i F} u$$

As seen, cell volume $V$ depends on the voltage $u$ and constants such as $q$, the cross section of the aperture; $\rho$, the specific electrical resistance of the suspension medium; $i$, the current employed; $F_k$, a geometric factor of the Coulter orifice; and finally the form factor $F$ of the cell particle. Form factor $F$ considers the electrical resistance of the particle and particle configuration during passage of the aperture. This factor can be determined experimentally. A pertinent aspect of electrical cell sizing is the pathway of particles during passage of the aperature. Because of the geometry of the electrical field

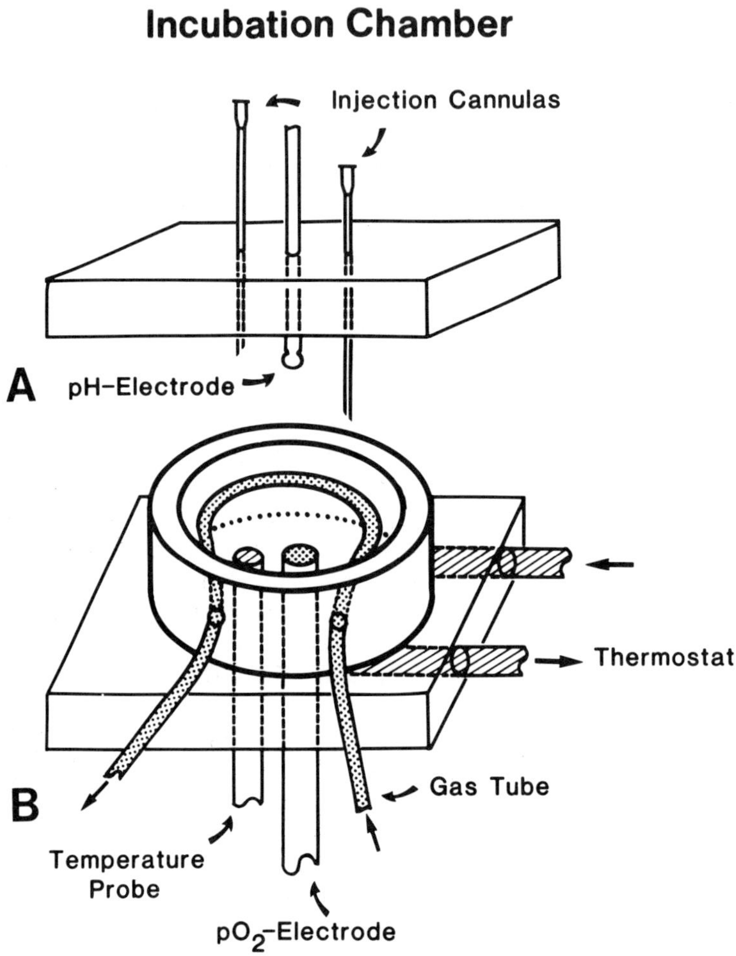


**Fig. 3-3.** Schematic drawing of the plexiglas test chamber used for incubation of suspended glial cells after harvesting from culture. The chamber is shown after opening: (**A**) insertion of the pH electrode and injection cannulas; (**B**) insertion of a temperature probe and the $Po_2$ electrode for continuous control during incubation. The medium in the chamber is oxygenated by a gaspermeable silicon rubber tube. The pH level is controlled by adjustment of $CO_2$ supply to bicarbonate-buffered medium. Temperature is held constant by a heat exchanger attached to the chamber. The chamber is placed in a plastic tent inflated with $N_2$ for induction of complete anoxia. From Kempski O, Chaussy L, Gross U, et al: Volume regulation and metabolism of suspended C6 glioma cells: an in vitro model to study cytotoxic brain edema. Brain Res 279:218. With permission.

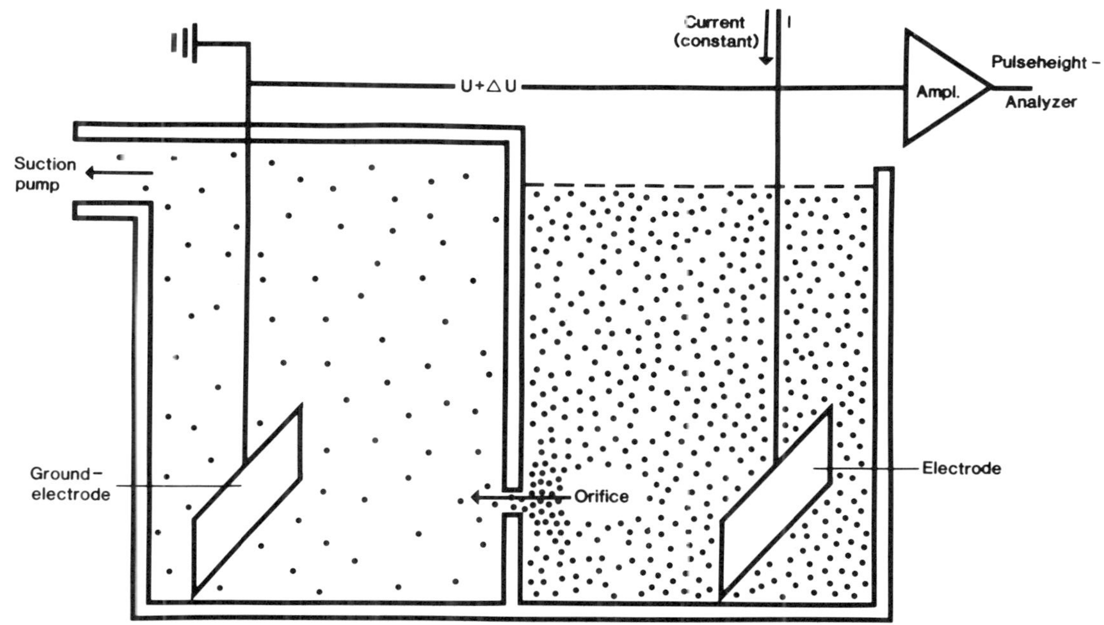


**Fig. 3-4.** Principle of volume determination of suspended particles by the Coulter method. Cell particles suspended in a chamber (right) are aspirated into the neighboring compartment by negative pressure. Passage of particles through the orifice imparts a sudden increase in resistance to a constant electrical current. The change of resistance is in proportion to the cross section and, hence, volume of the cell element. The abrupt rise of resistance produces a voltage pulse ($\triangle u$), which is amplified and processed for cell sizing. Modified after Kachel V: Basic principles of electrical sizing of cells and particles and their realization in the new instrument Metricell." J Histochem Cytochem 24(1):212, 1976. With permission.

across the aperature, it is important to allow cells to travel through the orifice along the center axis to obtain a homogenous voltage pulse. This is accomplished by hydrodynamic focusing of the particles by ensheathment of the suspension fluid with a particle free solution.[30] Electrical sizing is facilitated by a microprocessor attached to the system for control and display of an ongoing measurement, on-line impulse–height analysis and calibration, calculation of the particle size, and storage of data. Standard latex particles are employed for mechanical calibration. A measurement produces a distribution curve (histogram) of volume classes. The histogram peak (mode) characterizes the mean volume. The volume range may be specific for the cell type studied. Nonsynchronized cultured cells have a larger range of cell size according to the actual phase of the cell cycle than mature red blood cells, for instance. The volume histogram is normalized as Gaussian distribution for calculation of mode and standard deviation. Channel discrimination allows for simultaneous measurement of different cell populations, provided overlap in cell size is negligible.

## EXPERIMENTAL PROCEDURE

A control period of 30–60 minutes precedes the experimental phase, maintaining $O_2$ and $CO_2$ tensions constant as well as osmolarity and electrolyte concentrations. Cell volume and other parameters are repeatedly assessed. The experiments concern changes of osmolarity, effects of metabolic inhibitors or drugs, or withdrawal of $O_2$. In studies on cell volume response to an abnormal osmolarity (hypo- or hypertonicity) the medium was diluted or concentrated, however maintaining physiological $K^+$, $Ca^{++}$ and $Mg^{++}$ concentrations. The $O_2$ supply to the chamber was interrupted for studies on anoxia by blocking the silicon rubber tube used for oxygenation of the chamber. Induction of anoxia was enhanced by placement of the test chamber in a plastic tent inflated by $N_2$. Oxygen consumption of cells was polarographically measured in addition during brief discontinuation of the $O_2$ supply, utilizing the slope of the declining $Po_2$ as a parameter.

## VOLUME OF CULTURED NERVE AND GLIAL CELLS UNDER NORMAL AND ABNORMAL CONDITIONS IN VITRO

Cell volume of cultured cells may decline with increasing subcultivation. Heumann et al.[27] found a steady decrease of the cell volume in a neuroblastoma × glioblastoma hybrid cell line over 60 culture passages. This was associated with a corresponding loss of DNA; however, cell volume remained stable thereafter. When the steady state was reached, cell volume was 4900 $\mu^3$.[27] Cell volume of the parental C6 glioma and N18 TG2 neuroblastoma cells was 907.4 or 2268.5 $\mu^3$, respectively. The cell size of C6 glial cells found in other studies including of ourselves is surprisingly close. Kukes et al.,[33] employing histomorphometry plus cytocentrifugation, found a volume of 869 $\mu^3$. Volume measurements by Chan et al.[16] of cultured C6 glioma and neuroblastoma cells yielded higher values. This may be at attributed to the technique, specifically, isotope labeling with radioactive methylglucose and tritiated water, which rapidly penetrate cell membranes and $^{14}$C-inulin and polyethylene glycol as extracellular markers.

Volume of viable C6 glial cells suspended in isotonic medium (300 mOsm/l) ranged from 898 to 1033 $\mu^3$ (Metricell) during an observation period of 160 minutes and $F_{115}$ neuroblastoma cells from 979 $\pm$ 32 $\mu^3$ to 1083 $\pm$ $\mu^3$ within 300 minutes.[17,31] The values compare favorably with data of Olson and Holtzman[42] on astrocytes obtained from primary culture; they reported values of 1200–1350 $\mu^3$ under isotonic conditions. Taken together, quantitative estimates of cell volumes of nerve and glial cells in vivo and in vitro are in a reasonable agreement, even with comparison of methods as different as histomorphometry, cytocentrifugation, and electrical sizing. This may enhance confidence and reliability of in-vitro models for study of pathophysiological mechanisms of cell volume disturbances in cytotoxic brain edema.

## IN VITRO STUDIES ON CELL VOLUME CONTROL

Findings on volume response of suspended cells to an abnormal osmotic environment provide for an understanding on a cell-physiological basis of how the brain manages in vivo to adjust tissue volume in hypo- or hyperosmolar states. Actually, the cerebrum has a powerful capacity to compensate for changes in systemic osmolarity, such as on administration of distilled water.[2,6] Cells derived from CNS tissue, such as C6 glioma or F115 neuroblastoma normalize volume on suspension in hypotonic medium after transient swelling.[17,31] Respective findings are given in Fig. 3-5 demonstrating the response of cell volume of glial cells as a regression curve. The swift increase in cell volume on the hypotonic challenge is rapidly followed by recovery to the normal level within 30–60 minutes. The phenomenon is described as regulatory volume decrease (RVD). It has also been observed in other cell types, such as human lymphocytes, red blood cells of ducks and flounders, and Ehrlich ascites tumor cells.[13,14,24,28,47] Thus regulatory volume decrease appears to be a general phenomenon, furnishing cells with a powerful mechanism to respond to environmental osmotic changes. This may be particularly important in organisms living in water or in areas such as deserts with varying supply of drinking water.

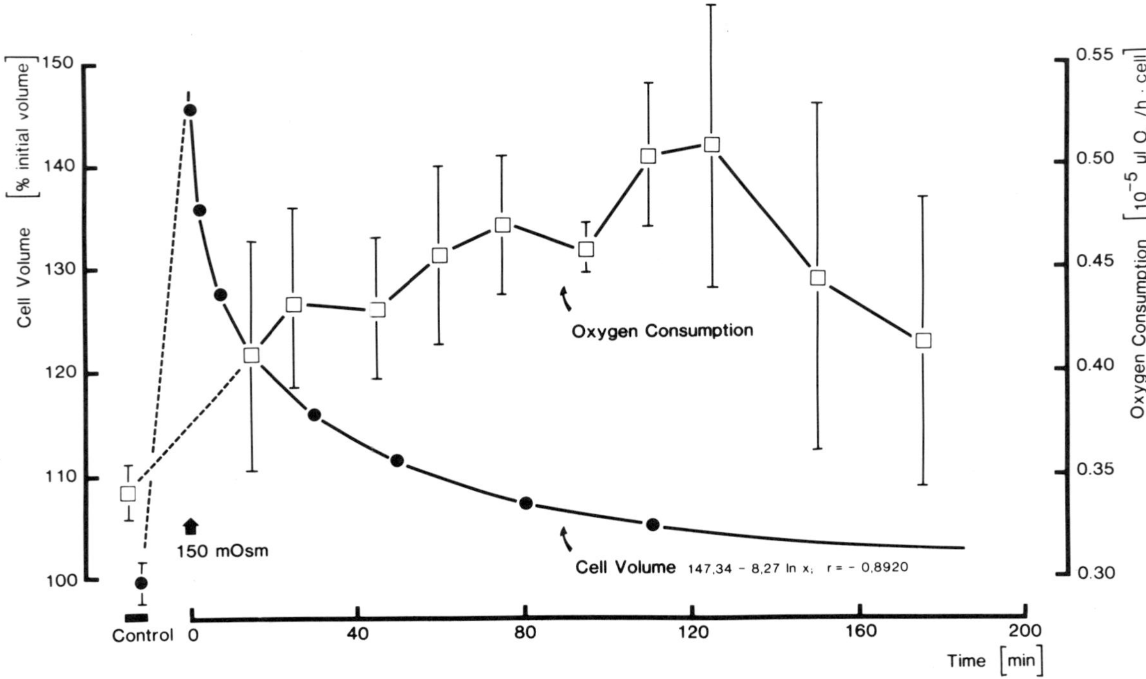


**Fig. 3-5.** Volume response of C6 glial cells on hypotonic exposure starting at time zero. Osmolarity was reduced from 300 to 150 mOsm/l by dilution of the medium with distilled water. Concentrations of $K^+$, $Ca^{++}$, and $Mg^{++}$ were maintained in the physiological range. The volume response is given in percent of the cell volume found in isotonic medium during a preceding control phase. The regression curve is based on 36 individual measurements. Cell volume reached a normal level again within 60–120 minutes, although hypotonicity was maintained. Cellular $O_2$ consumption was increased, reaching a maximum when cell volume became normal again. From Kempski O, Chaussy L, Gross U, et al: Volume regulation and metabolism of suspended C6 glioma cells: an in vitro model to study cytotoxic brain edema. Brain Rest 279:220. With permission.

Many studies were conducted for elucidation of the nature of cell volume adjustment under these circumstances. An elaborate model based on experimental data of transmembrane $K^+$, $Cl^-$, and proton fluxes was proposed by Cala[15] (Fig. 3-6). Hypotonically suspended cells loose or discharge $K^+$, $Cl^-$, and consequently water, thus allowing shrinkage back to normal. Electroneutrality is maintained by an exchange of $K^+$ against protons and $Cl^-$ against bicarbonate. Uptake of protons and bicarbonate does not increase the osmotic burden of the cell since both form carbonic acid, and consequently $CO_2$ plus water. It is not clear, however, whether the Cala mechanism conceived for red blood cells of Amphiuma also applies for cells of CNS tissue of higher vertebrates.

As seen in Figure 3-5, normalization of C6 glial volume involves energy metabolism as implied by the marked increase of $O_2$ uptake. Oxygen consumption of hypotonically suspended glial cells approached a maximum during the active phase of regulatory volume decrease and returned to lower levels after volume normalization was accomplished.[31] Regulatory volume decrease following hypotonic suspension was also found in F115 neuroblastoma cells, although the velocity of volume recovery appeared somewhat reduced.[17] The significance and high reproducibility of RVD in many cell types render the phenomenon an ideal subject to study general aspects of cell volume control pertaining also to mechanisms of cytotoxic cell swelling in the brain.

Additional experiments were conducted by combining hypotonic exposure of C6 glia with induction of energy failure, inhibition of $Na^+$-$K^+$-ATPase, and other methods. Inhibition of RVD is a virtually constant phenomenon after administration of ouabain to cells suspended in a hypotonic medium. Experiments in our laboratory failed to prevent normalization of volume of hypotoniclly suspended glial cells by ouabain,[31] whereas Rosenberg[47] reported reversible inhibition of the shrinking phase by ouabain. Interruption of the $O_2$ supply, together with inhibition of glycolysis with iodoacetate was found to prevent RVD.[38] Yet, suspension of glial cells under the same conditions in isotonic medium did not induce cell swelling, although a marked loss of intracellular $K^+$ was found to occur.[59] Maintenance of cell volume after complete shutdown of the cellular energy production may be explained by the nature of the experimental model. As mentioned, glial cells harvested from culture are suspended in a test chamber of a virtual infinite extracellular volume. Any cell response elicited by anoxia or by metabolic inhibition in vitro such as discharge of $K^+$ ions or glutamate, is effectively attenuated by dilution, whereas $K^+$ and glutamate would accumulate in vivo in the brain on account of the limited extracellular fluid volume. Consequently, swelling of cells in anoxia and other conditions could not occur in vitro, because effective concentrations of these factors, such as to affect membrane permeability as a mechanism of cell swelling, were never reached.

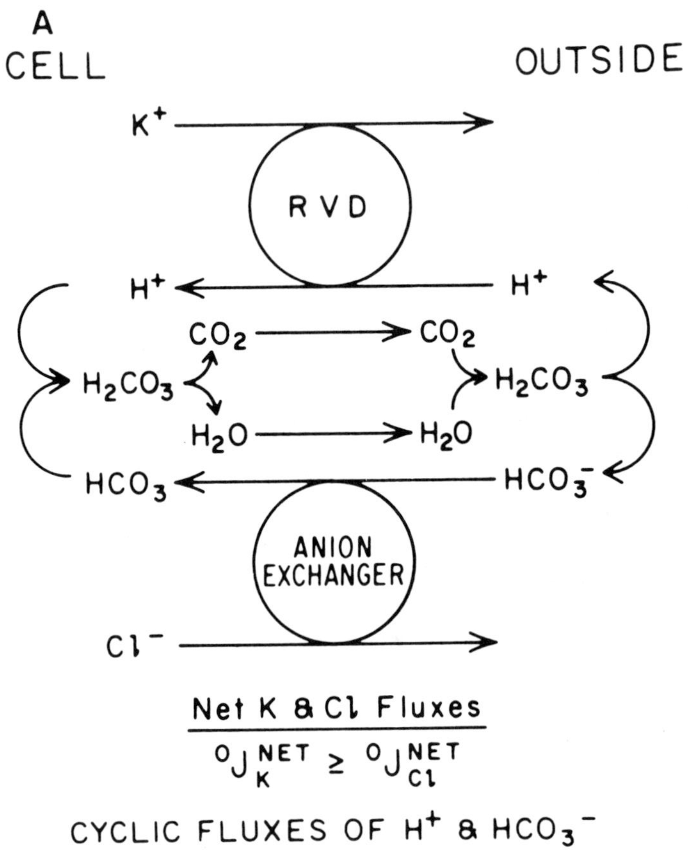


**Fig. 3-6.** Concept of mechanisms of regulatory volume decrease (RVD) of cells after hypotonic swelling. Obviously, cell volume normalization requires adjustment of intracellular osmolarity to that of the medium because of a high water permeability of cell membranes. This is accomplished by discharge of osmotic solutes, such as $K^+$ and $Cl^-$. Decrease of intracellular $K^+$ has been frequently observed under respective circumstances. A release of amino acids is discussed in addition. Electroneutrality is maintained by an obligatory exchange of $K^+$ against protons, and $Cl^-$ against bicarbonate. With the addition of $H^+$ and $HCO_3^-$, carbonic acid and water are formed without affecting cell osmolarity. It is currently not clear, however, whether the concept is valid for nerve and glial cells of higher vertebrates. From Cala PM: Cell volume regulation by flounder red blood cells in anisotonic media. J Gen Physiol 69:763. With permission.

This conclusion is in agreement with considerations of Van Harreveld[54] on the nature of ischemic cell swelling or after spreading depression.

Recently obtained findings by Ames and Nesbett[1] support this point. The authors subjected isolated retinas of rabbits in vitro to $O_2$ and substrate deprivation. Exposure of energy-deprived retinas to interstitial fluid obtained from ischemic retinas increased cell damage. Restriction of extracellular fluid had a similar effect, however, in relation to presence or absence of $Ca^{2+}$. The authors conclude also that changes in composition of extracellular fluid are a major determinant of ischemic damage of the brain.

A failure of cells to swell following anoxic exposure should not be viewed as a shortcoming but as a virtue of the experimental model. The in vitro model allows one to dissect a complex pathophysiological situation into pertinent components under control of many parameters. Resistance of cells to swell after complete shut down of energy metabolism may provide for a better understanding of factors responsible for the derangement of volume control under pathological conditions. We surmise that it is not anoxia per se inducing swelling but the response of exposed cells, such as their release of material into the extracellular space during anoxia. Potassium ions, or glutamate, may be considered. Evidently, the model is suited to study nature and threshold levels of potential factors accumulating in the extracellular space as a basis for arriving at an understanding of cell swelling mechanisms on a molecular level. Pertinent concepts on mechanisms of cell swelling under physiological and pathophysiological conditions of nerve and glial cells are condensed in Fig. 3-7.

In mechanism 2 (Fig. 3-7) swelling of cellular components, such as postsynaptic endings and glial cell processes is attributed to a release of excitatory transmitters raising membrane permeability to $Na^+$ ions. In mechanism 3 (Fig. 3-7) transmitters are cleared from the extracellular space by perisynaptic glial elements requiring metabolic energy. Uptake of glutamate occurs against a steep concentration gradient together with 2 moles of $Na^+$ per mole of glutamate. Hence intracellular osmolarity increases, causing influx of water, particularly if larger quantities of glutamate must be cleared. This is the case in anoxia or ischemia. In mechanism 4 (Fig. 3-7) cytotoxic cell swelling may result from release of free fatty acids, particularly arachidonate, which through disturbances of $Na^+$-$K^+$-ATPase inhibits active exchange of intracellular $Na^+$ against extracellular $K^+$. Eventually, cell swelling ensues. In mechanism 1 (Fig. 3-7) clearance of high extracellular $K^+$ involving carbonic anhydrase and specific anion transport systems may induce glial swelling, which is mediated through an exchange of bicarbonate versus chloride and $H^+$ against $Na^+$.[32] This is concluded from observations that removal of extracellular $Cl^-$ and inhibition of carbonic anhydrase by acetazolamide prevents swelling after exposure to high $K^+$ (Fig. 3-7).[10,11] Both Cl–$HCO_3^-$ and $Na^+$–$H^+$ antiporter systems of glial cells are postulated,

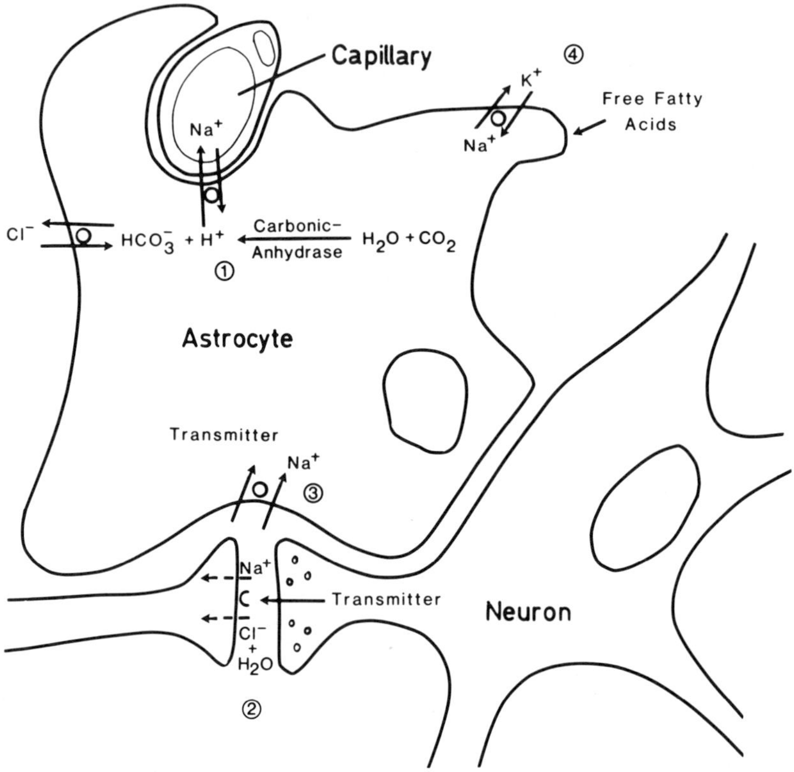


**Fig. 3-7.** Comprehensive model of nerve and glial volume changes under physiological and pathophysiological conditions. Hydration of carbonic anhydrase leading to formation of protons and bicarbonate may increase cell volume by their exchange against $Cl^-$ and $Na^+$ ions. The mechanism is considered to mediate swelling caused by high extracellular $K^+$ (1). Synaptic excitation associated with a release of transmitters increases $Na^+$ permeability of postsynaptic endings. Swelling results from an increased influx of $Na^+$ and $Cl^-$ together with water. Swelling of postsynaptic endings may provide for regional specificity of nerve cell circuits (2). Clearance of transmitters released during synaptic excitation (e.g., glutamate by perisynaptic glia) induces swelling by increase of cell osmolarity. Uptake of 1 *M* glutamic acid carries along 2 *M* $Na^+$. The process is most likely enhanced under pathological conditions, where extracellular glutamate reaches abnormally high levels (3). Finally, release of free fatty acids, arachidonic acid in particular, such as in cerebral ischemia, may induce swelling by interference with $Na^+$-$K^+$-ATPase of cell membranes disturbing normal Donnan equilibrium of ions between the intra-and extracellular compartment (4). From Kempski O: Cell swelling mechanisms in brain, in Baethmann A, Go KG, Unterberg A (Eds): Mechanisms of Secondary Brain Damage. London, Plenum Press, in press. With permission.

providing for 1:1 exchange of these ions. The systems obey saturation kinetics and can be inhibited pharmacologically. It should be mentioned, however, that the mechanisms 1–4 proposed in Fig. 3-7 are as yet interesting models. A definite role in cytotoxic cell swelling in the brain remains to be proved. Nevertheless, rapid advances in biochemistry, neurobiology, and cell culture techniques can be expected to uncover the mechanisms of cytotoxic swelling of cells in the near future. One should become aware of the fact that alterations of cell volume are not restricted to pathological conditions. Reversible swelling of neurons and glial elements may constitute an important physiological feature in maintenance of homeostasis. Extracellular clearance of material by glia may serve as an example. Moreover, formation of specific circuits between nerve cells involved in formation of fresh memory may be associated with reversible swelling of conducting axons to enhance selectivity of the network.

Swelling of cell elements in the brain becomes threatening at the moment when the influx of fluid causes an augmentation of brain mass leading to an increase of intracranial pressure. In addition, even without an increase of intracranial pressure, pathologically swollen nerve and glial elements may not be expected to function properly. As seen, analysis of cell volume of neurons and glial cells in physiological and pathological conditions has developed into a highly interesting field localized at the interface of basic sciences and clinical medicine.

## Acknowledgements

This work was supported by Deutsche Forschungsgemeinschaft: Ba 452/6-5. The authors are grateful for excellent technical and secretarial help provided by Ruth Demmer, Ulrike Goerke, and Friederike Helmes.

## REFERENCES

1. Ames A, Nesbett FB: Pathophysiology of ischemic cell death: III. Role of extracellular factors. Stroke 14(2):233–240, 1983
2. Arieff AI, Guisado R: Effects on the central nervous system of hypernatremic and hyponatremic states. Kidney Internat 10:104–116, 1976
3. Baethmann A, Van Harreveld A: Water and electrolyte distribution in grey matter rendered edematous with a metabolic inhibitor. J Neuropathol Exp Neurol 32:408–423, 1973
4. Baethmann A, Sohler K: Electrolyte- and fluid-spaces of rat brain in-situ after infusion with dinitrophenol. J Neurobiol 6:73–84, 1975
5. Baethmann A: Pathophysiological and pathochemical aspects of cerebral edema. Neurosurg Rev 1:85–100, 1978
6. Baethmann A: The mechanical, circulatory, osmotic, metabolic and toxic genesis of brain edema, in Ahnefeld FW, Bergmann H, Burri C, et al (Eds): Der Bewusstlose Patient, Berlin, Springer, 1979, pp 56–75
7. Bass NH, Hess HH, Pope A, et al: Quantitative cytoarchitectonic distribution of

neurons, glia, and DNA in rat cerebral cortex. J Compar Neurol 143(4):481–490, 1971
8. Benda P, Lightbody J, Sato G, et al: Differentiated rat glial cell strain in tissue culture. Science 161:370–371, 1968
9. Betz E: Vascular reactivity and ion homeostasis in heart and brain, in Zülch KJ, Kaufmann W, Hossmann KA, et al (Eds): Brain and Heart Infarct, Berlin, Springer, 1977, pp 10–18
10. Bourke RS: Studies of the development and subsequent reduction of swelling of mammalian. Cerebral cortex under isosmotic conditions in vitro. Exp Brain Res 8:232–248, 1969
11. Bourke RS, Kimelberg HK, Nelson LR, The effects of temperature and inhibitors on $HCO_3$-stimulated swelling and ion uptake of monkey cerebral cortex. Brain Res 105:309–323, 1976
12. Bourke RS, Kimelberg HK, Daze M, et al: Swelling and ion uptake in cat cerebrocortical slices: Control by neurotransmitters and ion transport mechanisms. Neurochem Res 8(1):5–24, 1983
13. Bui AH, Wiley JS: Cation fluxes and volume regulation by human lymphocytes. J Cell Physiol 108:47–54, 1981
14. Cala PM: Volume regulation by flounder red blood cells in anisotonic media. J Gen Physiol 69:537–552, 1977
15. Cala PM: Cell volume regulation by Amphiuma red blood cells. J Gen Physiol 82:761–784, 1983
16. Chan PH, Kerlan R, Fishman RA: Intracellular volume of osmotically regulated C-6 glioma cells. J Neurosci Res 8:67–72, 1982
17. Chaussy L, Baethmann A, Lubitz W: Electrical sizing of nerve and glia cells in the study of cell volume regulation, in Cervos-Navarro J, Fritschka E (Eds): Cerebral Microcirculation and metabolism. New York, Raven Press, 1981, pp 29–40
18. Choi BH, Lapham LW: Interactions of neurons and astrocytes during growth and development of human fetal brain in vitro. Exp Molec Pathol 24:110–125, 1976
19. Collewijn H, Schade JP: Changes in the size of astrocytes and oligodendrocytes during anoxia, hypothermia and spreading depression, in DeRobertis EDP, Carrea R (Eds): Biology of Neuroglia. Amsterdam, Elsevier, 1965, pp 184–195
20. Cornog JL, Gonatas NK, Feierman JR: Effects of intracerebral injection of ouabain on the fine structure of rat cerebral cortex. Am J Pathol 51:572–590, 1967
21. de Vellis J, Brooker G: Induction of enzymes by glucocorticoids and catecholamines in a rat glial cell line in Sato G (Ed): Tissue Culture of the Nervous System. New York, Plenum Press, 1973, pp 231–245
22. Fishman MC: Endogenous digitalis-like activity in mammalian brain. Proc Natl Acad Sci 76:4661–4663, 1979
23. Garcia JH, Kalimo H, Kamijo Y, et al: Cellular events during partial cerebral ischemia. Virchows Arch B Cell Pathol 25:191–206, 1977
24. Grinstein S, Clarke CA, Rothstein A: Activation of $Na^+/H^+$ exchange in lymphocytes by osmotically induced volume changes and by cytoplasmic acidification. J Gen Physiol 82:619–638, 1983
25. Harvey JA, McIlwain H: Excitatory acidic amino acids and the cation content and sodium ion flux of isolated tissues from the brain. Biochem J 108:269–276, 1968
26. Herschman HR, Grauling BP, Lerner MP: Nervous system-specific proteins in cultured neural cells, in Sato G (Ed): Tissue Culture of the Nervous System. New York, Plenum Press, 1973, pp 187–202
27. Heumann R, Valet G, Maison D, et al: Influence of the time in culture on cellular and neuronal properties of neuroblastoma × glioma hybrid cells. J Cell Sci 27:141–155, 1977
28. Hoffman EK, Simonsen LO, Lambert IH: Volume-induced increase of $K^+$ and $Cl^-$ permeabilities in Ehrlich ascites tumor cells. Role of internal $Ca^{++}$. J Membrane Biol 78:211–222, 1984
29. Hossmann KA: Development and resolution of ischemic brain swelling, in Pap-

pius HM, Feindel W (Eds): Dynamics of Brain Edema. Berlin, Springer, 1976, pp 219–227
30. Kachel V: Basic principles of electrical sizing of cells and particles and their realization in the new instrument "Metricell." J Histochem Cytochem 24(1):211–230, 1976
31. Kempski O, Chaussy L, Gross U, et al: Volume regulation and metabolism of suspended C6 glioma cells: An in vitro model to study cytotoxic brain edema. Brain Res 279:217–228, 1983
32. Kempski O: Cell swelling mechanisms in brain, in Baethmann A, Go KG, Unterberg A (Eds): Mechanisms of Secondary Brain Damage. London, Plenum Press, in press
33. Kukes G, Elul R, de Vellis J: The ionic basis of the membrane potential in a rat glial cell line. Brain Res 104:71–92, 1976
34. Ling EA, Paterson JA, Privat A, et al: Investigation of glial cells in semithin sections. I. Identification of glial cells in the brain of young rats. J Compar Neurol 149(1):43–72, 1973
35. Maier-Hauff K, Lange M, Schurer L, et al: Glutamate and free fatty acid concentrations in extracellular vasogenic edema fluid, in Go, KG, Baethmann A (Eds): Recent progress in the Study and Therapy of Brain Edema. New York, Plenum Press 1984, pp 183–192
36. Mayevsky A, Zeuthen T, Chance B: Measurements of extracellular potassium, ECoG and pyridine nucleotide levels during cortical spreading depression in rats. Brain Res 76:347–349, 1974
37. Meier-Ruge W, Gygax P, Iwangoff P, et al: The significance of pericapillary astroglia for cerebral cortical blood flow and EEG activity in Cervos-Navarro J (Ed): Pathology of Cerebral Microcirculation. Berlin, W de Gruyter, 1974, pp 235–243
38. Neu A Thesis. University of Munich, in preparation.
39. Norenberg MD, Lapham LW: The astrocyte response in experimental portal-systemic encephalopathy: An electron microscopic study. J Neuropathol Exp Neurol 33(3):422–435, 1974
40. Norton WT, Poduslo SE: Neuronal soma and whole neuroglia of rat brain: New isolation technique. Science 167:1144–1146, 1970
41. Okamoto K, Quastel JH: Tetrodotoxin-sensitive uptake of ions and water by slices of rat brain in vitro. Biochem J 120:37–47, 1970
42. Olson J, Holtzman D: Respiration and cell volume of primary cultured cerebral astocytes in media of various osmolarities. Brain Res 246:273–279, 1982
43. Palay SL, Chan-Palay V: Cerebellar Cortex. Berlin, Springer, 1974
44. Partin JC, Partin JS, Schubert WK, et al: Brain ultrastructure in Reye's syndrome. J Neuropathol Exp Neurol 34(5):425–444, 1975
45. Powell H, Swarner P, Gluck L, et al: Hexachlorophene myelinopathy in premature infants. J Pediatr 82:976–981, 1973
46. Reulen HJ: Vasogenic brain edema. New aspects in its formation, resolution and therapy. Br J Anaesth 48:741–751, 1976
47. Rosenberg HM, Shank BB, Gregg EC: Volume changes of mammalian cells subjected to hypotonic solutions in vitro: Evidence for the requirement of a sodium pump for the shrinking phase. J Cell Physiol 80:23–32, 1972
48. Schade JP, Ford DH: Basic Neurology. Amsterdam: Elsevier, 1971
49. Symon L, Branston NM, Strong AJ: Gradation of ischaemia with threshold flow levels for tissue function and structure in the brain, in Zulch KJ, Kaufmann W, Hossmann V, et al (Eds): Brain and Heart Infarct. Berlin, Springer, 1977, pp 150–158
50. Tasaki I, Iwasa K: Swelling of nerve fibers during action potentials. Upsala J Med Sci 85:211–215, 1980
51. Uemura E, Hartmann HA: RNA content and volume of nerve cell bodies in human brain. II. Subiculum in aging normal patients. Exp Neurol 65:107–117, 1979

52. Van Harreveld A, Crowell J, Malhotra SK: A study of extracellular space in central nervous tissue by freeze-substitution. J Cell Biol 25:117–137, 1965

53. Van Harreveld A: Brain tissue electrolytes, in Bittar EE (Ed): Molecular Biology and Medicine Series. London, Butterworths, 1966

54. Van Harreveld A: The extracellular space in the vertebrate central nervous system, in Bourne GH (Ed): The Structure and Function of Nervous Tissue. London, Academic Press, 1972, pp 447–511

55. Van Harreveld A, Fifkova E: Mechanisms involved in spreading depression. J Neurobiol 4(4):375–387, 1973

56. Van Harreveld A, Fifkova E: Involvement of glutamate in memory formation. Brain Res 81:455–467, 1974

57. Van Harreveld A, Fifkova E: Swelling of dendritic spines in the fascia dentata after stimulation of the perforant fibers as a mechanism of post-tetanic potentiation. Exp Neurol 49:736–749, 1975

58. Williams V, Grossman RG, Edmunds SM: Volume and surface area estimates of astrocytes in the sensorimotor cortex of the cat. Neuroscience 5:1151–1159, 1980

59. Zimmer M, Kempski O, Neu A, et al: Anoxic incubation of suspended glial cells. An in-vitro model of cerebral anoxia to study cytotoxic brain edema. Adv Neurosurg 12:271–273, 1984

*J. Gordon McComb*

# 4

# Normal Cerebrospinal Fluid Dynamics

Cerebrospinal fluid (CSF) suspends the brain and spinal cord in a watery medium and cushions the CNS from external force applied to the skull or vertebral column. CSF is essential to maintaining the normal homeostasis of the brain. A number of substances are actively transported in and out of the CNS by both the choroid plexus and parenchyma so as to keep the internal milieu constant. Passive removal of metabolic wastes and macromolecules is provided by the "sink action" of the CSF since continual CSF drainage will keep their concentrations low, producing a gradient by which they are cleared. The CSF within the ventricular cavities and subarachnoid space (SAS) is in continuity with and similar to the fluid in the extracellular spaces, as there is no restriction to free exchange of any of its constituents. Neurotransmitters within both the parenchyma and the ventricles, vital to normal activity of the CNS, can move by way of the CSF.[1] The multiple functions of CSF, coupled with its rapid turnover, indeed make it a "third circulation" was first referred to by Cushing.[5]

## CSF CIRCULATION

Cerebrospinal fluid circulation throughout the CNS is maintained primarily by the hydrostatic difference between the newly formed CSF within the ventricles and that at its sites of drainage. Less important are the factors associated with the pulsations of the brain and choroid plexus from the arterial tree, respiratory variations, change in bodily position, and ciliary action. Cerebrospinal fluid normally flows through the ventricular system to exit

BRAIN INSULTS IN INFANTS AND CHILDREN
0-8089-1723-4

from the fourth ventricle, through the midline foramen of Magendie and the paired lateral foramina of Luschka, into the basal cisterns at the base of the brain. Once having reached the SAS, CSF percolates through the various cisterns and spaces surrounding the brain and spinal cord to reach the ultimate sites of egress. For further understanding the pathophysiology of impaired CSF circulation, one must consider the normal mechanisms of CSF formation and absorption must be considered.

## CSF FORMATION

It is generally agreed that most CSF is formed within the ventricular system from either the choroid plexus, the ependyma, or the parenchyma. A method has not been developed to separate the function of the ependyma from that of the remainder of the parenchyma, so the role of the ependyma in bulk CSF formation is not known, although morphological considerations suggest that its contribution is insignificant. Results from isolated choroid plexus preparations would indicate at least that 80 percent of CSF production is from this source alone.[2] Evidence that the brain is the principal source of extrachoroidal CSF, amounting to possibly 10–20 percent of the total CSF production, has been shown in several studies. From a morphological standpoint the choroid plexus has characteristicss associated with secretory function and has been compared with the proximal renal tubule, as it can both secrete and absorb a number of substances. In contradistinction to the capillaries of the parenchyma, where tight junctions between endothelial cells constitute the blood–brain barrier, the capillaries of the choroid plexus are of the fenestrated type and devoid of tight junctions. Tight junctions are present at the apical side of the choroid epithelium, however, and constitute the blood–CSF barrier. Cerebrospinal fluid appears to be formed in a two-step process, the first of which is the formation of an ultrafiltrate of plasma through the non-tight-junction choroidal capillary endothelium by hydrostatic pressure into the connective tissue stroma beneath the epithelium of the villus. In the second step the ultrafiltrate is subsequently transformed into a secretion by an active metabolic process within the choroidal epithelium. Although the mechanism is not known, one model suggests that sodium potassium adenosine triphosphatase ($Na^+$-$K^+$-ATPase) pumps sodium into the basal side of the cell with water passively following by the osmotic gradient thus created. Carbonic anhydrase catalyzes the formation of bicarbonate inside the cell with hydrogen ion being sent back to the sodium pump as a counter ion with potassium. In a manner analagous to that involving the basal side of the epithelium, $Na^+$-$K^+$-ATPase located in the microvilli on the apical surface extrudes sodium into the ventricle followed by osmotically drawn water. Since the cells do not swell or shrink, the sum of the two processes must be in balance.[7]

Cerebrospinal formation averages 20 ml/h or 500 ml/day. An approximately threefold turnover of CSF occurs daily as the total volume of the CSF in the ventricles and SAS averages 150 ml. Under normal physiological conditions CSF formation can be considered independent of pressure. Markedly elevated intraventricular pressure will reduce CSF formation by diminishing the quantity of ultrafiltrate from the choroidal capillary. Formation of CSF in relation of the maturation process has been studied in several animal species but not in humans. The data indicated an increase in CSF production at a rate greater than can be accounted for by the correspondeding increase in choroid plexus or brain weight and may reflect more the maturation of the enzyme systems involved. Although the data are very limited, CSF production in infants as well as in older patients is reported to be in the normal adult range. Neurogenic control of CSF formation has only recently been investigated as previously it was not possible to separate the effects of choroidal blood flow from direct neurogenic stimulation of the choroidal epithelium. Studies show that stimulation of adrenergic fibers can acutely diminish CSF flow by 30 percent whereas stimulation of cholinergic pathways will increase CSF production by as much as 100 percent, without altering blood flow in the choroid plexus.[1]

Although it has long been suspected that oversecretion of CSF occurs in the presence of a choroid plexus papilloma, unequivocal evidence for this has been documented on only two occasions.[4,5] Evidence for overproduction of CSF in the absence of the choroid plexus papilloma does not exist.[3] Through its presumed action on cyclic adenosine monophosphate, cholera toxin has been reported to double the flow of CSF, a finding that has not been confirmed by another study. The apparent increase in CSF formation may be the result from plasma entering the ventricle following a breakdown of the blood–brain barrier rather than an increased CSF secretion rate. Drugs that reduce CSF formation do so by interferring with the entire cellular metabolic process or specific transport mechanisms. The action of acetazolamide (Diamox, manufactured by Lederle) on CSF production has been studied extensively. This agent decreases CSF production by interferring with the function of carbonic anhydrase and appears to significantly diminish CSF formation in humans both acutely and chronically. It has been noted that, because of the nature of formation versus absorption curve, a one-third reduction of normal CSF production would reduce the intracranial pressure by only 1.5 cm of water. This explains why Diamox or other agents that reduce CSF formation have not proved useful in control of hydrocephalus. These conclusions have focused in investigations into the pathogenisis of hydrocephalus on CSF absorption.

## CSF ABSORPTION

The absorption of CSF and its constituents depends on bulk flow in addition to passive or facilitative difusion and active transport of specific solutes. The rate of CSF absorption is pressure-dependent and relatively linear over a fairly wide physiological range. The resistance to flow diminishes at higher than normal physiological pressures and may relate to the opening of channels not available at lower pressures. The only proven force responsible for CSF absorption is that of a hydrostatic gradient. It has been firmly established that arachnoid villi drain CSF.[6] Those villi that are grossly visible termed *arachnoid granulations* or *Pacchionian bodies,* are functionally similar to those that are not. Controversy remains regarding the structure of the arachnoid villus as to the existence of open channels connecting the arachnoid side with the venous side, for the presence or absence of such channels would indicate a basic physiological difference in the manner in which CSF and its constituents drain. The open villus model would be solely pressure-responsive and allow for passive escape of macromolecules, whereas a villus covered by a continuous tight-junctioned endothelial membrane would add the factors of osmosis, diffusion, and filtration; macromolecules would require an active transport process to cross this barrier. The various anatomic studies are fairly evenly divided between these two possibilities. Discrepancy in morphological findings may relate in part or whole to the manner in which the villus is prepared for histological study; a zero pressure gradient between the arachnoid and venous sides of the villus during fixation would allow for its collapse, and as a result open channels would not be apparent. Considerations as to whether open channels exist and the size of such channels are pertinent only if the villus is virtually the exclusive location for bulk egress of CSF into the blood stream. If a significant fraction of CSF and its constituents are draining elsewhere, these considerations are less relevant.

Weed[6] acknowledged in his pioneering studies on CSF absorption, that some of his injected solutions, in addition to existing through the arachnoid villi, drained into the mucosa of paranasal sinuses, nasal mucosa, cranial nerve root sheaths, and cervical lymph nodes; he thought these routes were accessory. The idea that a portion of the CSF could and did drain through the lymphatic system was gradually relegated to obscurity, and standard text and teaching have limited CSF drainage solely to the arachnoid villus for more than a generation now. Several laboratory investigations would indicate that approximately half of the CSF normally drains into the lymphatics.[4] These observations are currently being confirmed in primates. Presently no studies show to what extent lymphatic drainage of CSF exists in humans, but some support for this concept comes from the clinical observation that parents of children with CSF-diverting shunts occasionally report nasal congestion and periorbital or facial swelling when the child's shunt becomes obstructed. The lymphatic drainage of CSF seems likely to play a role in the pathophysiology of hydrocephalus, as either an alternative pathway for drainage or a cause in cases of impaired access to the lymphatic system.

## REFERENCES

1. Cutler RWP, Sperrell RB: Cerebrospinal fluid: A selective review. Ann Neurol 11:1–10, 1982
2. Davson H: Physiology of the Cerebrospinal Fluid. London, Churchill, 1967, 445 pp
3. Fishman RA: Cerebrospinal Fluid in Diseases of the Nervous System. Philadelphia, Saunders, 1980, 384 pp
4. McComb JG: Recent research into the nature of cerebrospinal fluid formation and absorption. J Neurosurg 59:369–383, 1983
5. Milhorat TH: The third circulation revisted. J Neurosurg 42:628–645, 1975
6. Weed LH, McKibben PS: Pressure changes in the cerebrospinal fluid following ultravenous injection of solutions of various concentrations. Am J Physiol 48:512–530, 1919
7. Welch K: The principles of physiology of the cerebrospinal fluid in relation to hydrocephalus including normal pressure hydrocephalus, in Friedlander WJ (Ed): Current Reviews, Advances in Neurology, vol 13. New York, Raven Press, 1975, pp 247–332

*Derek A. Bruce*

# 5

# Cerebrovascular Dynamics

In the cerebral circulation, which is supplied through the two carotid and the two vertebral arteries, 10–15 percent of the cardiac output goes to the brain, and the total cerebral blood flow (CBF) in adults is 750 ml/min. This is a regional blood flow of 75–80 ml/100 g/min to the grey matter and approximately 25 ml/100 g/min to the white matter. Table 5-1 shows recent human CBF data in newborn children. The two major elements controlling blood flow to an organ are the resistance of the vessels and the pressure drop across the organ:

$$\text{CBF} = \pi r4 \frac{(P_1 - P_2)}{8\lambda L}$$

where $r$ is the arteriolar radius, $P_1 - P_2$ is the pressure drop across the bed, $\lambda$ is the viscosity, and $L$ is the length of the vascular bed. Since viscosity and length are generally unchanged, the major factors controlling CBF are radius and pressure drop. In the brain, $P_1 - P_2$ can be considered to be systemic arterial pressure (SAP) minus intracranial pressure (ICP).

## AUTOREGULATION

The brain vascular bed exhibits several kinds of autoregulation. Pressure autoregulation is defined as the ability to maintain CBF constant despite changes in SAP or ICP. Systemic arterial pressure minus ICP is defined as cerebral perfusion pressure (CPP). In a healthy brain, the pressure autoregulation curve (Fig. 5-1) shows a constant CBF with variations in CPP between 50 and 150 torr; whether these changes are induced by alterations in either

BRAIN INSULTS IN INFANTS AND CHILDREN
0-8089-1723-4

**Table 5-1** *CBF Studies in the Human Neonate*

| Subjects | Regional Blood Flow | Reference |
|---|---|---|
| Full-term newborns | 40 ml/100 g/min | 4 |
| Preterm newborns | 42 ml/100 g/min | 4 |
| Low-birth-weight newborns | 37 ml/100 g/min | 3 |
| Stressed prematures | 29.9 ml/10 g/min | 3 |
| Stressed prematures | 24.0 ml/100 g/min | 4 |

SAP or ICP. As the CPP is lowered, vasodilation occurs, and as CPP is increased, vasoconstriction occurs to maintain a constant CBF. The transduction mechanism that results in pressure autoregulation is not clear. It does not appear to be primarily a neurogenic mechanism, although changes in resting sympathetic tone of the cerebral vessels may affect the response to changes in $CO^2$ and the shape of the autoregulatory curve. An intrinsic myogenic mechanism appears to play a role, and it has recently been suggested that small changes in cerebral adenosine may be a chemical trigger for pressure autoregulation. Pressure autoregulation may be impaired by trauma, hypoxia, or ischemia either regionally or globally. Unfortunately, the loss or preservation of pressure autoregulation is variable when brain insults occur. Thus the use of a 50-torr CPP does not necessarily ensure a normal blood flow in a

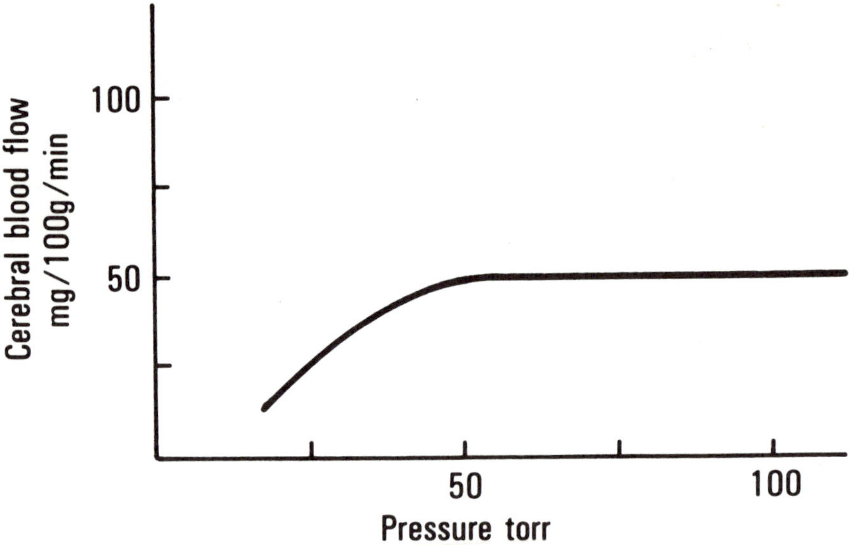


**Fig. 5-1.** Perfusion pressure (autoregulation intact).

diseased brain. If the CBF is passively responsive to CPP (loss of autoregulation), the CBF may be lower or higher than expected for any given CPP.[5] It is better to try and maintain a normal ICP of 15 to 20 torr and a normal or slightly elevated SAP for age in the intensive care unit rather than to opt for a fixed CPP. Cerebrovascular pressure autoregulation has been demonstrated in newborn animals, but the limits are unclear (i.e., the pressures above and below which a passive flow pressure situation occurs). It has been suggested that autoregulation is impaired by neonatal asphyxia. In animal experiments, however, the CBF is usually decreased with systemic hypoxia. Very little or nothing is known about the control of the cerebral circulation in the human premature or neonate.

### Metabolic Autoregulation

The cerebral circulation also manifests chemical or metabolic autoregulation. This is the ability of the local tissues to modify CBF to their metabolic requirements (i.e., as metabolism is increased, local cerebral blood flow also increases).[5] This occurs with many forms of regional brain activity from focal motor movements (e.g., finger tapping to seizures). The transduction mechanism here is also not totally clear. Such agents as pH, potassium, $K^+$, and $Ca^{++}$ will also produce changes in vessel caliber.[5] At present, small changes in cerebral adenosine content is a likely mechanism for local metabolic control of CBF. Whether other chemical compounds are also involved is not yet clear. This form of chemical autoregulation is apparently much more resistant to damage than is pressure autoregulation and is preserved until the terminal states of brain function. Acidotic brain secondary to tissue damage has a higher resting CBF and shows evidence of impairment of chemical control. The preservation of chemical autoregulation at a time when pressure autoregulation is defective can lead to cerebral damage, since if vasodilation is produced by a focal increase in tissue metabolities but the CPP is inadequate to deliver an increase in CBF, functional tissue ischemia may result.

The cerebral circulation is also responsive to changes of arterial blood gases. As $Pao_2$ decreases, there is no change in CBF until $Pao_2$ drops below 50 torr. Thereafter, there are marked increases in CBF with a further decrease in $Pao_2$ such that at an arterial oxygen pressure of 20–25 torr, CBF is increased threefold. The cerebral blood vessels are extremely responsive to changes in arterial $Paco_2$. For each 1-mm change in $Paco_2$, CBF changes by approximately 3–4 percent such that CBF doubles as $Paco_2$ changes from 20 to 40 torr.[5] Below a $Paco_2$ of 20 torr in adults, there is little or no further decrease in CBF. In children, however, the exact lower limits of $Paco_2$ response is unknown. Our own information suggests that it is lower than 20 torr.[6] In fetal and newborn animals, decreases in CBF with decreasing $Paco_2$ down to 12 to 15 torr have been reported.[2,3] The $CO_2$ responsiveness of the cerebral circulation is usually preserved until death, and $CO_2$ responses may, in fact, be enhanced following trauma in a specific group of patients. Whereas $CO_2$ responses are not abolished by alterations in sympathetic tone in the cerebral vessels, the slope of the $Pa_{CO_2}$/CBF curve is increased with sympathetic stimulation and decreased with sympathetic blockade.[7] Studies suggest that hyperventilation may contribute to the reconstitution of lost pressure autoregulation. In the noninjured brain, continued hyperventilation results in a gradual increase in CBF back to control levels over approximately 6 hours.[5] In the traumatized brain, this does not appear to occur, and indeed the $CO_2$ response may become enhanced over time. The best explanation is that under normal conditions metabolic control overcomes the local effect of the low $Pa_{CO_2}$ with resultant vasodilatation. Another contributing fact is that CSF pH gradually returns to its resting value despite continued hyperventilation due to the rather slow changes in CSF bicarbonate. In the injured brain, metabolism is generally decreased and thus there is a decreased stimulus for the accumulation of tissue metabolites that might produce vasodilatation and increased CBF.

## NEUROGENIC REGULATION

Cerebral vessels have both cholinergic and adrenergic supplies, and the neural network continues into the parenchymal vessels.[7] There is a little evidence, however, for a neurogenic control of the intraparenchymal vessels. On the other hand, it is clear that the major vessels (internal carotid and middle cerebral arteries) do respond to sympathetic stimulation by vasoconstriction. The cerebral vessels may be considered in two groups: the larger vessels that are under some neurogenic control and the small pial and intraparenchymal vessels whose major control is chemical change in the tissue.[7] Changes in $Pa_{CO_2}$, for example, affect primarily the intraparenchymal vessels. At this time, there is no clinical therapy directed to manipulation of the neurogenic control of CBF except is states of systemic hemorrhagic shock. Here alpha blockade has been shown to increase CBF presumably by decreasing large vessel constriction. The two portions of the cerebral circulation should work in series. Low perfusion pressure will primarily trigger vasodilatation to reduce resistance and increase flow, whereas tissue hypoxia will tend to produce an increase in the number of open capillaries. As the insult worsens, both mechanisms will act to improve tissue flow and prevent hypoxia and ischemia. If the large vessel system is constricted at a time when the intraparechymal vessels are dilating (e.g., by sympathetic stimulation), an inadequate increase in CBF will result in tissue ischemia. It can be seen that in the clinical setting focal changes in anatomic damage, variably disturbed autoregulation and different chemical milieus will result in a very heterogenous response of the cerebral circulation. It is impossible to predict under all circumstances what these changes will be, and the present guess is to try to normalize as many of the parameters as possible.

## REFERENCES


1. Bruce DA: Clinical reflections on brain stem injury in childhood, in Villani R, Papo I, Giovanelli M, et al. (Eds): Advances in Neurotraumatology. Excerpta Medica, Amsterdam, 1983, pp 74–78
2. Gregory GA, Org W, Tweed A, et al: The effects of severe alkalosis and hypoxaemia on cerebral metabolism in the newborn lamb. Anesthesiology 57:1724, 1982
3. Lou MC, Lassen NA, Friis-Hansen B: Impaired autoregulation of cerebral blood flow in the distressed newborn infant. J Pediatr 94:118–121, 1979
4. Ment LR, Duncan CC, Ehrenkray RA, et al: Intraventricular hemorrhage of the preterm neonate: Timing and cerebral blood flow changes. Ann Neurol 14:356, 1983
5. Siesjo BK: Cerebral circulation and metabolism. J Neurosurg 60:883–908, 1984
6. Swedlow D, Frewen T, Watcha W, et al: Cerebral blood flow, AJDO2 and CMRO2 in comatose children, in Go KG, Baethmann A (Eds): Brain Edema. New York, Plenum Press, 1984, pp 365–372

# PART II

# Basic Pathophysiology

*Andreas Unterberg*
*Alexander Baethmann*

# 6

# Secondary Changes in Brain Biochemistry with Brain Edema

Brain edema can be defined as an increase of cerebral tissue water causing an increase of tissue volume.[49] Brain edema by definition is thus associated with chemical changes of the affected tissue. Biochemical investigations on brain edema prove useful in enhancing our understanding of the complex process. Respective findings distinguish major prototypes (discussed in this chapter), such as vasogenic, cytotoxic, and osmotic.[37] Moreover, chemical analysis of the tissue is a reliable method for quantification of edema and, most importantly, for evaluation of the efficiency of treatment.

The survey on secondary changes in brain biochemistry with brain edema focuses on the chemical composition of edematous brain tissue under various conditions, disturbances of the extracellular environment, and the metabolic response of cerebral tissue to edema and discusses the pathophysiological role of mediator substances, which are considered to enhance the edema process. Investigations on mediator substances of brain edema acquire an ever increasing interest for good reasons. It may provide a basis for study of therapeutic modalities to influence their release and function as a rational form of treatment of edema and of associated functional disturbances.

## BIOCHEMICAL RESPONSE TO BRAIN EDEMA IN CEREBRAL TISSUE

### Chemical Composition of Edematous Brain Tissue

Although the increase of cerebral water content is a common denominator of brain edema, changes of tissue electrolytes (e.g. $Na^+$, $K^+$) may vary

BRAIN INSULTS IN INFANTS AND CHILDREN
0-8089-1723-4

according to the underlying cause. Breakdown of the blood–brain barrier is the predominant mechanism of formation of vasogenic brain edema. Dysfunction of the blood–brain barrier leading to an accumulation of plasma proteins in the affected parenchyma, even in distant areas, is confined to the site of the primary lesion, such as a tumor or a contusion, which is the port of entry of vasogenic fluid from the intravascular space.[36] Increase of water content is—except for a few modifications—always combined with an increase of $Na^+$, but less frequently with a decrease of $K^+$.[2,3,17,30,46–48,53] Function of the blood–brain barrier is maintained in cytotoxic edema of metabolic or toxic origin or in acute hyponatremia.[2] Fluid entering the cerebrum is confined to the intracellular compartment at the expense of a shrinking extracellular space. The mechanisms causing swelling of nerve and glial cells in cytotoxic edema are far from understood. However, an increase in membrane permeability to $Na^+$ ions allowing for enhanced influx along the downhill extra–intracellular gradient, inhibition of active $Na^+$ pumps, (e.g., $Na^+$-$K^+$-ATPase), and breakdown of energy metabolism providing fuel for the pumps as in anoxia are likely to play a major role (Baethmann,[2] Chapter III).

Studies of the chemical composition of edematous brain may help to understand the corresponding computer tomographical (CT) findings in patients. Computed tomographic scanning is based on measurement of tissue density, which in brain tissue is predominantly determined by water and lipids. Vasogenic brain edema such as around tumors appears as a hypodense area in the CT scan as a result of an increased tissue water content. Since tissue lipids simultaneously decrease in edematous areas, however, the effect of the edematous water uptake on tissue density becomes attenuated.[40,41] Comparative studies of water content and density in CT scans are useful for determination of threshold levels of accumulation of water for recognition of edema. Edema may be already detected at a water content of only 1.5 percent above normal. New generations of CT scanners may afford an even better resolution.[41]

### Disturbances of the Extracellular Milieu

Studies on alterations of the cerebral extracellular environment provide important qualitative and quantitative information on the level of homeostasis maintained by edematous brain tissue. Control of the chemical composition of the extracellular environment of nerve and glial cells is impressively tight in normal brain. Obviously, it is a basic requirement for the proper function of the cell elements. Studies on the chemistry of isolated vasogenic edema fluid obtained by various methods, such as centrifugation of edematous tissue or interstitial fluid drainage, revealed neurons and glial cells to be exposed to an abnormal environment in edematous brain tissue areas.[17,25,26,43] Protein, amino acid, and fatty acid concentrations of interstitial fluid are negligibly small under physiological conditions with an intact blood–brain barrier. Respective conclusions were drawn from comparative studies of normal CSF used as reference of extracellular medium. Both are in an equilibrium in the steady state. Concentrations of major constituents of CSF, plasma, and edema fluid are compared in Table 6-1. First attempts toward a chemical characterization of vasogenic edema fluid confirmed its intravasal origin, as seen from the rich content in plasma proteins and an electrolyte composition closer to that in plasma than normal CSF. As far as $K^+$ is concerned, respective concentrations in edema fluid seem even to exceed those in plasma (see Table 6-1).

An important question is whether and how the abnormal extracellular environment influences function or structure of the exposed cells. Interference with cellular function involving membrane permeability, repolarization after firing, and so on may be assumed from alterations of relevant electrolytes, such as $K^+$ ($K^+$ is markedly higher in edema fluid than in the normal interstitial space). Furthermore, neurotoxic compounds such as unsaturated free fatty acids are released in damaged brain and spread into perifocal tissue. This is true for certain aminoacids that function as excitatory, or inhibitory transmitter compounds. Concentrations of glutamate, aspartate, proline, taurine, and similar compounds are contrary to respective concentrations in plasma—very low in normal CSF.[43,52] Extracellular concentrations are increased in lesions involving blood–brain barrier damage; however, since intravascular fluid rich in aminoacids then has access to cerebral parenchyma.

**Table 6-1** *Chemical Composition of Vasogenic Edema Fluid as Compared to CSF and Plasma*

| | | Edema Fluid | CSF | Plasma |
|---|---|---|---|---|
| Albumin | (mg/100 ml) | 2900 | 20 | 3,600 |
| $Na^+$ | (mEq/l) | 129 | 146 | 152 |
| $K^+$ | (mEq/l) | 5–15 | 3.0 | 4.5 |
| $Cl^-$ | (mEq/l) | 102 | 124 | 111 |
| $Ca_{total}$ | (mEq/l) | NA* | 2.7 | 4.9 |
| $Ca^{2+}$ | (mEq/l) | NA | 2.3 | 2.9 |
| Glutamate | (mg/100 ml) | 4.4–15.4 | 0.22 | 1.62 |
| Glycin | (mg/100 ml) | NA | 0.11 | 1.54 |
| Proline | (mg/100 ml) | NA | 0.01 | 2.36 |
| Taurine | (mg/100 ml) | NA | 0.07 | 0.55 |
| Fatty acids, total | (mg/100 ml) | NA | 0.07 | 4–18 |
| Arachidonic acid | (mg/100 ml) | 0.06–0.1 | ND | 0.03 |

*Not available.

†Not detectable.

The data were compiled from Perry,[51] Gazendam,[25] Go,[26] Clasen,[18] and Maier-Hauff.[42–44]

Traumatic, or ischemic, destruction of cerebral parenchyma resulting in loss of material from irreversibly damaged cells has the same effect (see section on mediator compounds of brain edema). Permanent increase of extracellular concentrations of excitatory transmitter compounds, such as glutamate, may be viewed to upset homeostasis of cell volume control because of continuing increase of membrane permeability to $Na^+$ ions (see section on mediator compounds of brain edema).

Further studies are certainly required for an understanding of how disturbances of the extracellular environment affect cerebral function and metabolism. Nevertheless, evidence is accumulating that extracellular homeostasis is severely affected and, moreover that the degree of injury correlates with the degree of dysfunction. A point in case is the kallikrein-kinin system and glutamic acid, which are discussed in the respective sections on glutamic acid and the kallikrein-kinin system.

### Metabolic Response of Cerebral Tissue to Edema

Alterations of cerebral metabolism may be attributed not only to exposure of the parenchyma to edema, but also to the consequences, such as an increase of intracranial pressure leading to impairment of tissue perfusion. Clinical and experimental studies abound on tissue metabolism in conditions associated with cerebral edema.[23,29] Perifocal brain tissue samples were taken during neurosurgery from patients with focal lesions, such as cerebral tumors employing freeze-stop techniques for fixation of tissue metabolism.[55] Parameters of the energy state, such as phosphocreatine, ATP/ADP ratio, and the energy charge potential were less affected than glycolysis, which became considerably stimulated. This was concluded from a rise in lactic acid concentrations and lactate/pyruvate concentration ratios, respectively. More recently conducted studies by Sutton[58] have confirmed that vasogenic edema may only marginally affect the energy state of the tissue while definitely enhancing glycolysis. Regression analysis between the cerebral water content and glycolytic activity demonstrates a possible relationship between both parameters indicative of stimulation of glycolysis by edema. Yet, discrete disturbances of the microcirculation leading to patchy tissue hypoxia cannot be ruled out. Glycolysis is known to respond more sensitively to changes of cerebral $O_2$ supply than the energy state.[57]

## MEDIATOR COMPOUNDS OF BRAIN EDEMA

Mediator compounds are neurotoxic substances that are considered to become released from primary lesions, or to enter the brain through the broken blood–brain barrier together with vasogenic edema fluid. Mediator compounds may enhance the edema process by either increase of the blood–brain barrier damage or induction of microcirculatory disturbances or secondary cytotoxic swelling of nerve and glial cells. Mediator compounds may also be responsible for metabolic and functional disorders of cells in edematous tissue. Enhancement of blood–brain barrier damage and vasodilation secondary to release or activation of mediator compounds would promote further influx of edema fluid and eventually increase of intracranial pressure. Since necrotic brain or the intravascular compartment is the original source, a great number and variety of mediators may be conceived. Particularly interesting candidates are summarized in Table 6-2. These include lysosomal enzymes, biogenic amines, such as serotonin and histamine, glutamate, fatty acids, particularly arachidonic acid and its metabolites, and finally the kallikrein-kinin system.[8,9,19,22,27,32,35,38,45,66] Identification of a candidate as a mediator requires a damaging potential for nervous tissue, formation or release in conditions associated with brain edema in relation with the extent of damage, and finally attenuation of tissue damage (e.g., edema) by specific inhibition of the mediator. The latter may concern inhibition of mediator formation and of its pathophysiological function in the tissue. The following discussion is restricted to glutamate, arachidonic acid, and the kallikrein-kinin system, which appear particularly promising.

#### Glutamic Acid

The amino acid glutamate is a highly potent pharmacological and toxic compound, if administered to nerve and glial cells in vivo and in vitro in concentrations of 100 $\mu$M and above.[64] Extracellular glutamate concentrations are negligible (ca. 10–15 $\mu$M) in normal brain, whereas the amino acid is abundantly present in cells (ca. 15 mM). The intra-extracellular concentration ratio is approximately 1000:1. It is assumed that glutamate is released from necrobiotic cells with gross damage of cell membranes in a focus from where it is carried along with the bulk of edema fluid into distant perifocal areas. If concentrations are sufficient, glutamate may induce secondary cell swelling, or even necrosis. It has indeed been demonstrated that high concentrations of glutamate cause cell swelling, probably by increasing $Na^+$ permeability of cell membranes.[1,28] Extracellular concentrations of 8 mM or higher led even to necrosis of nerve and glial cells in exposed cerebral tissue.[63] Cerebral administration of glutamate in vivo by ventriculocisternal perfusion or superfusion of cerebral cortex induces cytotoxic brain edema, that is, an increase of intracellular water content, resulting in shrinking of the extracellular compartment.[33,54] Cytotoxic swelling was ascertained in vitro in studies on cell volume response of C6 glial cells to administration of glutamate.[34]

A further level of evidence of a mediator function of glutamate was obtained in investigations on vasogenic edema secondary to cold injury.

**Table 6-2** *Brain Edema Factors*

| | |
|---|---|
| Enzymes | Fatty acids |
| Lysosomal enzymes | Arachidonic acid and metabolites |
| Proteolytic enzymes | Prostaglandins |
| Biogenic amines | Leukotrienes |
| Serotonin | Free radicals |
| Histamine | Kallikrein-kinin system |
| Amino acids | |
| Glutamate | |

According to Baethmann.[3]

Maier-Hauff et al[43] studied concentrations of glutamate in extracellular edema fluid obtained by interstitial fluid drainage according to the method of Gazendam et al[25] and Go.[26] Glutamate concentrations found in perifocal edema fluid were approximately 10 times that present in the extracellular space under normal circumstances. Normal CSF was employed as a reference. The increase of glutamate did not result from the influx of plasmalike fluid through the broken barrier into brain carrying glutamate, but from a release of damaged cells in the primary lesion. This is supported by the level of glutamate concentrations simultaneously determined in plasma, which was significantly lower than in edema fluid. Additional damage by an increase of intracranial pressure causing cerebral ischemia was found to dramatically raise extracellular glutamate in edema fluid. Concentrations of 1000 $\mu M$ or higher were attained under these circumstances.[43] Since threshold concentrations of only 100–200 $\mu M/l$ are considered for induction of cell swelling, the observations provided solid evidence for the concept that release of glutamate mediates secondary cytotoxic swelling in conditions associated with acute vasogenic edema. Whether inhibition of release or of the pathological functions of glutamate by specific antagonists atttenuates edema and other forms of cerebral damage remains to be seen, however.

### The Kallikrein-Kinin System

Bradykinin and kallidin are active peptides of the kallikrein-kinin system, which are cleaved by the proteolytic enzyme kallikrein from its precursors, the kininogens. The components of the system are natural constituents in plasma, although inhibited under physiological conditions.[20,21,24] Components of the kallikrein-kinin system are also found in brain tissue, but at markedly lower levels.[56] The system is activated in tissues by inflammation, coagulation, injury, and other insults. Exposure of cerebral parenchyma to bradykinin by ventriculocisternal perfusion to by-pass the blood–brain barrier was shown to increase the water content of gray and white matter.[59] Experimental findings demonstrate, moreover, that both extra- and intravascular administration of kinins induce selective opening of the blood–brain barrier for small molecules, such as $Na^+$-fluorescein.[60] Investigations on cerebral tissue impedance made obvious that the uptake of fluid into the parenchyma secondary to administration of kinins involves the extra- rather than the intracellular space.[61] Focal trauma to the brain, such as cold injury, is associated with penetration of kininogens from the intravascular compartment into the primary lesion as well as into perifocal tissue. Formation of kinins was always found in focal tissue areas. In perifocal edematous brain, formation of kinins could be less extensive, or even absent. However, disturbances of cerebral blood flow secondary to an increase of intracranial pressure always led to marked enhancement of kinin formation in perifocal brain.[42] Amounts of kinins formed in cold injured brain are sufficient for infliction of damage, including enhancement of blood–brain barrier opening.

Recent evidence is available that specific inhibition of formation of kinins significantly attenuates edema. Respective studies were again conducted in a standardized cold lesion model of vasogenic edema.[62] Aprotinin or soybean trypsin inhibitor was employed for treatment as polyvalent protease inhibitors. Both antagonize kallikrein, the enzyme that catalyzes formation of kinins. Treatment with inhibitors commenced 15 minutes after induction of trauma. The traumatized hemisphere of control animals (rabbits) receiving physiological saline only increased in weight by 13 percent 24 hours after lesion. Treatment with aprotinin led to a reduction of hemispheric swelling to only 10 percent. Reduction of brain swelling was associated with a smaller increase of cerebral water content in traumatized brain. The findings can be considered as an important piece of evidence for identification of the kallikrein-kinin system as mediator in vasogenic edema. Specific inhibition of the kallikrein-kinin system can be expected to benefit clinical treatment by enhancing specificity.

### Arachidonic Acid and Its Metabolites

Arachidonic acid and other polyunsaturated fatty acids are natural constituents of cell membrane phospholipids and are thus abundantly present in cerebral parenchyma. Bazan[4–7] observed that acute insults such as cerebral ischemia and epileptic seizures cause activation of lipolysis involving phospholipase $A_2$ and $C$. Enhancement of lipolysis has been also confirmed in focal lesions leading to vasogenic brain edema.[43] Moreover, cerebrospinal fluid obtained from patients with cerebral hemorrhage had detectable levels of arachidonate.[44] Arachidonic acid was shown to accumulate in pure vasogenic edema fluid collected by interstitial fluid drainage from cold injured cerebrum. Concentrations in the order of $10^{-4}$ $M$ were found in this material, which is approximately two times the level found in simultaneously drawn plasma samples.[43] Accumulation of arachidonic acid in interstitial edema fluid must be attributed to enhancement of lipolysis in damaged brain. Penetration of fatty acids through the damaged blood–brain barrier is less significant.

The damaging potential of arachidonic acid in cerebral tissue is considerable, involving cytotoxic effects on nerve and glial cells and lesions in cerebral vessels. Cytotoxic effects caused by arachidonic acid have been studied by Chan and Fishman.[10,11,14,15] The authors have demonstrated that exposure of brain slices to unsaturated fatty acids in vivo induces cell swelling, together with an increase of lactic acid. Administration of arachidonic acid also results in an increased volume of cultured glial cells in association with an intracellular accumulation of $Na^+$ and loss of $K^+$. Increase of cell volume on exposure to arachidonic acid occurred in a dose-dependent manner.[13] Various molecular mechanisms are considered, such as inhibition of $Na^+$-$K^+$-ATPase and uncoupling of oxydative phosphorylation.[15,16,31] The mechanisms may suffice for induction of cytotoxic cell swelling. Release of arachidonic acid into the extracellular space of cerebral parenchyma is proposed as a mechanism of structural damage of cerebrovascular endothelium. Kontos[39] studied endothelial surfaces of cerebral vessels following topical administration of arachidonic acid or its metabolites. Arachidonic acid as well as prostaglandin $G_2$ led to formation of endothelial lesions. This agrees perfectly with experimental findings of gross opening of the blood–brain barrier to fluorescein isothiocyanate (FITC)–dextran studied by fluorescence microscopy during administration of arachidonic acid to exposed cerebral cortex.[65]

It is not entirely clear, however, whether arachidonic acid itself, or metabolites of the cascade, such as prostaglandins, leukotrienes, or free radicals are responsible. Experimental evidence assigns a major role to free radicals. Incubation of cerebral tissue with unsaturated fatty acids in vitro raises concentrations of superoxide radicals and lipid peroxides.[11] Formation of free radicals may be considered as a final step of the cascade leading to cytotoxic swelling and stimulation of glycolysis.[12] Furthermore, generation of free radicals is considered instrumental for induction of cerebrovascular lesions.[39] This is concluded from the observation that inhibition of prostaglandin and free-radical synthesis by indomethacin prevents formation of endothelial lesions in the presence of arachidonate. As with glutamate, arachidonic acid and metabolites of the cascade are strong contestants for a mediator function in edema. It remains again to be shown whether specific inhibition of release of the fatty acid and its pathological mechanisms benefit treatment. Corticosteroids and barbiturates may be a case in point. Both were reported to interfere with the arachidonic acid cascade at different levels. Other substances that influence fatty acid metabolism, including indomethacin, were, however, uneffective on brain edema.[50] Nevertheless, research on inhibitors of lipolysis and subsequent metabolic steps may prove worthwhile for the development of specific therapeutic methods of cerebral damage.

## SUMMARY AND CONCLUSIONS

Brain edema can be characterized as an increase of tissue water content together with an accumulation of $Na^+$ and frequently a decrease of $K^+$. Loss of potassium is particularly prominent in intracellular, that is, cytotoxic, brain edema. In vasogenic brain edema, extracellular homeostasis becomes outmaneuvered by a massive spillover of intravascular fluid into the cerebral parenchyma. Mediator compounds normally not present, or very low, rise in interstitial fluid to abnormal levels. Increase in $Ca^{2+}$, $K^+$, and amino and free fatty acids can be expected on the basis of respective concentrations in plasma. Increase of $K^+$, glutamic acid, and free fatty acid concentrations was confirmed by studies on pure isolated edema fluid. Accumulation of glutamate and arachidonate in edema fluid can be attributed to a release from cerebral tissue rather than to transport from the intravascular compartment.

Cerebral edema is associated with enhancement of glycolysis, whereas parameters of the energy state, such as the energy-charge potential and ATP concentrations appear to be less affected. It is open to debate, however, whether inhomogeneities of tissue perfusion evolving with edema are responsible for stimulation of glycolysis. Attempts of cerebral tissue to reestablish homeostasis is likely to constitute an extra burden on energy metabolism.

Biochemical research concerning mediator compounds, which are formed in damaged cerebral tissue or enter the brain through the broken barrier has important perspectives for improvement of current forms of treatment. Mediator compounds may enhance the edema process on various routes, such as by increasing damage to the blood–brain barrier or by induction of microcirculatory disturbances or cell swelling. An understanding of the nature and mechanisms of chemical mediator compounds is a requirement for the development of better methods of treatment.

The kallikrein-kinin system, glutamic acid, and free fatty acids appear particularly promising among the many factors studied. Specific inhibition of formation of kinins attenuates cerebral edema. Respective findings may be expected in the future from studies on arachidonate and glutamic acid. However, it would be simple-minded to assume involvement of few mediator compounds only in view of the enormous complexity of processes occurring in damaged brain tissue.

**Acknowledgments**

This work was supported by Deutsche Forschungsgemeinschaft: Ba452/6-5. The technical and secretarial help of Ruth Demmer, Ulrike Goerke, Friederike Helmes, and Barbara Stöpfel is gratefully acknowledged.

## REFERENCES

1. Ames A, Tsukada Y, Nesbett FB: Intracellular $Cl^-$, $Na^+$, $K^+$, $Ca^{++}$, $Mg^{++}$ and P in nervous tissue; response to glutamate and to changes in extracellular calcium. J Neurochem 14:145–159, 1967
2. Baethmann A: Pathophysiological and pathochemical aspects of cerebral edema. Neurosurg Rev 1:85–100, 1978
3. Baethmann A, Oettinger W, Rothenfulsser W, et al: Biochemical aspects of cerebral edema, in Mrsulja BB, Rakic LM, Klatzo I, et al. (Eds): Pathophysiology of Cerebral Energy Metabolism. New York, Plenum Press, 1979, pp 189–209
4. Bazan NG: Effects of ischemia and electroconvulsive shock on free fatty acid pool in the brain. Biochim Biophys Acta 218:1–10, 1970
5. Bazan NG: Changes in free fatty acids of brain by drug-induced convulsions, electroshock, and anesthesia. J Neurochem 18:1379–1385, 1971
6. Bazan NG, Rodriguez de Turco EB: Membrane lipids in the pathogenesis of brain edema. Phospholipids and arachidonic acid, the earliest membrane components changed at the onset of ischemia. Adv Neurol 28:197–205, 1980
7. Bazan NG, Politi E, Rodriguez de Turco EB: Endogenous pools of arachidonic acid-enriched membrane lipids in cryogenic brain edema, in Go KG, Baethmann A (Eds): Recent Progress in the Study and Therapy of Brain Edema. New York, Plenum Press, 1984, pp 203–212
8. Bingham WG, Paul SE, Sastry KSS: Effects of cold injury on six enzymes in rat brain. Neurology 21:649–660, 1969
9. Bulle HP: Effects of reserpine and chlorpromazin in prevention of cerebral edema and reversible cell damage. Proc Soc Exp Biol Med 94:553–556, 1957
10. Chan PH, Fishman RA: Brain edema: Induction in cortical slices by polyunsaturated fatty acids. Science 201:358–360, 1978
11. Chan PH, Fishman RA: Transient formation of superoxide radicals in polyunsaturated fatty acid-induced brain swelling. J Neurochem 35:1004–1007, 1980
12. Chan PH, Yurko M, Fishman RA: Phospholipid degradation and cellular edema induced by free radicals in brain cortical slices. J Neurochem 38:525–531, 1982
13. Chan PH, Fishman RA: Alterations of membrane integrity and cellular constituents by arachidonic acid in neuroblastoma and glioma cells. Brain Res 248:151–157, 1982
14. Chan PH, Fishman RA, Longar S, et al: The role of arachidonic acid in cellular brain edema, in Sun GY, Bazan NG, Wu JY, et al (Eds): Neural Membranes. Clifton NJ, Humana Press, 1983, pp 141–152
15. Chan PH, Kerlan R, Fishman RA: Reduction of $\gamma$-aminobutyric acid and glutamate uptake and $(Na^+ + K^+)$-ATPase activity in brain slices and synaptosomes by arachidonic acid. J Neurochem 40:309–315, 1983
16. Chefurka W: Oxydative phosphorylation in in-vitro aged mitochondria: I. Factors controlling the loss of the DNP-stimulated ATP-ase activity and respiratory control in mouse liver mitochondria. Biochemistry 5:2887–3903, 1966
17. Clasen RA, Sky-Peck HH, Pandolfi S: The chemistry of isolated edema fluid in experimental cerebral injury, in Klatzo

I, Seitelberger F (Eds): Brain Edema. New York, Springer, 1967, pp 536–553

18. Clasen RA, Bezkorovainy A, Pandolfi S: Protein and electrolyte changes in experimental cerebral edema. J Neuropathol Exp Neurol 41:113–128, 1982
19. Clendendon NR, Allen N, Ito T, et al: Response of lysosomal hydrolases of dog spinal cord and cerebrospinal fluid to experimental trauma. Neurology 28:78–84, 1978
20. Erdös EG: The kinins. A status report. Biochem Pharmacol 25:1563–1569, 1976
21. Erdös EG (Ed): Bradykinin, kallidin, and kallikrein, in Handbook of Experimental Pharmacology XXV, Suppl, Berlin, Springer, 1979, pp 427–487
22. Fenske A, Sinterhauf K, Reulen HJ: The role of monoamines in the development of cold-induced edema, in Pappius HM, Feindel W (Eds): Dynamics of Brain Edema. Berlin, Springer, 1976, pp 150–154
23. Frei HJ, Wallenfang T, Pöll, W, et al: Regional cerebral blood flow and regional metabolism in cold induced edema. Acta Neurochirurg 29:15–28, 1973
24. Frey EK, Kraut H, Werle E: Das Kallikrein-Kinin-System und seine Inhibitoren. Stuttgart, Ferdinand Enke, 1968
25. Gazendam J, Go KG, van Zanten AK: Composition of isolated edema fluid in cold-induced brain edema. J Neurosurg 51:70–77, 1979
26. Go KG, Gazendam J, van Zanten AK: Influence of hypoxia on the composition of isolated edema fluid in cold-induced brain edema. J Neurosurg 51:78–84, 1979
27. Gross PM: Cerebral histamine: Indications for neuronal and vascular regulation. J Cereb Blood Flow Metabol 2:3–24, 1982
28. Harvey JA, McIlwain H: Excitatory acidic amino acids and the cation content and sodium ion flux of isolated tissues from the brain. J Biochem 108:269–274, 1968
29. regions around brain tumors, in Harper AM, Jennett WB, Miller JD, et al (Eds): Blood Flow and Metabolism in the Brain. Edinburgh, Churchill Livingston, 1975, pp 1341–1342
30. Hossmann KA: Development and resolution of ischemic brain swelling, in Pappius HM, Feindel W (Eds): Dynamics of Brain Edema. Berlin, Springer, 1976, pp 219–227
31. Hulsman WC, Elliott WB, Slater EC: The nature and mechanism of action of uncoupling agents present in mitochoudrial preparations. Biochim Biophys Acta 39:267–276, 1960
32. Joo F: Significance of adenylate cyclase in the regulation of the permeability of brain capillaries, in Mrsulja BB, Rakic CM, Klatzo I, et al (Eds): Pathophysiology of Cerebral Energy Metabolism. New York, Plenum Press, 1979, pp 211–237
33. Kempski O: The localization of glutamate induced brain edema. Medical Thesis, School of Medicine, Ludwig Maximilians University, Munich, 1982
34. Kempski O, Gross U, Baethmann A: An in-vitro model of cytotoxic brain edema: Cell volume and metabolism of cultivated glial and nerve-cells, in Driesen W, Brock M, Klinger M (Eds): Advances in Neurosurgery, vol 10. Berlin, Springer, 1982, pp 254–258
35. Khattab FI: Alterations in acid phosphatase bodies (lysosomes) in cat motoneurons after asphyxiation of the spinal cord. Exp Neurol 18:133–140, 1967
36. Klatzo I, Wisniewski H, Smith DE. Observations on penetration of serum-proteins into the central nervous system, in De Robertis EPD, Carrea R (Eds): Biology of Neuroglia, Progress Brain Research, vol 15, 1965, Elseveier Publishing Co., Amsterdam pp 73–88
37 Klatzo I: Neuropathological aspects of brain edema. J Neuropathol Exp Neurol 26:1–14, 1967

38. Kobrine AI, Doyle T: Role of histamine in posttraumatic spinal cord hyperemia and the luxury perfusion syndrome. J Neurosurg 44:16–20, 1976
39. Kontos HA, Wei EP, Povlishock JT, et al: Cerebral arteriolar damage by arachidonic acid and prostaglandin $G_2$. Science 209:1242–1245, 1980
40. Lanksch W, Öttinger W, Baethmann A, et al: CT-findings in brain edema compared with direct chemical analysis of tissue samples, in Pappius HM, Feindel W (Eds): Dynamics of Brain Edema. Berlin, Springer, 1976, pp 283–287
41. Lanksch W, Baethmann A, Kazner E: Computed tomography of brain edema, in De Vlieger M, De Lange SA, Beks JWF (Eds): Brain Edema. New York, John Wiley & Sons, 1981, pp 67–98
42. Maier-Hauff K, Baethmann A, Lange M, et al: The kallikrein-kinin system as mediator in vasogenic brain edema, part 2: Studies on kinin formation in focal and perifocal brain tissue. J Neurosurg 61:97–106, 1984
43. Maier-Hauff K, Lange M, Schürer L, et al: Glutamate and free fatty acid concentrations in extracellular vasogenic edema fluid, in Go KG, Baethmann A (Eds): Recent Progress in the Study and Therapy of Brain Edema. New York, Plenum Press, 1984, pp 183–192
44. Maier-Hauff K, Baethmann A, Vogt W, et al: Mediator compounds in CSF of neurosurgical patients with raised intracranial pressure, in Piotrowski W, Brock M, Klinger M (Eds): Advances in Neurosurgery, vol 12. Berlin, Springer, 1984 pp 302–306
45. Osterholm JL, Bell J, Meyer R, et al: Experimental effects of free serotonin on the brain and its relation to brain injury. Parts I–III. J Neurosurg 31:408–421, 1969
46. Pappius HM, McCann WP: Effects of steroids on cerebral edema in cats. Arch Neurol 20:207–216, 1969
47. Pappius HM, Gulati DR: Water and electrolyte content of cerebral tissue in experimentally induced edema. Acta Neuropathol 18:89–102, 1971
48. Pappius HM: Effects of steroids on cold injury edema, in Reulen HJ, Schürmann K (Eds): Steroids and Brain Edema. Berlin, Springer, 1972, pp 57–63
49. Pappius HM: Fundamental aspects of brain edema, in Vinken PJ, Bruyn GW (Eds): Handbook of Clinical Neurology, vol 16, pt I: Tumors of the Brain and Skull. Amsterdam, North-Holland Publishing Company, 1974, pp 167–185
50. Pappius HM, Wolfe LS: Some further studies on vasogenic edema, in Pappius HM, Feindel W (Eds): Dynamics of Brain Edema. Berlin, Springer, 1976, pp 138–143
51. Perry TL, Jones RT: The aminoacid content of human cerebrospinal fluid in normal individuals and mental defectives. J Clin Invest 40:1363–1372, 1961
52. Perry TL, Hansen S, Kennedy J: CSF amino acids and plasma–CSF amino acid ratios in adults. J Neurochem 24:587–589, 1975
53. Reulen HJ, Medzihradsky F, Enzenbach R, et al: Electrolytes, fluids and energy metabolism in human cerebral edema. Arch Neurol 21:517–525, 1969
54. Rothenfusser W: The significance of glutamate as a brain edema factor. Medical Thesis, School of Medicine, Ludwig Maximilians University Munich, 1982
55. Schmiedek P, Baethmann A, Sippel G, et al: Energy state and glycolysis in human cerebral edema. The application of a new freeze-stop technique. J Neurosurg 40:351–364, 1974
56. Shikimi T, Kema R, Matsumoto N, et al: Studies on kinin-like substances in brain. Biochem Pharmacol 22:567–573, 1973
57. Siesjö BK, Nielsson L, Rokeach M, et al: Energy metabolism of the brain at reduced cerebral perfusion pressures and in arterial hypoxemia, in Brierley J, Meldrum BS (Eds): Brain Hypoxia. London, Spastics International Medical Publ, 1971, pp 79–93
58. Sutton LN, Welsh F, Bruce DA: Bioenergetics of acute vasogenic edema. J Neurosurg 53:470–476, 1980
59. Unterberg A, Baethmann A: The kallikrein-kinin system as mediator in vaso-

genic brain edema, part 1: Cerebral exposure to bradykinin and plasma. J Neurosurg 61:87–96, 1984
60. Unterberg A, Wahl M, Baethmann A: Effects of bradykinin on permeability and diameter of pial vessels in-vivo. J Cereb Blood Flow Metabol 4:574–585, 1984.
61. Unterberg A, Hack U, Baethmann A: Blood flow, metabolism and function of the brain during cerebral administration of bradykinin, in Dietz H, Brock M, Klinger M (Eds): Advances in Neurosurgery, vol 13. Berlin, Springer, in press.
62. Unterberg A, Dautermann C, Müller-Esterl W, et al: Inhibition of the kallikrein-kinin system in traumatic brain swelling, in Baethmann A, Go KG, Unterberg A (Eds.) Mechanisms of Secondary Brain Damage (in press).
63. Van Harreveld A, Fifkova E: Light- and electronmicroscopic changes in central nervous tissue after electrophoretic injection of glutamate. Exp Molec Pathol 15:61–81, 1971
64. Van Harreveld A: The extracellular space in the vertebrate central nervous system, in Bourne HG (Ed): The Structure and Function of Nervous Tissue, New York, Academic Press, 1972, pp 447–511
65. Wahl M, Unterberg A, Baethmann A: Effects of arachidonic acid on blood–brain barrier function, in Dietz H, Brock M, Klinger M (Eds): Advances in Neurosurgery, vol 13. Berlin, Springer, in press.
66. Westergaard E: Enhanced vesicular transport of exogenous peroxidase across cerebral vessels, induced by serotonin. Acta Neuropathol 32:27–42, 1975

*J. Gordon McComb*

# 7

# Impaired Cerebrospinal Fluid Circulation: Alternative Pathways

Hydrocephalus is a net accumulation of cerebrospinal fluid (CSF) and occurs following an imbalance between CSF formation and absorption. In almost all instances hydrocephalus develops after an increase in the resistance to CSF absorption and at some point the CSF pressure is elevated, which may or may not be maintained, depending on subsequent compensatory forces.[2] With the one very rare exception of CSF overproduction from a choroid plexus papilloma, all hydrocephalus is obstructive;[1,4] therefore, the terms "obstructive" and "nonobstructive hydrocephalus" have been supplanted by those of communicating and noncommunicating hydrocephalus.[4] By definition, noncommunicating hydrocephalus indicates impairment of CSF flow within the ventricular system, while in communicating hydrocepalus, the obstruction is distal to the ventricles. Improved methods for treating hydrocephalus have made the distinction between the two types less essential, but significant etiologic differences exist. Noncommunicating hydrocephalus results from such lesions as aqueductal occlusion, obstruction of the outlets of the fourth ventricle, masses within or adjacent to the ventricular system, and hemorrhage and infection within the ventricular system.[3] Communicating hydrocephalus is usually associated with subarachnoid hemorrhage, meningitis, and spread of tumor within the subarachnoid space (SAS). Occasionally, extra-axial masses encroach upon the SAS directly or indirectly, increasing the resistance to CSF absorption and producing a communicating type of hydrocephalus. Obstruction of the venous drainage from the brain alone most likely does not produce hydrocephalus. Hydrocephalus can also be classified

BRAIN INSULTS IN INFANTS AND CHILDREN
0-8089-1723-4

as congenital or acquired, but such a distinction has no meaning in terms of the pathophysiological process.[5]

The incidence of congenital hydrocephalus occurring alone is about 1/1000 live births, whereas hydrocephalus associated with spina bifida cystica (myelomeningocele) is present in 1–3/1000 live births.[5] Few causes of congenital hydrocephalus are known, but a small number appear to result from maternal infection (cytomegalovirus; toxoplasmosis; and possibly mumps, rubella, varicella, etc.), nutritional disorders (experimently produced by hypo- and hypervitaminosis A), teratogenesis (radiation, lysergic acid dielthylamide), and genetic factors (X-linked). The X-linked form of congenital hydrocephalus occurs only in males and accounts for approximately 1 to 2 percent of the total number. There appears to be a slightly increased risk for isolated congenital hydrocephalus to be present in subsequent siblings compared to the general population. The incidence risk is much higher if hydrocephalus is associated with spina bifida cystica. Most acquired forms of hydrocephalus result from infection, tumors, trauma, and vascular lesions.[1,2]

## ALTERNATE CSF PATHWAYS

A question debated for some time is whether CSF can be absorbed by the brain. The penetration of substances into the periventricular region of hydrocephalic animals has been well documented. With the event of the computerized tomographic (CT) scanning, periventricular hypodensity may be noted in the presence of hydrocephalus and has been shown to be the result of CSF migrating into the area surrounding the ventricles in the face of increased intraventricular pressure.[5] Its presence in the parenchyma, indicative of migration, does not necessarily equate with absorption. Bulk flow of CSF is usually measured by the clearance of various reference macromolecules, such as albumin, which by necessity would have to enter the lumen of the blood vessel and be removed by the systemic circulation. It has been shown that the cerebral capillaries have a very low permeability to albumin and that most of any given quantity of albumin injected into the brain can be recovered from the lymph and CSF, with very little being left to the blood.[6] In addition to the impermeability of the capillaries to various reference markers, the clearance of which is the measure of CSF absorption, it has been pointed out that as absorption occurs in response to a pressure drop, requiring a higher pressure outside the lumen of the capillary than inside, which obviously would lead to capillary collapse and preclude absorption. The extracellular space in the brain, which amounts to 15 percent, readily allows fluid flow in the parenchyma. This flow of fluid within the parenchyma is present under normal physiological conditions, and its velocity and direction are responsive to changes in hydrostatic and osmotic pressure gradients. Macromolecules injected into the CSF of the ventricles or SAS have been observed to readily penetrate the extracellular space of the parenchyma and vice versa. Evidence thus supports the contention that the brain, rather than absorbing CSF, is acting as a conduit for fluid to move from the ventricles to the SAS or into the prelymphatic channels of the blood vessels.[3]

The choroid plexus might also possibly be involved in absorption of the CSF. Ventricular fluid can enter the subependymal extracellular space and once there could flow into the stroma of the choroid plexus, where absorption could take place at the choroidal capillaries since these capillaries are fenestrated and do not have tight junctions like those in the parenchyma. The role of choroid plexus CSF absorption in hydrocephalus is not known.[3]

Drainage of CSF appears to take place from the SAS surrounding the cranial and spinal nerve root sleeves with entry into the lymphatic system. Studies have shown that an outer arachnoid barrier layer exists between the SAS and dura and functions as the blood–CSF barrier at this location. At higher than normal pressures the barrier layer can be disrupted with resultant penetration of macromolecules into the extracellular space of the dura mater and dural lymphatic channels. At unphysiologically high pressures, disruption of this arachnoid barrier layer may allow for significant absorption of CSF.[3]

Production of CSF in hydrocephalus is either normal or near normal.[4,6] In compensated hydrocephalus the rate of absorption must equal the rate of formation or approximately 500 ml/day, and in the uncompensated state, only a small fraction of the total amount secreted is retained; thus the overwhelming majority of CSF output is still absorbed. As CSF formation is relatively constant, the change in resistance to absorption determines CSF pressure and whether the hydrocephalus is progressive. Impairment of CSF absorption in communicating hydrocephalus could occur at some or all of the following sites: the arachnoid villus, the lymphatic channels associated with the cranial and spinal nerves, lymphatic channels in the adventitia of the cerebral vessels, or the arachnoid membrane.[3] If CSF outflow from the ventricles is blocked (i.e., noncommunicating hydrocephalus), absorption could still take place through the blood vessel adventitia, the stroma of the choroid plexus, and passage of CSF through the extracellular space of the cortical mantle to reach the brain surface. Assuming complete ventricular blockage, which is not always the case, additional ways for CSF to exit the ventricles would be by way of the dilated spinal cord central canal or through a fistula opening created by a rupture of the ventricular system into the SAS at such locations as the lamina terminalis or suprapineal recess.[3]

## VENTRICULOMEGALY

The rate of ventricular enlargement will depend on the degree to which the resistance to absorption has increased and the distensibility of the ventricular system. Expermental acute complete obstruction of the fourth ventricle in primates produces a rapid dilatation of the lateral and third ventricles in the first 3 hours followed by a 3-hour period of less rapid enlargement. After 6 hours the ventricles very slowly increase in size, reaching a gross steady state in a few days.[4] The ependymal cells lining the ventricles become thinned and disrupted, periventricular edema develops, and tracers placed into the ventricular CSF migrate into the periventricular white matter.[6] Cortical changes secondary to hydrocephalus affect almost exclusively the white matter, especially that surrounding the ventricles, whereas the gray matter of both the cortex and the deep nuclear masses is spared.[6] The severity and duration of the elevated pressure within the ventricles determine the chronic changes that follow and include progressive axonal disintegration, secondary myelin degeneration, and finally reactive gliosis that lead to irreversible tissue damage and atrophy. Clinical experience as documented by CT scanning and animal studies has shown that decompressing the dilated ventricular system in acute hydrocephalus will result in a very rapid reconstitution of the cortical mantle (rebulking of the parenchyna). The mechanism by which this occurs is poorly understood.[4]

## CLINICAL IMPLICATIONS OF VENTRICULOMEGALY

Most congenital forms of hydrocephalus are of the noncommunicating type, with obstruction at the Sylvian aqueduct accounting for more than two-thirds of this group. Most obstructions at the aqueduct, usually referred to as *aqueductal stenosis*, are characterized by either gliosis or forking of this structure. An overgrowth of the subependymal glia occurs in aqueductal gliosis, and although the cause is rarely known, this gliosis may be the result of a post inflammatory ependymitis. A forked aqueduct divides into several blind channels surrounded by normal brain, as there is no excess of subependymal glial tissue. Aqueductal forking is more frequently noted in conjunction with other congenital anomalies, specifically myelomeningocele, and is more likely developmentally related. The frequency of the site at which obstruction occurs within the ventricular system corresponds well to the anatomic locations where it is narrowed. Since the Sylvian aqueduct is the most constricted region, it has the highest incidence of blockage. In decreasing order of frequency, obstruction also occurs at the outlets of the fourth ventricle, the intraventricular formina of the Monro third ventricle, and finally a portion of the lateral ventricles. Obstruction may occur at more than one location, as may be case with myelodysplasia since the ever-present Chiari II malformation may impede CSF flow at the aqueduct, at the outlets of the fourth ventricle, or in the basal cisterns of the posterior fossa. Following intraventricular hemorrhage or meningitis with ventriculitis the obstruction can develop both within and outside the ventricles and probably often is a combination of both. It has also been suggested that dilatation of the ventricular system in communicating hydrocephalus might compress the SAS, thereby producing a secondary block to CSF absorption as well.[2,5] The age of the patient, the duration of the elevated intracranial pressure (ICP), and most importantly the rate at which the ICP (ICP is used here synonymously with intraventricular pressure for simplification) rises—which, in turn, is a function of the change in resistance to absorption—will characterize the clinical findings associated with hydrocephalus.[4] The younger the infant, the more readily the cranial vault can expand in response to elevated ICP. Below about 2 years of age an abnormal increase in head circumference in response to elevated ICP associated with hydrocephalus is the rule, whereas this ability is progressively reduced in the child and is not at all a factor in the older child or adult. The infant with obvious hydrocephalus will have a prominent forehead (bossing). If aqueductal stenosis is present, the posterior portion of the skull will be underdeveloped, whereas in an infant with a Dandy-Walker malformation, the same region can be disproportionately large. Suture separation, mainly sagittal and coronal, will occur and is easily palpable in the infant.[2]

If the skull is percussed, a "cracked pot" or a "ripe watermelon" sound can be elicited with significant hydrocephalus. The anterior fontanel will be full and tense and will remain so even when the infant is held upright and is quiet. Venous blood directed from the dural sinuses by way of the emmissary veins distends the scalp veins to an abnormal degree and is accentuated when the infant cries. As the infant's head is large, control is poor. Development is often delayed or even regressive. Feeding may be poor and weight gain inadequate. Irritability is common, and the infant's cry may be shrill. Esotropia is a frequent ophthalmologic finding and results from a lateral rectus palsy secondary to stretching of the sixth nerve. The eyes may deviate downward ("setting sun" effect). Upward gaze and accommodation can be impaired from compression of the gaze centers in the midbrain region by the dilated posterior third ventricle. Gaze evoked nystagmus is also common. Papilledema and optic atrophy are rarely present as the expanding cranium ameliorates the elevation of ICP. Tone and reflexes are increased, especially in the lower extremities, and are thought to relate to a stretching of the corticospinal fibers transversing the dilated ventricular system. These symptoms may be marked, absent, or somewhere in between and relate to the degree to which ICP is elevated. In some cases the only clinical evidence for progressive hydrocephalus is an abnormal increase in head circumference without fullness in even the anterior fontanel. In premature infants the ventricles have been found to progressively dilate for several weeks before the head circumference begins to enlarge at an abnormal rate.[2]

In the older child, adolescent, or adult, in whom the cranial sutures are not separable, the onset of hydrocephalus will not produce abnormal enlargement of the head and the anterior fontanel will long since have closed. Clinical manifestations of hydrocephalus will once again depend on the rate and height of the ICP elevation. A rapid rise in ICP in acute hydrocephalus is accompanied by headache, nausea, vomiting, and progressive deterioration in mental function followed by coma and ultimately death if not treated. Vital sign changes develop only after compression of the medulla (Cushing response), at which time irreversible changes are beginning. Death usually ensues from respiratory failure. Seizures are very uncommon. Decerebrate posturing, which may be mistaken for convulsions (so-called cerebellar fits), may occur prior to death. On the other hand, if the hydrocephalus is chronic and very slowly progressive, clinical changes will occur over a course of months or years. The intelligence quotient (IQ) will become impaired, and verbal performance will be less affected than motor performance. Coordination becomes progressively worse, with truncal ataxia becoming more pronounced than limb ataxia. Similar to the infant, tone and reflexes are increased most in the lower extremities. Papilledema or optic atrophy may be present, as is gaze-evoked nystagmus. A wide variety of endocrine and metabolic abnormalities may develop and reflect impairment of normal hypothalamo-pituitary function.[2,4,5]

In the older child or adult whose head circumference is near or above the 98th percentile and in whom CT scanning shows a marked enlargement of the ventricles, hydrocephalus obviously will have developed prior to closure of the sutures, indicating a chronic process that was not recognized previously. The patient may have none or all of the features described above.[4]

Accurately measured, serial head circumferences continue to be one of the most valuable parameters in assessing an infant or child with hydrocephalus. The head circumference needs to be recorded on a head growth chart, after multiple measurements with a good cloth or steel tape to assure that the maximum circumference has been obtained. The head circumference will not be abnormally large in the older child or adult who develops hydrocephalus after the cranial sutures have effectively closed. However, progressive hydrocephalus beginning before the closure of cranial sutures will prevent complete fusion of the sutures and allow continued excessive head enlargement even in the older child. Continued abnormal head enlargement in the older child with the presumed diagnosis of "arrested" hydrocephalus will prove this diagnosis to be in error.[2]

## DIAGNOSTIC APPROACH TO VENTRICULOMEGALY

Computed tomographic scanning is for the most part the definitive diagnostic procedure as it is highly accurate and noninvasive.[4] The resolution attainable with the newest generation of CT scanners is impressive and in most cases is the only study needed for diagnosis and appropriate therapy. The site and nature of the obstruction to CSF flow is often discernable. With aqueductal stenosis the lateral and third ventricles will be dilated, but not the fourth ventricle or the subarachnoid spaces. With communicating hydrocephalus the entire ventricular system is dilated, as well as the subarachnoid spaces. There are, however, several additional points worth mentioning. Communicating hydrocephalus with dilatation of the ventricular system and subarachnoid spaces can produce a picture on a CT scan that is indistinguishable from cerebral atrophy. It is not uncommon for a radiologist, who infrequently interprets pediatric CT scans, to make the diagnosis of "cerebral atrophy" even though on clinical examination the infant's head circumference is greater than the 98th percentile, the anterior fontanel full, and all other hallmarks of raised intracranial pressure present. Often it is not possible to accurately distinguish whether fluid on the surface of the infant brain is in the subarachnoid or subdural space. Such a fluid collection is not uncommon and may or may not be associated with a very mild ventricular dilatation. The fluid accumulation is usually present primarily over the frontal lobes and relates to the fact that the infant is usually scanned in the brow-up position. The fluid collection is of concern only if it is of considerable volume. A relatively small fluid collection not associated with any clinical findings of note is of no consequence.[5]

With more routine use of magnetic resonance (MR) the etiology of hydrocephalus may be more readily ascertained. This form of neurological imaging permits a better resolution and evaluation of the brainstem and periaqueductal regions.

## REFERENCES


1. Fishman RA: Cerebrospinal Fluid in Diseases of the Nervous System. Philadelphia, Saunders, 1980, 380 pp
2. Matson DD: Neurosurgery of Infancy and Childhood, 2 ed, Springfield, Charles C Thomas, 1969, p 934
3. McComb JG: Recent research into the nature of cerebrospinal fluid formation and absorption. J Neurosurg 59:369–383, 1983
4. Milhorat TH: Hydrocephalus and the Cerebrospinal Fluid. Baltimore, Williams & Wilkins, 1972, p 237
5. Shapiro K, Marmaron A, Partnoy H: Hydrocephalus. New York, Raven Press, 1984, p 401
6. Welch K: The principles of physiology of the cerebrospinal fluid in relation to hydrocephalus including normal pressure hydrocephalus, in Friedlander WJ (Ed): Current Reviews. Advances in Neurology, vol 13. New York, Raven Press, 1975, pp 247–332

*Derek A Bruce*

# 8

# Cerebrovascular Dynamics following Brain Insults

The changes in cerebrovascular control mechanisms and cerebral blood flow vary depending on the insult. The most obvious insults that primarily affect cerebral blood flow (CBF) are those involving vessel occlusions. Trauma, infection, hypoxia, and any condition causing elevated intracranial pressure (ICP), however, can all result in changes in cerebral blood flow (CBF) and cerebrovascular control mechanisms.

## CBF IN INFANTS AND CHILDREN

In the neonate and premature baby, there is minimal information available on either the normal resting CBF and its control or what occurs under pathological conditions. The presence of germinal matrix hemorrhage is associated with a decreased CBF. It has also been suggested that pressure autoregulation is lost in the distressed newborn. This is not proven, but several studies do confirm the presence of the low CBF.[7,8] Hypoxia in newborn and fetal animals produces a marked increase in CBF and can occur despite a low $Pa_{CO_2}$ (i.e., the hypoxic drive is able to overcome the $CO_2$ affect), although in some studies there has been a selective decrease in CBF in the frontal lobes, particularly in the deep white matter.[5] This low flow has been suggested as the cause of periventricular encephalomalacia. There is no procedure applicable to the clinical care of the newborn because of the lack of information; however, arterial pressure should be maintained in the normal or slightly elevated range for age and large oscillations in arterial and intracranial pressure avoided. In

BRAIN INSULTS IN INFANTS AND CHILDREN
0-8089-1723-4

experimental studies it is clear that intermittent elevations and decreases in ICP can abolish pressure autoregulation in a progressive fashion.[9]

Normal cerebral blood flow in the child is approximately 20 percent higher than in the adult and appears to reach adult levels somewhere in adolescence.[2,3] Cerebral metabolic rate for oxygen ($CMRO_2$) is also elevated in the younger child.[2,3] As mentioned in Chapter 5, pressure autoregulation, metabolic autoregulation, and $CO_2$ responses are all present in the child. The exact shape of the CBF/$PaCO_2$ response curve is not known. In newborn and premature animals, the $CO_2$ response is less for each millimeter of change in $PaCO_2$ than in the adult animal.[11] In children, clinical experience suggests that the level at which the CBF/$CO_2$ response curve becomes flat is lower than in the adult, but there are no good systematic studies of $CO_2$ response available.[2,3]

## CEREBRAL BLOOD FLOW IN ANOXIA AND ISCHEMIA

Following anoxia and ischemia, the initial response of the CBF is that of hyperemia.[11] During the anoxia or ischemia, acidotic metabolites accumulate in the brain, producing vasodilatation.[5,10] When the tissue perfusion is restored, it is into dilated vessels and thus the hyperemia.[11] Pressure autoregulation is frequently abolished by ischemia and an acidotic extracellular space leads not only to vasodilation and hyperemia but to defective pressure autoregulation.[9,11] Most experimental studies of prolonged ischemia show that initial reperfusion is adequate if a good perfusion pressure is established, but in cases of prolonged ischemia there is a gradual drop in cerebral blood flow.[9,11] Whether this is the cause of secondary damage or is simply the result of cellular injury and decreased metabolism is unclear. The best evidence is that the postischemic hypoperfusion is the result of poor cellular recovery and decreased metabolism rather than the cause of it. From a therapeutic standpoint, the best approach following global cerebral ischemia (e.g., cardiac arrest) is to reestablish an adequate arterial perfusion pressure possibly on the high side for age as early as possible in the course of resuscitation. Despite multiple experimental studies there are not yet any drugs that have been shown to be consistently effective in improving the outcome from experimental ischemia that are yet at the stage of being applied to our patients.

## CEREBRAL BLOOD FLOW IN TRAUMA

The best studied alterations in CBF are those following head trauma.[6,10] In adults comatose as a result of head trauma, the usual finding is of decreased CBF and appropriately decreased metabolism.[6,10] These findings demonstrate intact chemical autoregulation, decrease in cerebral metabolic rate due to the trauma, and secondary decrease in CBF. Chemical autoregulation thus appears to be fairly resistant to trauma. Pressure autoregulation, on the other hand, may be defective globally or regionally or may be intact throughout. Adult studies have failed to correlate, the type of mechanism, CT scan or Coma Score with predictable loss or preservation of pressure autoregulation.[10] Initially, CBF studies in children suggested that normal or increased CBF was a common finding despite a low $CMRO_2$ and coma.[2,12] This relative or actual state of excess CBF over metabolic needs represents hyperemia.[2,12] Recent studies in adults have also shown hyperemia in up to 50 percent of patients.[10] Significantly, in adults the hyperemia is most frequently unilateral, whereas in children it is generally bilateral.[12] In both groups of patients the ICP is more likely to be elevated than in patients who do not have a hyperemia. The increased blood flow is believed to be due to decreased vascular resistance and vasodilatation and, therefore, associated with an increase in intracerebral blood volume, which may contribute to the elevated ICP. There is no substantive evidence yet available as to whether pressure autoregulation is present or defective in patients with hyperemia. In children, the lack of variation in ICP with variation in arterial pressure suggests, but does not prove, that autoregulation is intact. Recent studies in head-injured children suggest that those with early-onset hyperemia may also have unusually high metabolism for their conscious state in the absence of frank seizure activity.[12] At the present time, it is unclear whether the hyperaemic state is associated with cerebral hypermetabolism. Clearly it is important that this be clarified since, if metabolism is the driving force, therapy to decrease metabolism may be more appropriate than therapy to decrease flow. If the flow is the uncontrolled variable, however, efforts to lower blood flow would seem more appropriate.

There is a group of children who appear very similar to adults in terms of low blood flow and metabolism.[1,6,10] In general, children with a pattern of diffuse swelling on CT scan, small ventricles, and perimesencephalic cisterns are more likely to have initially high CBF.[2,3] Those with a pattern of diffuse axonal injury with corpus callosum hemorrhage or brainstem hemorrhage or those with severe subarachnoid hemorrhage are more likely to have decreased cerebral blood flow and metabolism.[12] Children with epidural or subdural hematomas may have increased or decreased CBF depending on the size of the mass, level of the ICP, and the presence or absence of autoregulation.[12] Carbon dioxide responses appear to be well preserved following trauma. Children who are admitted to hospital in coma rarely demonstrate evidence of cerebral edema on early CT scan but frequently exhibit a pattern of diffuse swelling on CT scan that is associated with increased CBF.[2] The early treatment for such children is thus endotracheal intubation and moderate hyperventilation to $Paco_2$ of 25–30 torr. This will decrease the cerebral blood volume and flow rapidly. The emergency use of mannitol, unless the clinical picture is highly suggestive of an expanding mass (e.g., epidural hematoma), is discouraged because mannitol may further increase CBF and potentially can elevate ICP before lowering it through its dehydrating effect. Following head trauma, $CO_2$ responses are usually well preserved and may even be enhanced; thus changes in $CO_2$ are a rapid and effective way to lower ICP.[12] Following anoxia or ischemia, especially if there is tissue necrosis and low tissue pH, $CO_2$ responses may be abolished, and thus hyperventilation may not be an effective means of controlling ICP.[12] Chemical metabolic autoregulation is usually preserved with brain injuries short of tissue infarction but may not be adequate to ensure tissue perfusion in the face of complex brain trauma. If a seizure occurs in a patient with elevated ICP or low systemic arterial pressure, the CBF may not increase despite local vascular dilatation, and thus functional tissue ischemia may result, producing further cellular damage. In mature animals the critical thresholds at which CBF becomes inadequate for electrical activity and tissue integrity are shown in Table 8-1. It seems likely that these values can be applied to the child, but unclear whether they can be applied to the premature or newborn infant.

Disturbances of cerebrovascular control mechanisms following brain insults in children are only now being defined. Comparison with data derived from adult patients seems to be appropriate in some cases but not others. The status of pressure autoregulation has not been studied. Carbon dioxide responses are preserved or even enhanced following trauma but may be lost in infarcted tissue. Metabolic autoregulation may be disturbed by head trauma or function inadequately when seizures or increased metabolism are superimposed on other disturbances such as elevated ICP. Since CBF measurements are not available in most patients, the question arises as to what other techniques may be appropriate to help define disturbances of the cerebral circulation in the clinical setting. One simple method involves measurement of arterial jugular difference for oxygen. This is the balance between CBF and cerebral metabolism and may be a useful way of monitoring changes in this balance. Similarly, monitoring of intracranial pressure and arterial pressure

**Table 8-1** *Thresholds for Ischemic Effect on Electrical Activity, $K^+$, and $Ca^+$ Release*

| Activity | CBFML/100 gm/min |
|---|---|
| Electrical | 16 |
| $K^+$ Release | 10 |
| $Ca^+$ Release | 10 |
| Infarction | 10 |

*May be additives effects of flow and time

will permit an adequate perfusion pressure to be maintained and hopefully a normal ICP and blood pressure. Sophisticated analysis of electrical activity from the EEG or from evoked responses has not proved as helpful as hoped in defining the early stages of inadequate cerebral perfusion. Prolongation of the latency of the somatosensory-evoked response does occur with CNS ischemia and has been valuable in subarachnoid hemorrhage patients. Unfortunately, the sensitivity has not yet been adequate to permit its widespread use in the hospital intensive care unit as a monitoring device. Brainstem auditory-evoked responses are relatively resistant to trauma and to changes in the cerebral circulation and, once again, have not proved very helpful as early monitors of herniation. Current best therapy is thus to monitor those physiological parameters available for monitoring and attempt to maintain a normal state of arterial pressure. This involves maintaining steady intracranial pressure, keeping adequate oxygenation as stable as possible, and any specific therapy for underlying problems. Medications that might be used systemically to support the severely brain traumatized patient (e.g., vasopressors) fortunately have little effect on resting blood flow.[4] Norepinephrin in the face of a damaged blood–brain barrier can produce increases in cerebral metabolism that may be deleterious if blood flow cannot be increased appropriately. Otherwise, there is little concern for cross-reaction between systemically delivered medication and cerebrovascular response.

## REFERENCES


1. Bruce DA: Langfitt TW, Miller JD, et al: Regional cerebral blood flow, intracranial pressure and brain metabolism in comatose patients. J Neurosurg 38:131–144, 1973
2. Bruce DA, Alavi A, Bilaniuk LT, et al: Diffuse cerebral swelling following head injuries in children: The syndrome of "malignant brain edema." J Neurosurg 54:170–178, 1981
3. Bruce DA: Clinical reflections on brain stem injury in childhood, in Villani R, Papo I, Giovanelli M, et al (Eds): Advances in Neurotraumatology. Excerpta Medica, Amsterdam, 1983, pp 74–78
4. Goddard-Finegold J, Donley DK, Baffone GJ, et al: Phenobarbitol lowers mean arterial pressurure but does not blunt resting cerebral blood flow or the autoregulatory response to moderate hypovolemic hypertension. Ann Neurol 14:358, 1983
5. Gregory GA, Org W, Tweed A, et al: The effects of severe alkalosis and hypoxaemia on cerebral metabolism in the newborn lamb. Anesthesiology 57:1724, 1982
6. Langfitt TW, Obrist WD: Cerebral blood flow and metabolism after intracranial trauma. Progr Neurol Surg 10.14–48, 1981
7. Lou MC, Lassen NA, Friis-Hansen B: Impaired autoregulation of cerebral blood flow in the distressed newborn infant. J Pediat 94:118–121, 1979
8. Ment LR, Duncan CC, Ehrenkray RA, et al. Intraventricular hemorrhage of the preterm neonate: Timing and cerebral blood flow changes. Ann Neurol 14:356, 1983
9. Miller JD, Stanek A, Langfitt TW: Concepts of cerebral perfusion pressure and vascular compression during intracranial

hypertension. Prog Brain Res 35:411–432, 1971

10. Obrist WD, Langfitt TW, Jaggi JL, Cruz J, et al: Cerebral blood flow and metabolism in comatose patients with acute head injury. Relationship to intracranial hypertension. J Neurosurg 61:241–253, 1984

11. Siesjo BK: Cerebral circulation and metabolism. J Neurosurg 60:883–908, 1984

12. Swedlow D, Frewen T, Watcha W, et al: Cerebral blood flow, $AJDo_2$ and $CMRo_2$ in comatose children, in Go KG, Baethmann A (Eds): Brain Edema. New York, Plenum Press, 1984, pp 365–372

# PART III

# Basic Neuroradiology and the Pediatrician

*Robert A. Zimmerman*

# 9

# Normal Cranial Computed Tomography

The impact of cranial computed tomography (CT) in the evaluation of the pediatric patient has been the ability to directly demonstrate the cerebral parenchyma, the subarachnoid space, and the ventricular system.[1]

## RADIOLOGICAL ANATOMY

Normal brain morphology can be demonstrated by direct sectioning in the transverse plane [Fig. 9-1(**A**) and (**B**)] and in the cooperative patient, in the coronal plane provided that motion is not a problem (Fig. 9-2) and that artifacts from fillings in the teeth do not degrade the image quality. In the patient who is not sufficiently cooperative for direct coronal sections, multiple overlapping transverse sections of sufficient thinness (5 mm) can be obtained and then reconstructed by computer algorithms into coronal, transverse, or paraxial (oblique) sections. In addition to depicting the gross morphology of the brain parenchyma, CT also shows well the structure of the cranium, orbits[5] (Fig. 9-2), paranasal sinuses, and cranial base[4] (Fig. 9-3). Resolution achieved is comparable to, and often superior to that obtained with conventional plane radiographic studies (skull films). In general, the expense of the CT scan is sufficiently greater than that of studies such as the skull radiograph that the information to be derived should be considered relative to its cost. In the situation of head injury where brain damage or extracerebral hematoma is suspected, CT provides the best and most inexpensive[2] current imaging modality available.

BRAIN INSULTS IN INFANTS AND CHILDREN
0-8089-1723-4

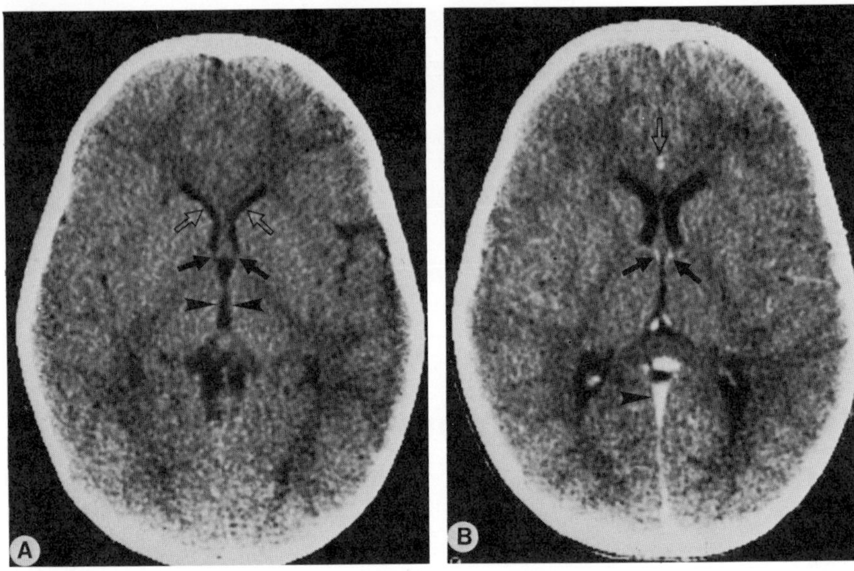


**Fig. 9-1.** **(A)** CT section in the transverse plane of the brain demonstrating the brain and the lateral ventricles (*light arrows*), the foramina of Monro (*large dark arrows*), and third ventricle (*smaller dark arrows*); **(B)** CT section following intravenous contrast. The top center arrow points to the anterior cerebral arteries. The two large black arrows point to the initial segments of the internal cerebral veins. The single black arrow points to the vein of Galen and straight sinus.

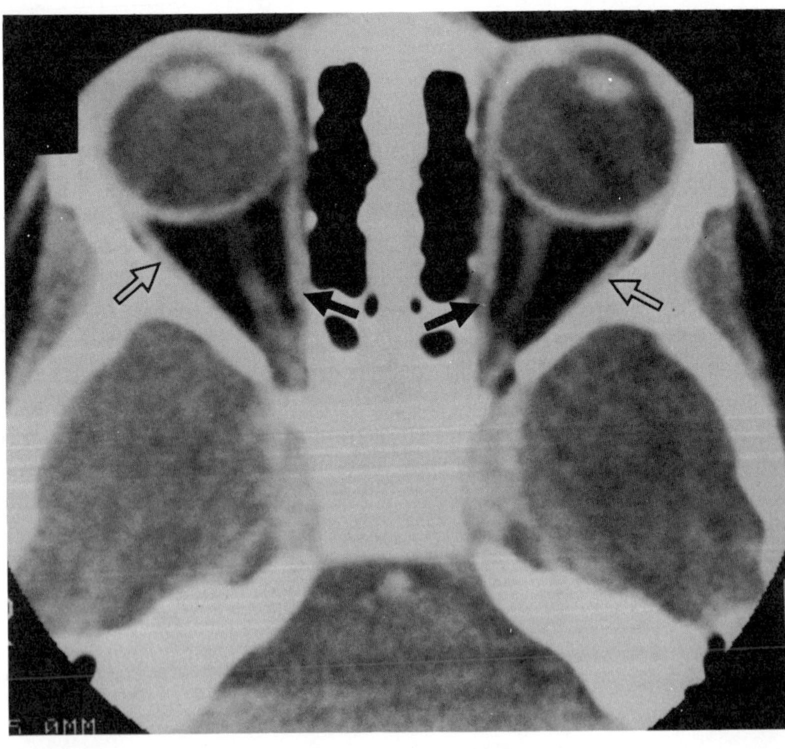

**Fig. 9-2.** CT of the orbits demonstrating the globles and the lateral (*light arrows*) and medial (*dark arrows*) rectus muscles.

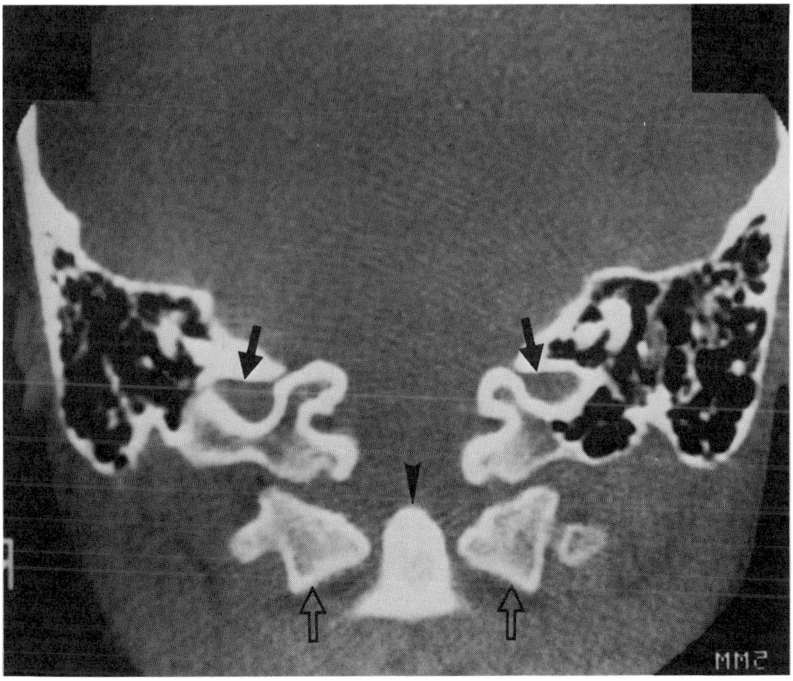


**Fig. 9-3.** Coronal CT section of the cranial base. The odontoid process (*center, black arrows*), the lateral masses of CI (*light arrows*), and the jugular foramen (*black arrows*) are seen.

## TECHNICAL ASPECTS

Most CT examinations are done in the transverse or axial plane.[3] This is usually in a plane parallel to a line drawn from the lateral canthus of the orbit through the external auditory meatus. In special situations the plane of section may be changed relative to this orbital meatal (OM) line. It is preferable to do the sections in the OM plane because of the ease of reproducing similar slices if anatomic reexamination is required. Slice thickness is usually variable from 1.5 to 10 mm. Depending on the part examined and the urgency of the examination, slice thickness can be varied. Routine examination of the older child's supratentorial brain is usually adequate with 10-mm-thick CT sections (Fig. 9-1). Examination of the posterior fossa usually requires thinner CT sections (5 mm). Examination of the temporal bone for evidence of fracture requires sections on the order of 1.5 mm thick. If reconstruction of sagittal or coronal images is to be done, thin or overlapping thin sections are desirable. For a small area of interest, 1.5-mm sections can be done, but for a large area of interest the time required to complete the study by such thin sections would be prohibitive. Thin CT sections are of value in solving the problem of volume averaging. Volume averaging can be illustrated in the following manner. If a small hematoma measuring 2 mm in size is present within a 10-mm-thick CT slice, the representative density seen on the CT image is the average between the 2-mm hematoma and the surrounding normal or edematous brain. In all likelihood, the hematoma would not be discerned as an area of increased density. Spatial resolution is another consideration. The pixel size will usually be on the order of $1 \times 1$ mm but can be made even smaller.

Computed tomography demonstrates the difference in absorption x-rays passing through tissues. This is a reflection of the electron density of the different tissues.[4] The skull is made up of compact bone and absorbs a great deal of the x-ray and is represented on the CT scan as white. Bone measures many hundreds of Houndsfield units (HU). Calcification is less dense than that in bone, and a retracted blood clot is less dense than calcification. A retracted blood clot measures on the order of 50–90 HU. Gray matter is more dense than white matter. The unmyelinated white matter of the newborn infant is less dense than the myelinated white matter seen after age 2. Less dense than the unmyelinated white matter is the cerebrospinal fluid (CSF). Arbitrarily, CT scanners have as their zero (0 HU), the density of CSF. Fat is less dense than CSF, and air is less dense than fat. Tissues of decreased density are represented as dark shades of gray or black. Brain parenchyma is represented as intermediate shades of gray [(Fig. 9-1(**A**) and (**B**)]. With the modern fourth generation CT scanners, therefore, differentiation can routinely be made between the calvarium, subarachnoid space, cortical gray matter, white matter, ventricular system, and any physiological calcifications such as those occurring in the pineal or choroid plexus.

## CLINICAL CONSIDERATIONS

Most patients suffering from head injury will be studied by the plain CT examination only. Intravenous injection of iodinated radiographic contrast media has two effects. First, it increases the iodine content of the blood pool. The cerebral blood vessels, both arteries, and the veins become of greater density and hence are more identifiable on the CT scan [Fig. 9-1(**B**)]. Second, portions of brain tissue in which there has been a disturbance of the blood–brain barrier are identified. Disruption of the tight junctions of the endothelium allows the leakage of the iodine-containing contrast media into the damaged tissue. This produces the phenomenon called *contrast enhancement*. With the use of both the history and anatomically delineated information, contrast enhancement can be used to characterize brain tumors (Fig. 9-4), abscesses and other abnormalities. Relative to head trauma, contrast

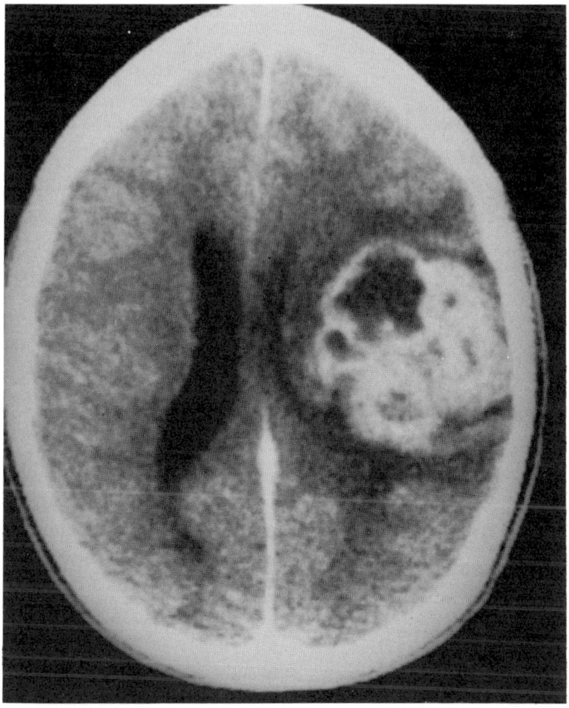

**Fig. 9-4.** CT following contrast revealing a large hemispheric brain tumor.

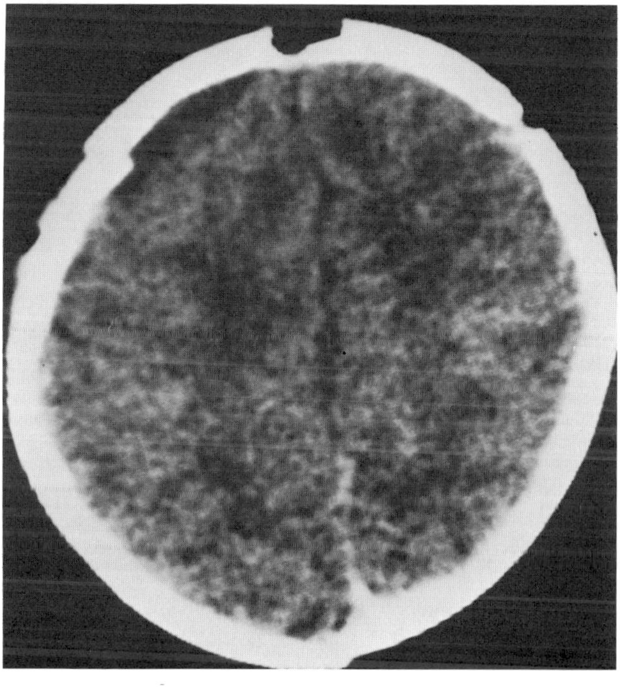

**Fig. 9-5.** Hypodensity of the white matter of the brain seen on CT scan of the newborn.

enhancement can be used to demonstrate inward displacement of cortical blood vessels by extracerebral collections, displacement of cerebral blood vessels by herniating portions of the brain such as the temporal lobes, and membranes associated with chronic subdural or epidural hematomas.

## CT AND THE CHILD

The brain of the newborn and young infant is different from that of the older infant and child. Myelination of the white matter occurs primarily during the first 8 months of life. In the newborn, therefore, the white matter of the brain appears hypodense (Fig. 9-5). As myelination progresses, the white matter appears more dense [Fig. 9-1(**A**) and (**B**)]. During the first year of life the subarachnoid space (including the basilar cisterns) is prominent (Fig. 9-6). During the second year of life, the subarachnoid space assumes proportions more characteristic for the remainder of childhood.

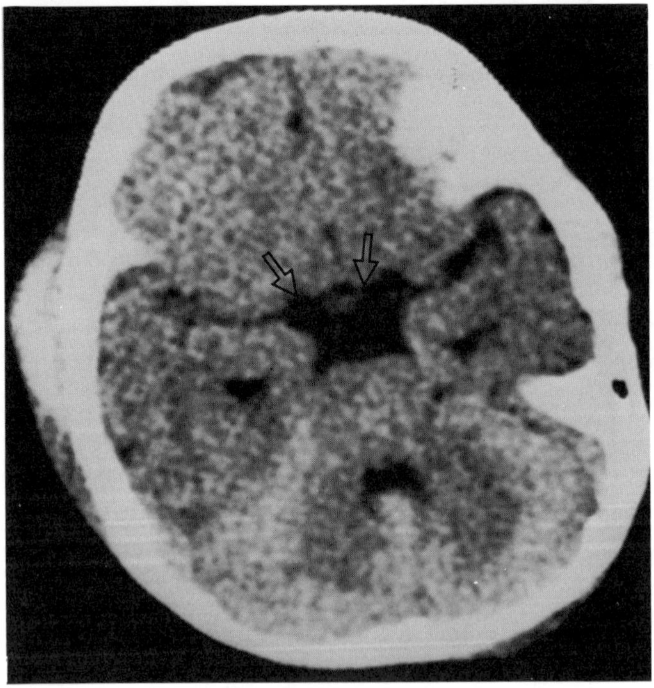

**Fig. 9-6.** Prominence of the subarachnoid space in the suprasellar cisterns seen on a CT scan during the first year of life.

## REFERENCES

1. Ferry PC: Computed cranial tomography in children. J Pediatr 96:961-967, 1980
2. Jacobsen HH, Kragsholm M, Holm C: The economy of the EMI scanner. Neuroradiology 11:183–184, 1976
3. Norman D, Korobkin M, Newton TH (Eds): Computed tomography. University of California Press, Berkeley, CA, 1977
4. Ter Pogossian MM: Computerized cranial tomography: Equipment and physics. Semin Roentgenol 12:34–25, 1977
5. Wende S, Aulich A, Nover A, et al: Computed tomography of orbital lesions. Neuroradiology 13:123–134, 1977

*Raul Bejar*
*Ronald Coen*

# 10

# Normal Cranial Ultrasonography in Neonates

Brain damage in the immature infant is a common event. Intraventricular subependymal hemorrhages (IVH/SEHs) occur in 40–75 percent of premature infants less than 34 weeks of gestation. Multifocal necrosis of the white matter (paraventricular necrosis, periventricular leukomalacia) develops in 15–20 percent of infants weighing less than 2000 g at birth. These lesions are associated with increased mortality and abnormal neurological and intellectual development.[1–4,7–9,13]

Our comprehension about these brain lesions increased significantly with the use of computerized tomography (CT) and recently with the development of ultrasonic procedures to study the infant's brain through the fontanels and sutures with real-time echoencephalography (RTE). RTE is a nonionizing bedside technique very well tolerated by small and ill infants. It allows early and frequent studies of the population at risk. Several authors have shown the clinical utility of RTE. The correlation of the ultrasonic diagnosis with clinical, autopsy, and CT scan findings has been accurate.[1–3,5,6,10–12]

## TECHNIQUE

### Supratentorial Compartment

The supratentorial structures may be visualized in several planes through the anterior, posterior, and mastoid fontanels. The most useful views are coronal, modified coronal, sagittal, and parasagittal (Fig. 10-1).

BRAIN INSULTS IN INFANTS AND CHILDREN
0-8089-1723-4

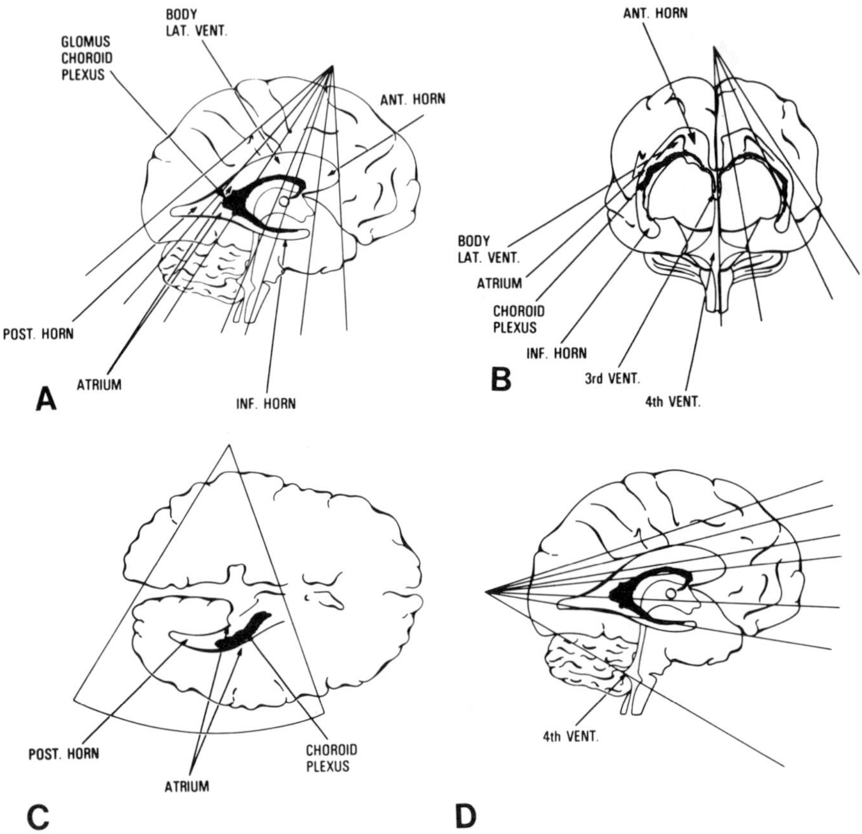


**Fig. 10-1.** Schematic representation of brain slices used to study the supratentorial compartment: **(A)** coronal studies; **(B)** sagittal and parasagittal studies; **(C)** mastoid fontanel studies (axial plane); **(D)** posterior fontanel studies (axial plane). Note that the posterior horn is devoid of choroid plexus. Studies through the posterior fontanel provide anatomic views similar to those obtained with CT. Note also the distance of the different brain structures from the anterior fontanel in the various planes.

### *Coronal and Modified Coronal Studies*

Coronal views of the brain are obtained when the transducer is positioned on the anterior fontanel and the scanning plane follows the coronal suture (Fig. 10-1). The transducer should be centered in the suture line to avoid bone interference. The anatomic structures visualized in these planes are shown in Figure 10-2.

Images obtained with coronal scans should be symmetrical. The bones and the middle cerebral arteries in the Sylvian fissures provide the anatomic

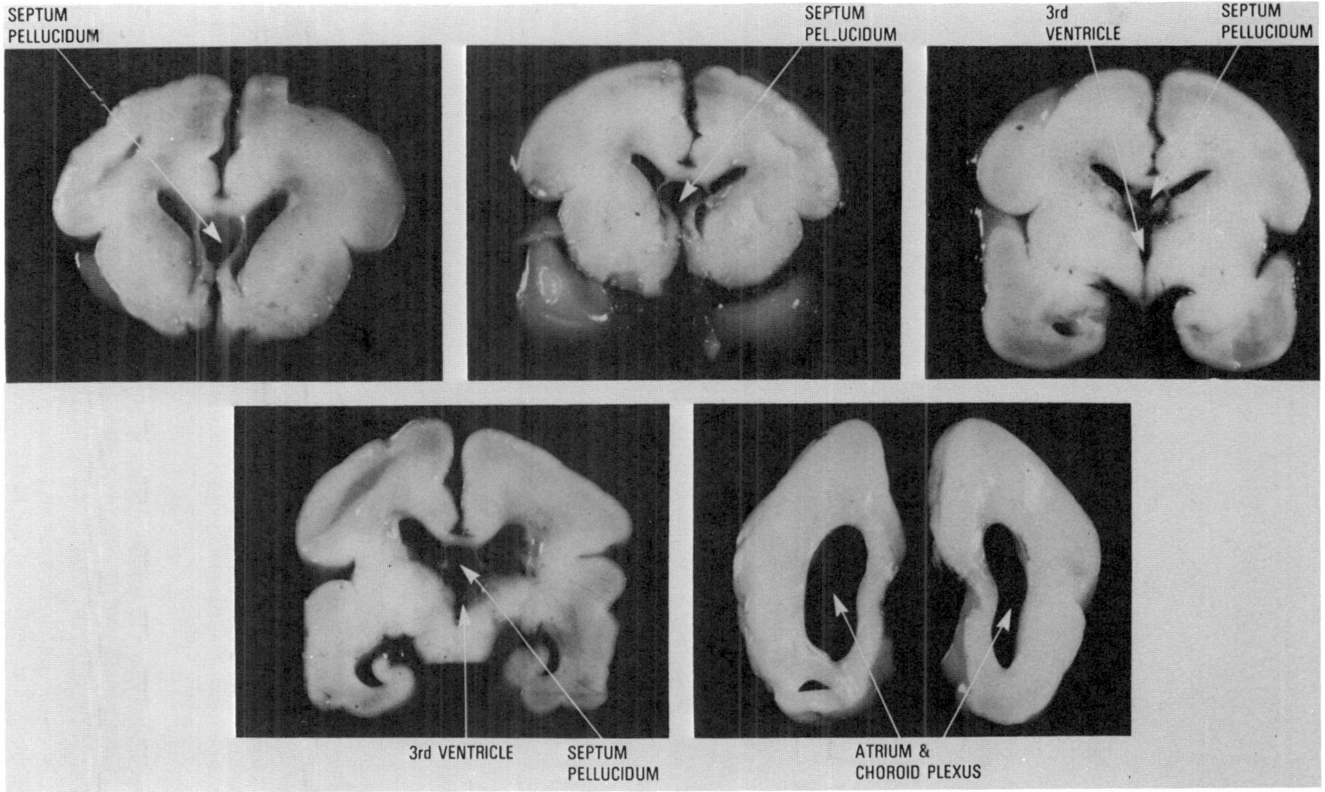


**Fig. 10-2.** Anatomy of an immature brain in the coronal plane.

bases for determining symmetry. The bones and arteries should be approximately the same size bilaterally (Fig. 10-3).

When a symmetrical image is obtained, the transducer is angled anteriorly and posteriorly to complete visualization of the lateral ventricles, the third ventricle, and the white matter (Figs. 10-1 and 10-3).

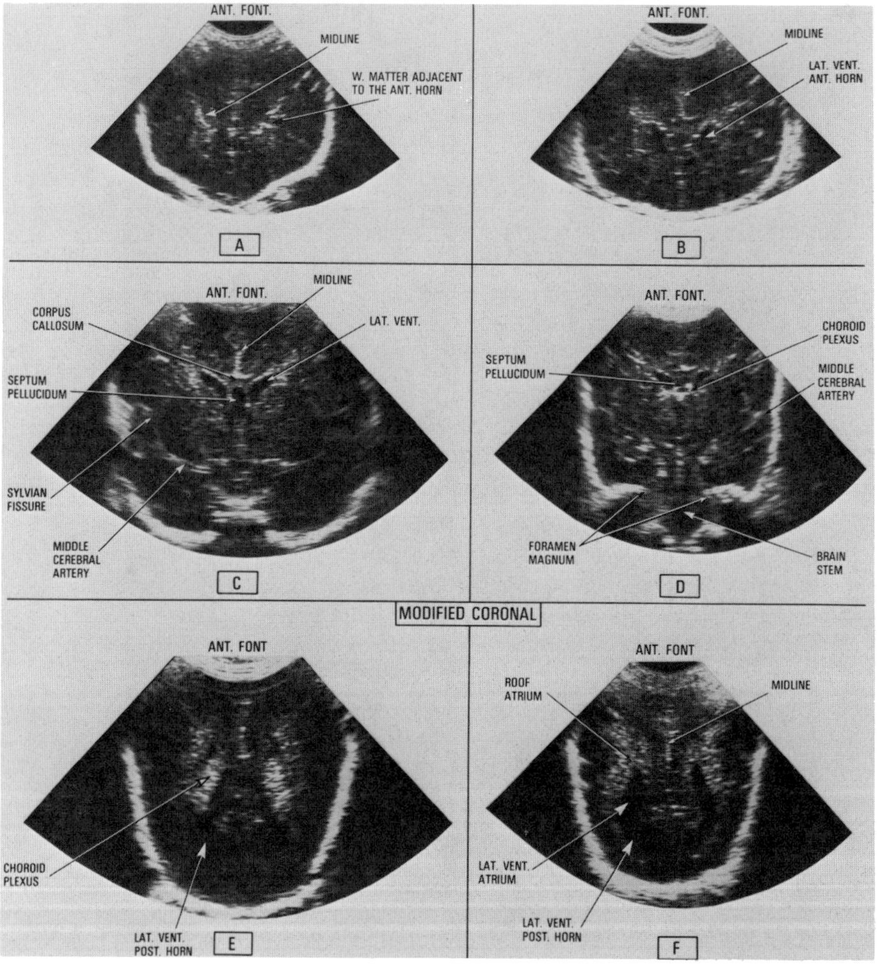


**Fig. 10-3.** Normal ultrasound studies in the coronal and modified coronal planes: **(A–D)** coronal studies; **(E, F)** modified coronal studies. Note the shape and size of the ventricles in the different views and the relationship of the ventricular cavities to the septum pellucidum and the choroid plexus. The choroid plexus is absent in the most anterior views. The surface of the brain is seen in the third picture. This is a normal finding in very tiny infants since they usually have large subarachnoid spaces.

The lateral ventricles appear as nonechogenic cavities about 2 mm wide. In the anterior cuts the ventricles are slit-shaped, and as the transducer is angled posteriorly they become "commalike." Their width increases to 3–6 mm in the modified coronal views. The highly echogenic tissue at the base of the ventricle is the choroid plexus. The septum pellucidum appears as a cyst between the bodies of the lateral ventricles (Fig. 10-3). In the coronal view the third ventricle is not observed under normal conditions. Occasionally it may appear as a very echogenic slit in the midline immediately below the lateral ventricles. The choroid plexus extends from the lateral into the third ventricle and appears as an echodense mass in the midline (Fig. 10-3).

Coronal studies also show the basal ganglia and the periventricular white matter. The caudate nuclei lie below the external walls and floor of the bodies and anterior horns of the lateral ventricles. The caudate nucleus may have higher echogenicity than the rest of the brain parenchyma, particularly in very small infants. It should not be mistaken with subependymal hemorrhages (SEHs) (Fig. 10-3).

***Sagittal and Parasagittal Studies***

Sagittal and parasagittal views are obtained by positioning the transducer in the center of the anterior fontanel with the scanning plane following the sagittal suture (Fig. 10-1). These views provide the most extensive anatomic description of the brain.

The "straight" sagittal plane shows the midline structures, including the infratentorial compartment. The midline should be visualized before performing right and left parasagittal views. The sagittal plane serves as the guide to determine whether a parasagittal cut corresponds to the right or left side (Fig. 10-4).

Three parasagittal studies should be performed. One close to the midline shows the anterior horn, the body of the ventricle, the choroid plexus, and the thalamus and the head of the caudate nucleus (Fig. 10-4). The ventricular cavity is narrow and nonechogenic. The floor of the ventricle is determined by the boundary between the highly echogenic choroid plexus and the low echogenic thalamus. The space between the floor and the roof of the ventricular body is normally anechoic. It has a height of less than 7 mm at midthalamus. The choroid plexus is a small (2–3 mm) and very echogenic structure lying against the thalamus. The plexus appears to end in the thalamic–caudate groove, the most common place where SEHs begin. The floor of the ventricle ventral to the groove is formed by the head of the caudate nucleus, which has a slightly higher density than the round thalamus (Figs. 10-2 and 10-4).

The second parasagittal cut is more lateral and includes the entire ventricular cavity. Since the posterior half of the lateral ventricles is more exterior than the anterior part, the transducer should be slightly rotated

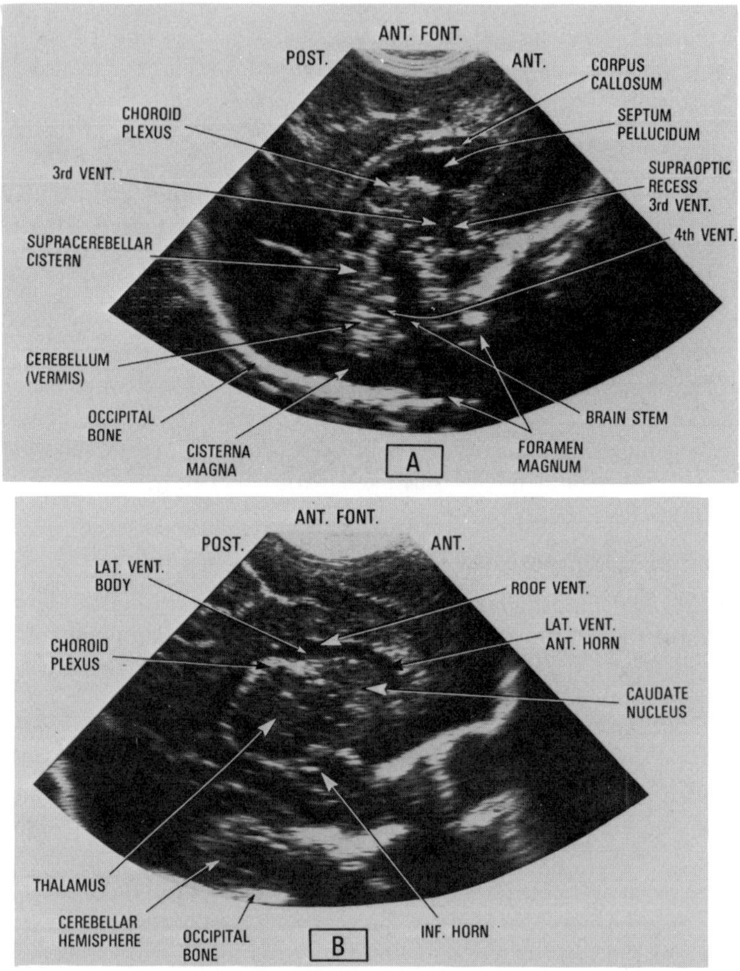


**Fig. 10-4.** Normal ultrasound studies in the sagittal and parasagittal planes: (**A**) sagittal (midline); (**B**) parasagittal (close to midline); (**C**) parasagittal (ventricular plane); (**D**) parasagittal (lateral wall). Note the size and shape of the ventricular cavities in the various planes. Compare the echogenicity of the thalamus, choroid plexus, caudate nucleus, and cerebellum. Note the appearance of the normal paraventricular white matter and the absence of choroid plexus in the anterior and posterior horns.

counterclockwise to form an acute angle with the sagittal suture anteriorly. When the plane of the ventricle comes into view, it is possible to observe the ventricular horns and the choroid plexus, including the glomus, the thalamus, and the caudate nucleus (Fig. 10-4).

The most exterior parasagittal view cuts the brain lateral to the ventricular cavity through the paraventricular white matter (Fig. 10-4). This study is

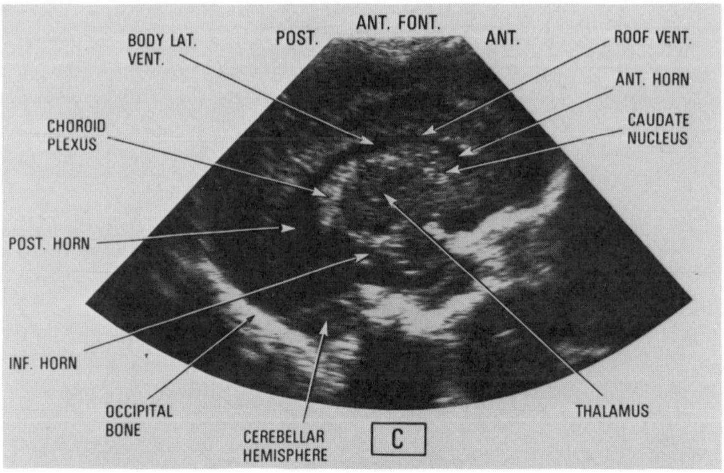


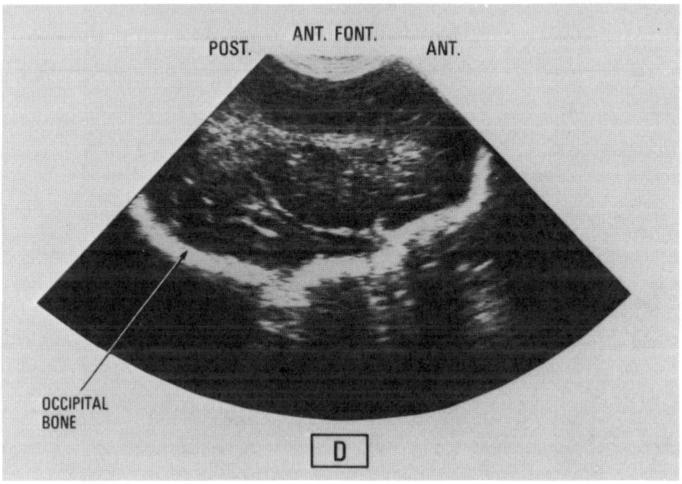


(**Fig. 10-4.** Continued)

important for diagnosis of intraparenchymal hemorrhages, porencephaly, and multifocal necrosis of the white matter.

*Axial Studies*

An axial view of the brain is obtained by scanning through the mastoid fontanel and the temporol-occipital suture. The posterior horn, the atrium, and the glomus of the choroid plexus are visible in this plane. This view is used to follow the size of the atria and posterior horns, since these are the first structures to dilate in posthemorrhagic hydrocephalus. The choroid plexus partially fills the atrium at this level and rarely extends into the occipital horn (Fig. 10-5). Using the choroid plexus as a reference to obtain the same

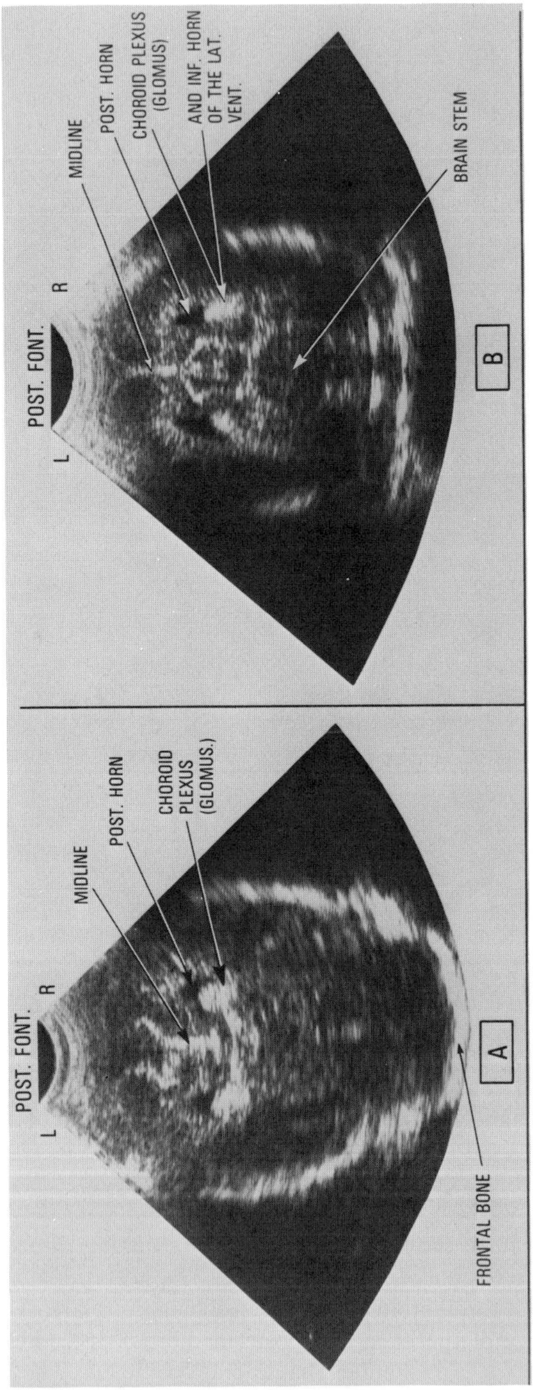

POST. FONT.
L
R
MIDLINE
POST. HORN
CHOROID PLEXUS (GLOMUS.)
FRONTAL BONE
A
POST. FONT.
L
R
MIDLINE
POST. HORN
CHOROID PLEXUS (GLOMUS)
AND INF. HORN OF THE LAT. VENT.
BRAIN STEM
B

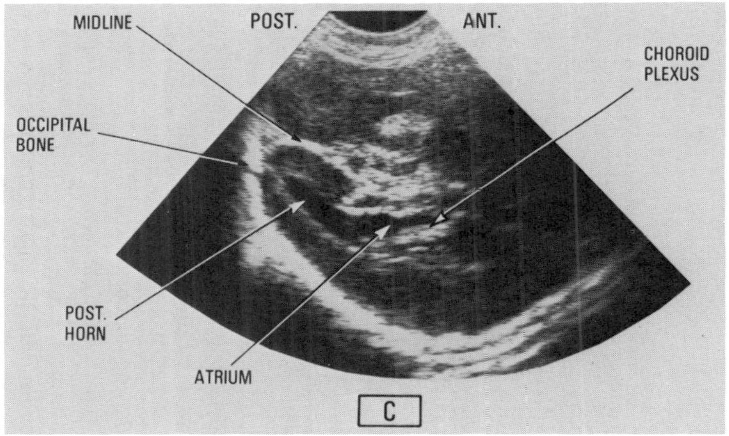


**Fig. 10-5.** Normal ultrasound studies in the axial plane: (**A, B**) posterior fontanel studies; (**C**) mastoid fontanel studies. Note the shape of the posterior horns and atria and their relationship to the choroid plexus. The choroid plexus rarely enters the occipital horns. There is always a small space between the choroid plexus and the lateral walls of the atria. This space may disappear when there is an IVH or a choroid plexus hemorrhage.

anatomic view in this plane, it is possible to serially assess and accurately measure the ventricular size.

The axial plane also is visualized through the posterior fontanel. The posterior horns appear as small anechoic triangles with the vertex oriented posteriorly. The base of the triangle is very echogenic and corresponds to the glomus of the choroid plexus. This view must be completely symmetrical. Symmetry is assured by using the cranial bones as reference. One slice through the posterior horns and the atria and a lower cut through the posterior horns and the temporal horns should be made (Fig. 10-5). If the fontanel is enlarged, multiple views of the brain similar to that obtained with a CT scan may be outlined (Fig. 10-1).

The ventricles should be visualized from the posterior fontanel. This fontanelle is closer to the occipital horns than the anterior fontanel. These horns will thus lie in the focal distance of the transducer and a greater amount of energy will reach them, thereby increasing the sensitivity and precision of the technique. This is relevant because it lends itself to the detection of small quantities of blood in the posterior horns and helps to differentiate intrachoroidal hemorrhages from a normal choroid plexus.

## Infratentorial Compartment

This compartment is studied in four planes: sagittal (midline), parasagittal, modified coronal, and coronal. The sagittal, parasagittal, and modified coronal planes are viewed from the anterior fontanel. Views of the coronal plane are obtained from the mastoid fontanel and the occipitotemporal suture. The anatomic structures observed in the four planes are represented in Figs. 10-6 and 10-7.

In the sagittal plane midline the corpus callosum, the septum pellucidum, the choroid plexus, the third ventricle with the supraoptic recess, the brainstem, the vermis of the cerebellum, the fourth ventricle, the cisterna magna, and the supracerebellar and the quadrigeminal cisterns are visualized (Figs. 10-6 and 10-7).

The corpus callosum appears as two parallel lines separated by a thin nonechogenic space. The septum pellucidum is a cyst and consequently is anechoic. The brainstem has low echogenicity, with a very dense anterior border produced by echoes from the basilar artery. The cerebellar vermis is very echodense and is separated from the occiptal bone by a anechoic space (approximately 1 cm), the cisterna magna. The other cisterns also are anechoic spaces located above and behind the cerebellum. The fourth ventricle appears as a small "v" (3 mm high) with the vertex oriented posteriorly inside the vermis and limited anteriorly by the brainstem (Fig. 10-7).

After visualization of the midline, the transducer is moved slightly to the right or left side to view the parasagittal structures. The tentorium and the hemispheres of the cerebellum are imaged clearly. The cerebellar hemispheres

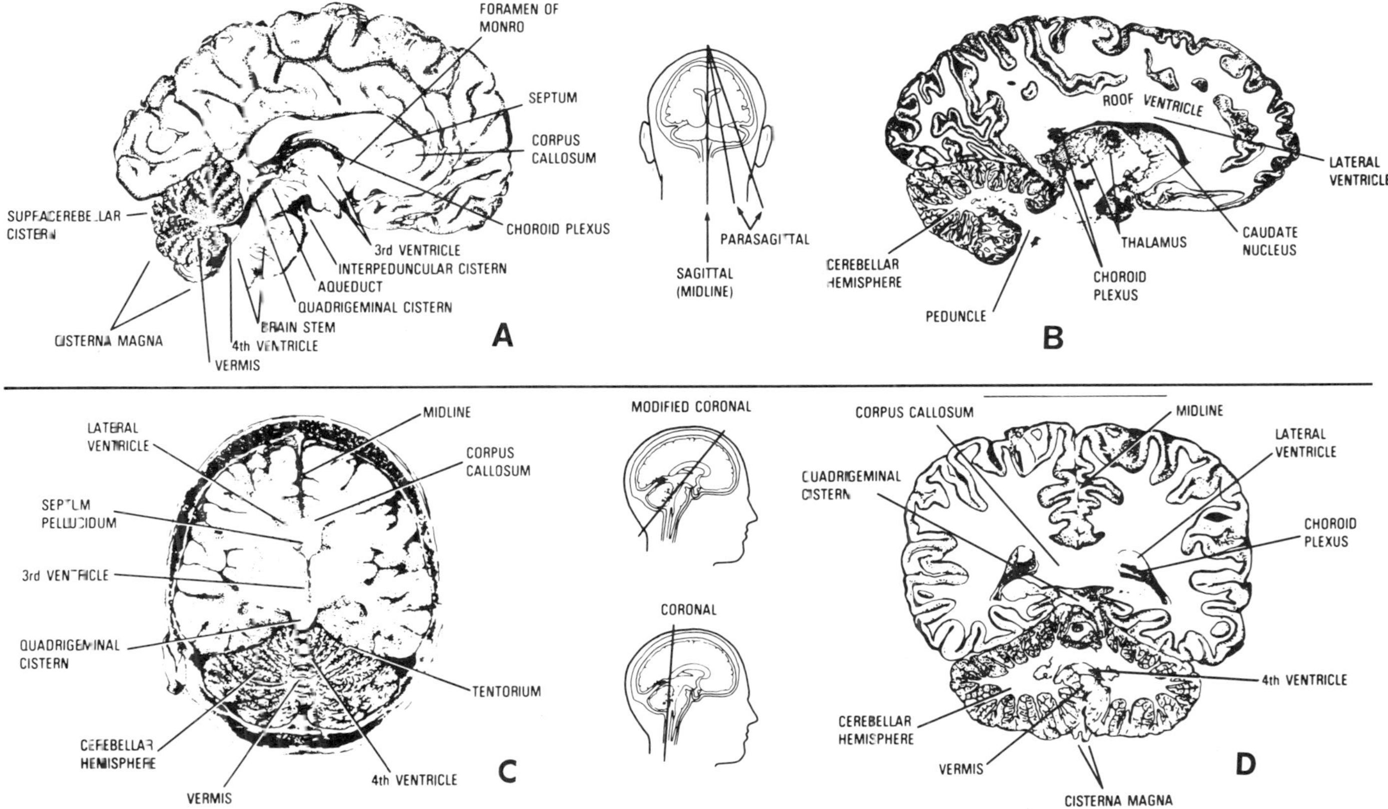


**Fig. 10-6.** Schematic representation of the anatomy in the different planes used to visualize the posterior fossa: (**A**) sagittal plane (anterior fontanel), midline sagittal; (**B**) sagittal plane (anterior fontanel), parasagittal; (**C**) modified coronal plane (anterior fontanel); (**D**) coronal plane (temporal bone).

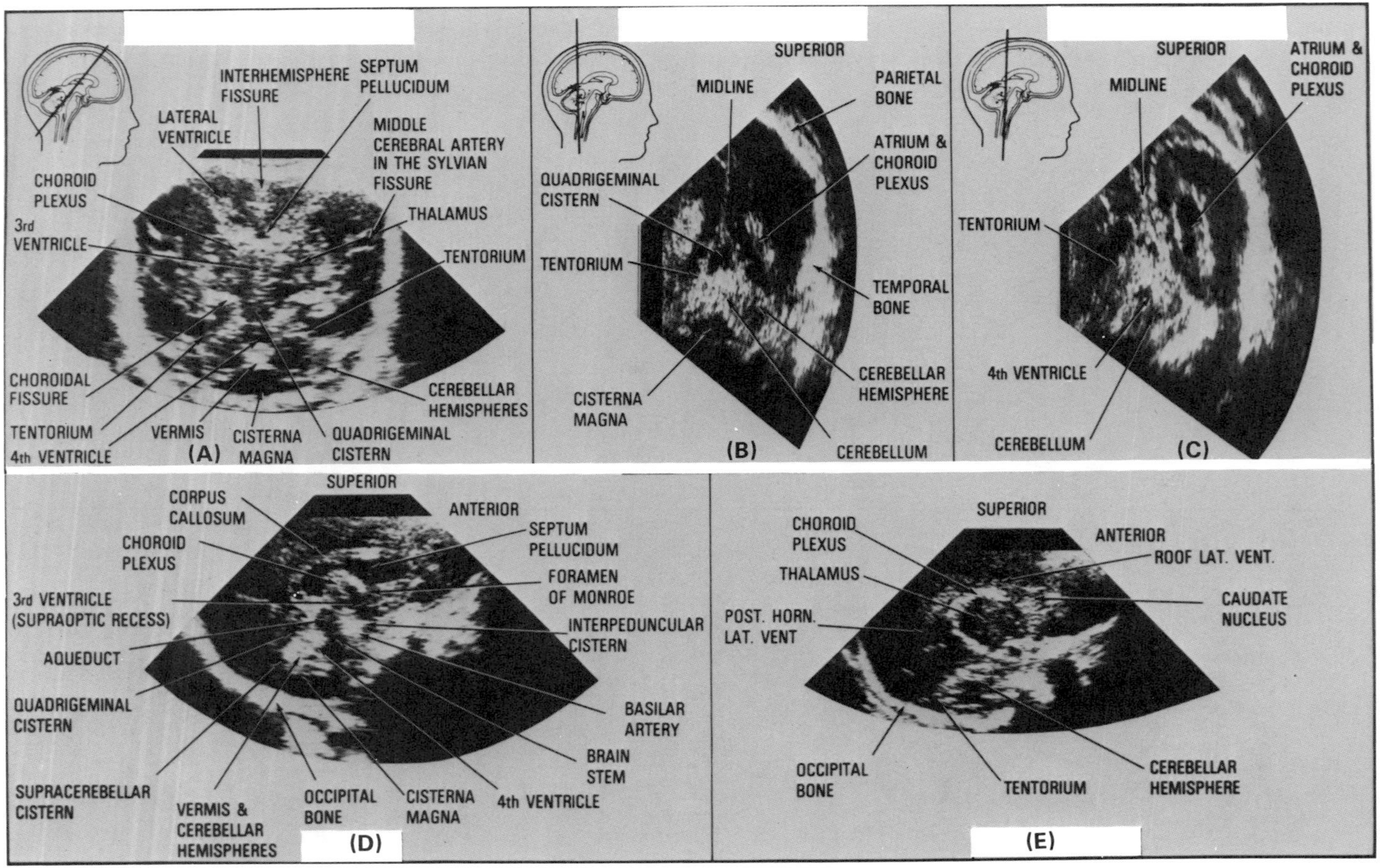
INTERHEMISPHERE FISSURE
SEPTUM PELLUCIDUM
LATERAL VENTRICLE
MIDDLE CEREBRAL ARTERY IN THE SYLVIAN FISSURE
CHOROID PLEXUS
THALAMUS
3rd VENTRICLE
TENTORIUM
CHOROIDAL FISSURE
CEREBELLAR HEMISPHERES
TENTORIUM
4th VENTRICLE
VERMIS
CISTERNA MAGNA
QUADRIGEMINAL CISTERN
(A)
SUPERIOR
MIDLINE
PARIETAL BONE
ATRIUM & CHOROID PLEXUS
QUADRIGEMINAL CISTERN
TENTORIUM
TEMPORAL BONE
CEREBELLAR HEMISPHERE
CISTERNA MAGNA
CEREBELLUM
(B)
SUPERIOR
MIDLINE
ATRIUM & CHOROID PLEXUS
TENTORIUM
4th VENTRICLE
CEREBELLUM
(C)
SUPERIOR
CORPUS CALLOSUM
ANTERIOR
CHOROID PLEXUS
SEPTUM PELLUCIDUM
FORAMEN OF MONROE
3rd VENTRICLE (SUPRAOPTIC RECESS)
INTERPEDUNCULAR CISTERN
AQUEDUCT
QUADRIGEMINAL CISTERN
BASILAR ARTERY
BRAIN STEM
SUPRACEREBELLAR CISTERN
VERMIS & CEREBELLAR HEMISPHERES
OCCIPITAL BONE
CISTERNA MAGNA
4th VENTRICLE
(D)
SUPERIOR
CHOROID PLEXUS
ANTERIOR
ROOF LAT. VENT.
THALAMUS
CAUDATE NUCLEUS
POST. HORN. LAT. VENT
OCCIPITAL BONE
TENTORIUM
CEREBELLAR HEMISPHERE
(E)

have lower echodensity than the vermis. Occasionally the hemispheres appear as nonenchodense structures with moderate echogenic surfaces (Fig. 10-7).

The modified coronal plane is visualized from the anterior fontanel. A symmetrical view of the middle cerebral arteries and the bones should be obtained first. The transducer is then moved posteriorly to a 30–40° angle between the scanning and the axial planes. The bodies of the lateral ventricles, the third ventricle, and the posterior fossa should come into view (Fig. 10-7). The tentorium, the vermis, the fourth ventricle, the cerebellar hemispheres, and the cisterna magna also are seen. The vermis is a very echodense midline structure. The fourth ventricle appears as a small anechoic space (2–3 mm) in the midline anterior to the vermis. The cerebellar hemispheres have low echogenicity and are contiguous with the echodense vermis. The cisterna magna is a round semicircular nonechogenic space located between the cerebellum and the bone (Fig. 10-7).

The coronal slice of the posterior fossa is obtained by placing the transducer on the mastoid fontanel and/or the occipitotemporal suture immediately behind the ear. The scanning plane is perpendicular to the axial plane. The tentorium, the cerebellar hemisphere, the cisterna magna, the supracerebellar cistern, and the fourth ventricle are visualized (Figs. 10-6 and 10-7). After a view of the posterior fossa is obtained in the true coronal plane, the transducer is moved anteriorly to form an acute angle with the axial plane, bringing into view the fourth ventricle and the brainstem. The fourth ventricle appears as a small equilateral triangle (3 × 3 mm) inside the cerebellum. The most ventral aspect of the supracerebellar cistern also comes into view above the cerebellum (Fig. 10-7).

The coronal scan is important for study of the posterior fossa. This compartment is the most distant structure from the anterior fontanel. When the posterior fossa is scanned from the anterior fontanel, the infratentorial compartment is outside the focal length of the transducer and only a small portion of the ultrasonic energy will reach this area. The infratentorial structures are visualized with greater resolution when they are scanned from the mastoid fontanel. Pathology in this compartment (e.g., subarachnoid and intracerebellar hemorrhages) are observed more precisely.

## CONCLUSION

Three-dimensional ultrasonographic scans of the newborn brain have been used since 1979 in the Infant Special Care Center of the University of

**Fig. 10-7.** Real time echoencephalography images of the four planes in normal preterm infants: (**A**) modified coronal plane; (**B**) coronal plane (posterior); (**C**) coronal plane (anterior); (**D**) sagittal plane, midline; (**E**) parasagittal plane. In the midline sagittal study (**D**) the vermis and the internal part of the cerebellar hemispheres may be visualized together because of the width of the ultrasound slice.

California, San Diego. Thousands of studies have been performed without complications even in very ill immature infants.

This technique has permitted quick and easy serial assessment of IVH/SEHs, hydrocephalus, porencephaly, subarachnoid hemorrhages, multifocal necrosis of the cerebral white matter, brain atrophy, ventriculitis, and malformations. Real-time echoencephalography has replaced CT as the primary technique for diagnosis of these complications in newborn infants, thereby reducing the exposure to ionizing radiation.

## REFERENCES


1. Babcock D: Cranial Ultrasonography of Infants. Williams & Wilkins, Baltimore, 1981
2. Babcock D, Han B: The accuracy of high resolution real-time ultrasonography of the head in infancy. Radiology 139:664, 1981
3. Bejar R, Curbelo V, Coen R, et al: Diagnosis and follow-up of intraventricular and intracerebral hemorrhages by ultrasound studies of infant's brain through the fontanelles and sutures. Pediatrics 66:661, 1980
4. Dykes FD, Lassara A, Ahmann P, et al: Intraventricular hemorrhage: A prospective evaluation of ethiopathogenesis. Pediatrics 66:42, 1980
5. Grant E, Schellinger D, Richardson J: Real-time ultrasonography of the posterior fossa. J Ultrasound Med 2:73, 1983
6. Harwood-Nash D, Flodmark O: Diagnostic imaging of the neonatal brain: Review and protocol. Am J Neurol 3:103, 1982
7. Lebed M, Schifrin B, Waffran F, et al: Real-time B scanning in the diagnosis of neonatal intracranial hemorrhage Am J Obstet Gynecol 142:851, 1982
8. Levene MI, Wigglesworth JS, Dubovitz V: Hemorrhagic periventricular leukomalacia in the neonate: A real-time ultrasound study. Pediatrics 71:794, 1983
9. Levinton A, Gilles F: Acquired perinatal leukoencephalopathy. Ann Neurol 16:1, 1984
10. Pape K, Bennet-Britton S, Szymonowicz W, et al: Diagnostic accuracy of neonatal brain imaging: A postmortem correlation of computed tomography and ultrasound scans. J Pediatr 102:275, 1983
11. Papile L, Burstein J, Burstein P, et al: Incidence and evolution of subependymal and intraventricular hemorrhage: A study of infants with birth weights less than 1500 gm. J Pediatr 92:529, 1978
12. Rumack C, Johnson M: Role of computed tomography and ultrasound in neonatal brain imaging. J Comp Tomogr 7:17, 1983
13. Volpe JJ: Neurology of the Newborn, Philadelphia, Saunders, 1981

*Robert A. Zimmerman*

# 11

# Computed Tomography and Head Trauma

Emergency room radiological evaluation of the acute pediatric head injury patient, if at all indicated, is usually limited to a cursory examination of the skull and cervical spine. More extensive evaluation in order to detect extra cerebral hematoma or parenchymal brain damage requires the use of computed tomorgaphy (CT).[7] High-resolution CT with thin section also gives good anatomical detail of the cranial base, cervical spine, and facial structures [Fig. 11-1 (A)]. In the patient likely to incur significant intracranial injury, skull radiographs are often canceled or postponed and the CT scan obtained.[8] Prior to mobilization of the patient for the CT scanner, it is desirable to exclude possibility of an unstable fracture of the cervical spine. This can often be done with a single lateral cervical spine radiograph that is adequately exposed. This should demonstrate the region from the cranial base to the bottom of the seventh cervical vertebral body.

Evaluation of the head-injured patient by CT is directed at detecting the nature of the underlying pathological process. Computed tomography can delineate changes within the brain parenchyma, subarachnoid space, and ventricular system and can demonstrate abnormalities of the blood–brain barrier following intravenous (IV) injection of iodinated contrast material. Serial CT examinations can demonstrate morphological changes that evolve out of the initial trauma.

## SKULL FRACTURES

Depending on the severity of the trauma and the forces acting to protect the patient, the skull may be fractured. Fracture of the calvarium does not

BRAIN INSULTS IN INFANTS AND CHILDREN
0-8089-1723-4

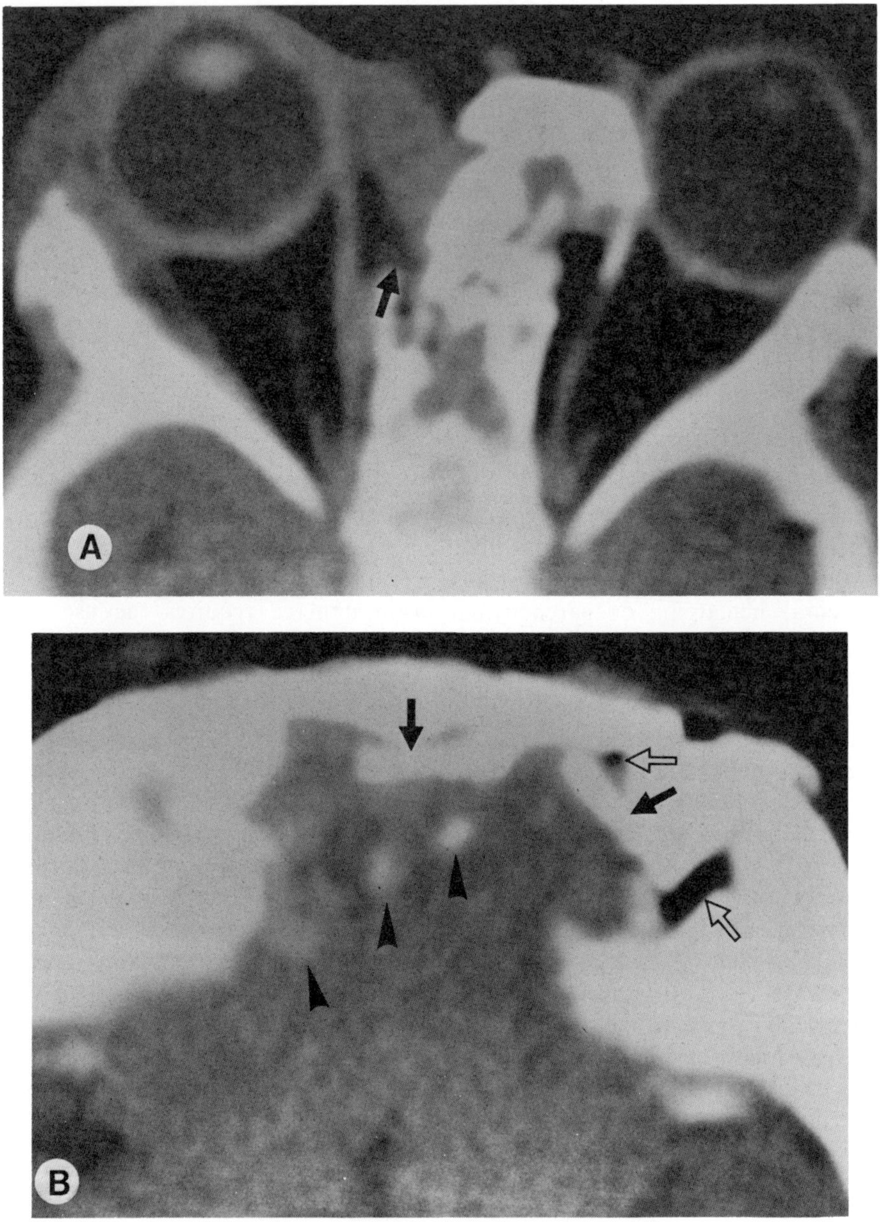


**Fig. 11-1.** Comminuted displaced fracture of the nose in a 2-year-old child struck by parent with hammer: (**A**) CT showing hemorrhage surrounding the right globe but the globe is intact—the nose is displaced to the left, with a fracture extending from the lamina papyracea (arrow) through the ethmoid air cells and through the nasal cavity to the other side; (**B**) higher section showing depressed fracture of frontal bone (arrow), hemorrhagic contusion (arrowheads), and pneumocephalus (open arrows).

necessarily imply presence of extra cerebral hematoma or cerebral traumatic pathology. In a series of 570 pediatric patients examined with skull radiographs there were 49 fractures, for an incidence of 8.25 percent.[6] Of these fractures, only two were considered significant, in that they changed medical management. Thus the incidence of significant fractures was 0.35 percent.[6] A significant fracture is one that alters management and includes the depressed fractures in which the fragment is locked under the inner edge of the adjacent intact calvarium (Fig. 11-2), depressed fractures over the major dural venous sinuses, fractures associated with the presence of intracranial air or foreign body, and cases in which the fracture passes through air-containing spaces such as the paranasal sinuses and mastoid air cells. A fracture that involves these air-containing spaces or one that is associated with a laceration of the overlying scalp presents the risk of intracranial infection. Skull radiographs

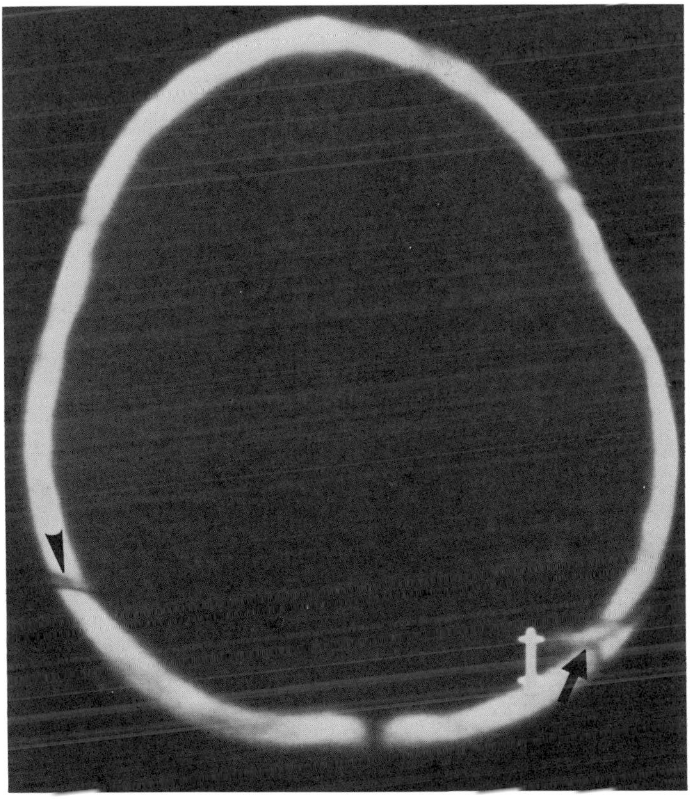

**Fig. 11-2.** Skull fracture in an 18-month-old child. Linear parietal fracture (arrowhead); contralateral—note depressed fracture (arrow).

usually suffice to identify convexity skull fractures in the patient, but do not manifest serious evidence of brain injury. Fractures of the temporal bone and cranial base are infrequently demonstrated by conventional skull radiographs.[3] Pluridirectional tomography or still better, CT, is more accurate in the demonstration of basilar skull fractures.

The dura mater is closely applied to the cranial base. This is especially true in the young infant and pediatric patient. Fractures that disrupt the cranial base usually disrupt the dura mater. This allows cerebrospinal fluid (CSF) to enter the middle-ear cavity, to exit through the tympanic membrane if it has been disrupted, or to exit by the eustachian tube into the nasopharynx. Otorrhea and rhinorrhea have an incidence of about 0.5 percent each in hospitalized pediatric head trauma patients.[9] Air may enter the intracranial cavity through such fractures, producing pneumocephalus, which may lodge in either the epidural, subdural, subarachnoid, intraparenchymal, or intraventricular space. Although pneumocephalus was thought to be uncommon in the pre-CT era, CT with its sensitivity to differences in tissue absorption by x-ray can detect minimal amounts of intracranial air as focal areas of hypodensity (dark relative to brain tissue) [Fig. 11-1 (**B**)]. Amounts as small as 0.5 ml may be seen with CT.[5] The presence of pneumocephalus is of concern because of the danger of intracranial infection.

Depressed fractures occur most frequently in the parietal and frontal region [Fig. 11-1 (**B**)]. Failure of the bone to rebound may be due to interlocking of the edge of the depressed fracture under the adjacent intact calvarial margin. With inward displacement of the fracture fragment, the underlying dura can be torn and the cerebral cortex contused. Harwood-Nash et al.[4] observed 23 percent of pediatric patients studied to have cerebral contusions under depressed fractures. Computed tomography is an ideal means for evaluating the depressed fracture and demonstrating the degree of depression (Fig. 11-2) and whether there is contusion of the underlying cortex [Fig. 11-1 (**B**)]. Skull radiographs taken tangential to the site of depression are also useful in the demonstration of the depressed fragment.

## EXTRACEREBRAL HEMATOMAS

### Epidural Hematomas

In the series by Zimmerman and Bilaniuk,[10] fractures were found to be associated with epidural hematomas in 91 percent. Bleeding into the epidural space occurs as a result of laceration of either a dural blood vessel, such as the middle meningeal artery, or a dural venous sinus such as the superior sagittal sinus. Although fractures frequently cross the middle meningeal arterial groove, they rarely injure the artery and produce epidural hematomas. Rapidity with which the epidural hematoma increases in size depends on whether the source of bleeding is artery or vein. Similarly, the location of the epidural hematoma also depends on the site of bleeding. Arterial epidural hematomas originating from the anterior or posterior division of the middle meningeal artery occur in the temporoparietal region and are the single most common type of epidural hematoma (66 percent).[2] Epidural hematomas occurring at the cerebral convexity or in the frontal pole usually relate to tears of the superior sagittal sinus, and epidural hematomas that occur in the posterior fossa or interoccipital region usually relate to tears of the confluence of the venous sinuses at the torcular Herophili or tears of the transverse sinus.

Most often the acute epidural hematoma is a biconvex configuration (Fig. 11-3), with its anterior–posterior extent demarcated by the binding of

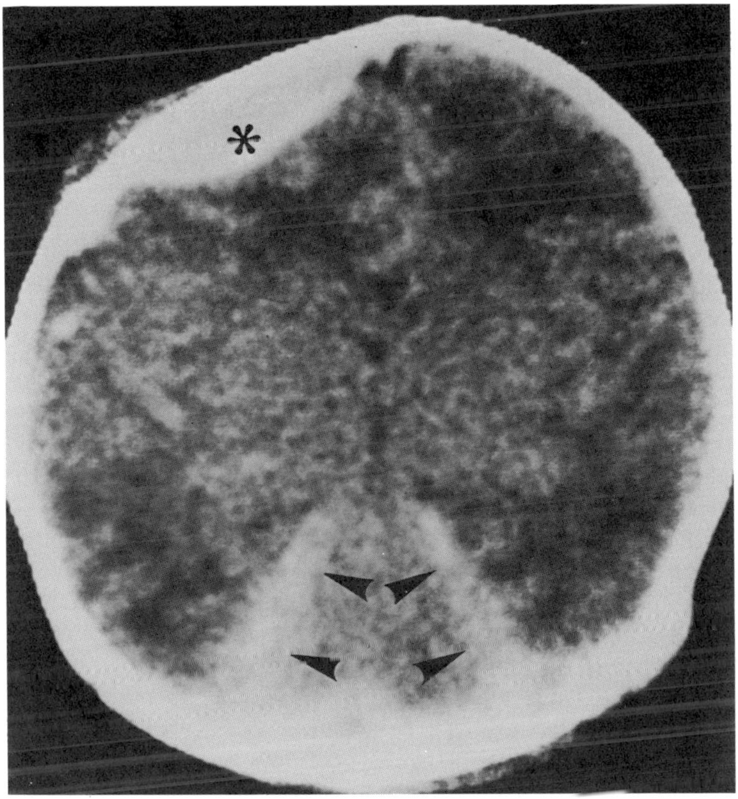

**Fig. 11-3.** Acute epidural hematoma. Acute peritentorial hemorrhage following traumatic delivery with forceps injury. Right frontal bone is flattened with a biconvex hyperdense blood clot in the epidural space underlying it (star, *). Hemorrhage outlines the leaves of the tentorium (arrowheads). It is likely that the hemorrhage is within the leaves of the tentorium.

the dura at the suture margins.[10] In the acute phase there may be identified in some a lucent swirl, which has been linked to the presence of less dense blood that is actively being extravasated within a surrounding denser retracting clot. Presence of this is of concern and suggests a need for immediate surgery. In the series by Zimmerman and Bilaniuk[10] those patients with hematomas that were associated with arterial bleeding had larger hematomas, presented earlier, and were more likely to have other traumatic lesions such as intracerebral hematomas and acute subdural hematomas. These were the patients with the highest mortality and the greatest morbidity. The subacute epidural hematoma is one that is homogenously dense throughout, suggesting clot retraction throughout. These tend to be of moderate size, with the patient presenting one or more days after injury. In such cases the patient is often awake and shows a high incidence of venous-origin epidural bleeding. Chronic epidural hematomas are usually of venous origin, are biconvex in configuration, have a contrast-enhancing inner membrane, and have contents that are mixed or of decreased density.

### Acute Subdural Hematomas

Acute subdural hematomas may arise from the rupture of a bridging cerebral vein, from cortical laceration, or from cortical arterial injury. Those seen immediately after injury are commonly associated with underlying brain damage and carry a significant incidence of morbidity and mortality.[1] A small proportion of adolescents are seen with small acute subdural hematomas, without evidence of cerebral parenchymal injury, and do quite well with or without surgery. Computed tomography shows a peripheral crescentic blood collection of increased density that conforms to the shape of the cerebral hemisphere [Fig. 11-4 (**A**)].[8] It should be noted that in the child with hydrocephalus or porencephaly, both acute and chronic subdural hematomas may present with bizarre appearances due to the collapse of the underlying ventricle or porencephalic cyst.

Equal in frequency to the lateral convexity acute subdural hematoma in the series by Dolinskas et al.[1] were acute interhemispheric subdural hematomas [Fig. 11-4 (**B**)]. Both occurred in about 5 percent of head-injured pediatric patients. The acute interhemisphere subdural hematomas appeared to develop as a result of laceration of bridging cerebral veins that extend from the medial aspect of the cerebral hemispheres into the superior sagittal sinus.[11] In most instances patients have been in the first years of life, and it was thought that the hematomas arose as a result of a whiplash shaking injury. Whiplash shaking injuries are one manifestation of child abuse. Predisposing to the rupture of the veins is the weak support provided by the cervical musculature to the infantile head that permits the head to snap back and forth with shaking. Associated with the acute intrahemispheric subdural hematoma

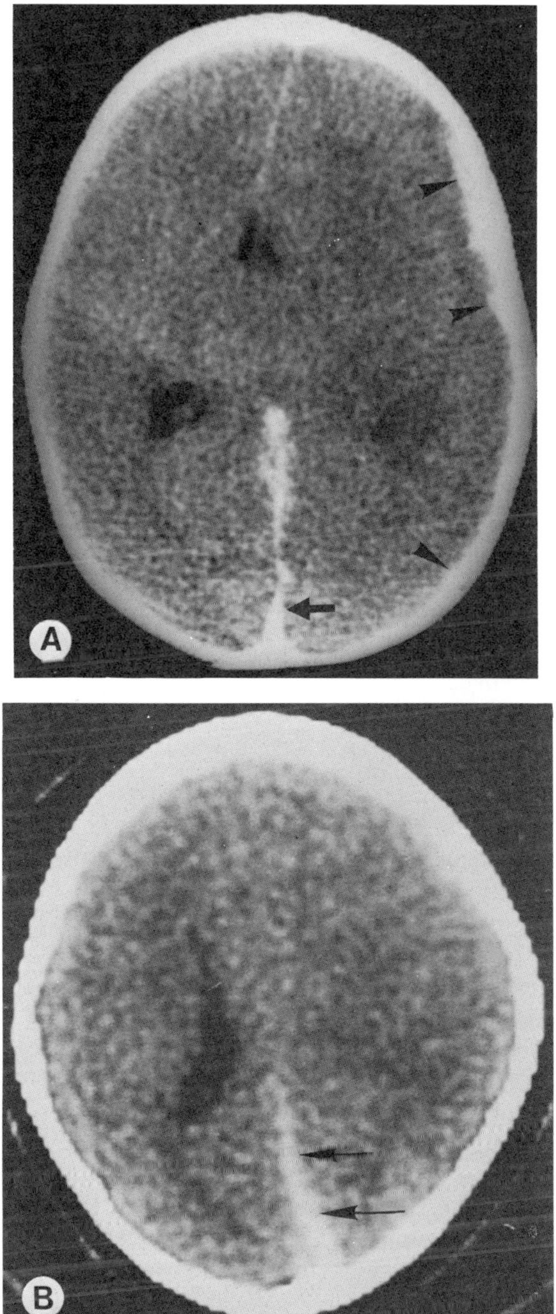


**Fig. 11-4.** (**A**) A small peripheral area of blood density (*arrowheads*) encompasses the left hemisphere. The ventricles are displaced, and there is mass effect greater than that attributed to the subdural. Note the presence of blood within the interhemispheric fissure between the occipital lobes (*arrow*). (**B**) An 18-month-old postwhiplash shaking injury shows acute interhemispheric subdural hematoma (*arrows*). Ventricle on side of hematoma is obliterated.

has often been the presence of retinal hemorrhages and the absence of skull fractures. A beaten child has a stigmata of not only bruises and skull fracture, but often of cerebral contusions, intracerebral hematomas, and lateral acute-convexity subdural hematomas.

## PARENCHYMAL BRAIN INJURY

### Cerebral Contusion

Contusions involve the gyral crests maximally and to a lesser extent, the underlying white matter. Although most contusions are hemorrhagic, the hyperdensity of the blood may be obscured by value-averaging of the brain and bone. The early hypodensity on the CT represents nonhemorrhagic areas of brain necrosis [Fig. 11-1 (**B**)].[12] Within several days of injury, edema will develop and the area may become more hypodense with associated increase in mass effect. If the hemorrhage did not form a hematoma, the admixture of the low-density edema with blood may lead to the whole area being hypodense in appearance. The danger of cereberal herniation is greatest at the time of the development of edema.

### Intracerebral Hematoma

Direct injury to a penetrating blood vessel within the brain parenchyma or extensive bleeding at the site of a contusion leads to formation of an intracerebral hematoma. Intracerebral hematomas are most common in the frontal and temporal lobes, as are hemorrhagic contusions. With enlargement of the hematoma and dissection along the white matter axon pathways, the hematoma may rupture into the ventricle. Hematomas appear as areas of increased density, often homogenously solid in appearance (Fig. 11-5) and measure on the order of 50–90 Houndsfield units (HU). Intracerebral hematomas are relatively less frequent in pediatric patients (3 percent) than are hemorrhagic contusions (16 percent).[7] Delayed intracerebral hematomas may occur 1–7 days following injury. These represent a relatively unusual complication of trauma and occur most often at the site of contusional or ischemic brain damage. Removal of an extracerebral mass such as a compressive acute subdural hematoma that has tamponaded the intraparenchymal vascular injury site has been implicated in some cases with delayed intracerebral hematoma formation. This form of intracerebral hematoma is an important and treatable etiology of secondary deterioration of the posttraumatic patient.

### Shearing Injury

As a result of sudden deceleration of an automobile, the brain may be abruptly accelerated. A shearing force can be applied to the white matter

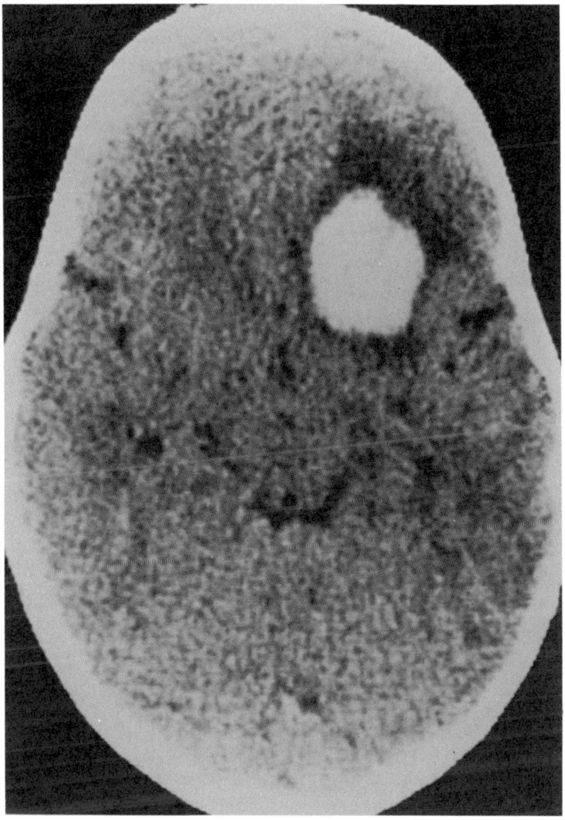

**Fig. 11-5.** Intracerebral hematoma is present in the inferior left frontal lobe surrounded by edema.

axons that radiate throughout the brain so that axonal rupture will occur. If the rupture is associated with injury to an accompanying blood vessel, hemorrhage might be indicated at this site on the CT. The most common site for hemorrhagic manifestations of the shearing injury is the corpus callosum (Fig. 11-6), at the gray–white matter junctures of the cerebral hemispheres, within the peri-third ventricular nuclear gray matter and internal capsule, and in the upper brainstem. Recognition of these characteristic hemorrhages is important because they signify much greater underlying nonhemorrhagic brain damage.[13]

### Cerebral Swelling

Swelling of the cerebral hemisphere may occur as a result of axonal enlargement (cytotoxic edema), as a result of distention of the cerebral

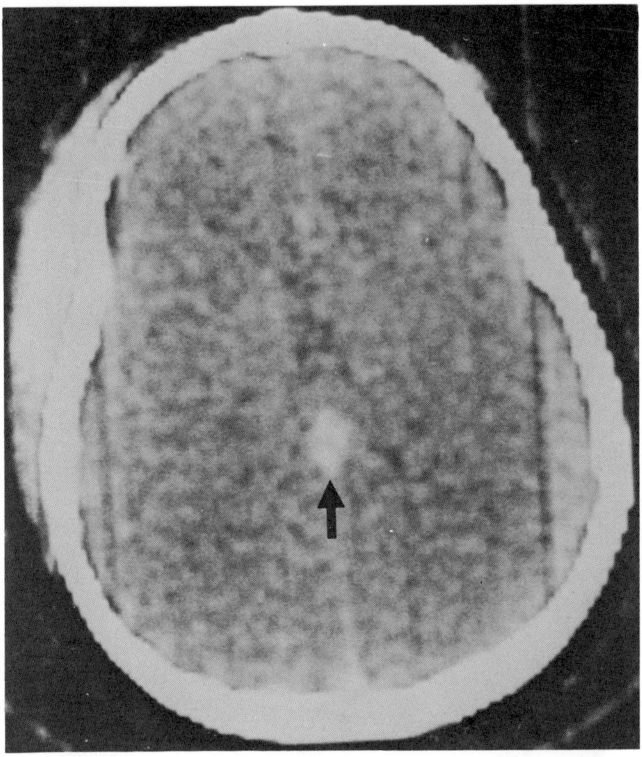

**Fig. 11-6.** Shearing injury. Eight-year old male involved in motor vehicle accident. Ventricles compressed by cerebral swelling. Focal hemorrhage in splenium of corpus callosum (*arrow*).

vascular blood pool, or possibly to some extent as a result of cerebral edema. The pediatric patient appears to be prone to development of cerebral swelling.[14] Compression of the lateral and third ventricles and perimesencephalic cisterns is the initial CT appearance (Fig. 11-7). This occurs frequently without evidence of other brain injury in the form of extracerebral hematoma or intraparenchymal hemorrhagic lesion. Sequential CT studies over the course of hospitalization show a resolution of the swelling with transitory enlargement of the extracerebral cerebrospinal fluid (CSF) spaces, often with an eventual return to a normal CT appearance. In the acute phase, when the swelling is present, the cerebral white and gray matter appears of normal to slightly increased density. This is distinct from the patient with vasogenic edema, in which the increased water content of the white matter produces an area of hypodensity.

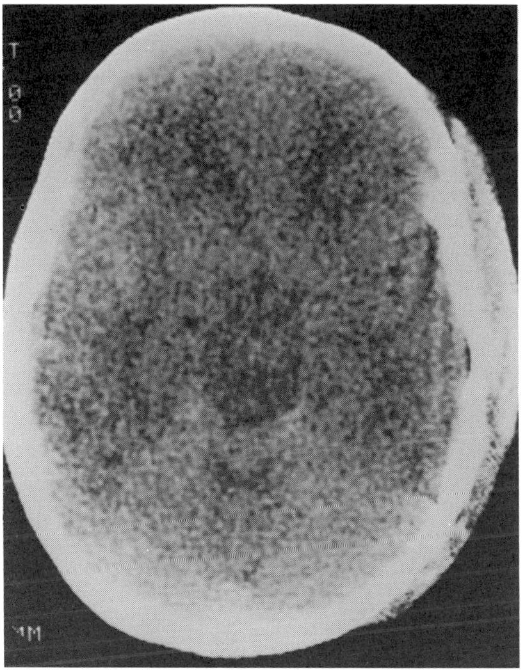

**Fig. 11-7.** Cerebral swelling. Ventricles and subarachnoid space are obliterated by the bilateral swelling of the cerebral hemispheres.

## REFERENCES


1. Dolinskas CA, Zimmerman RA, Bilaniuk LT, et al: Computed tomography of post-traumatic extracerebral hematomas: Comparison to pathophysiology & Responses to therapy. J Trauma, 19:163–169, 1979
2. Hardman JM: The Pathology of traumatic brain injuries, in Thompson RA, Green JR (Eds): Advances in Neurology, vol 22. New York, Raven Press, 1979, pp 15–50
3. Harwood-Nash DC: Fractures of the petrous and tympanic parts of the temporal bone in childhood: A tomographic study of 35 cases. Am J Roentgenol 101:151–155, 1971
4. Harwood-Nash DC, Hendrich EB, Hudson AR: The significance of skull fractures in children. Radiology 101:151, 1971
5. Osborn AG, Daines JH, Wing SD, et al: Intracranial air on computerized tomography. Neurosurgery 48:355–359, 1978
6. Roberts F, Shopfner CE: Plain skull roentgenograms in children with head trauma. Am J Roentgenol 114:230–240, 1972
7. Zimmerman RA: The effectiveness of skull plain films in the evaluation of traumatic coma. J Neuroradiol 10:145–148, 1983
8. Zimmerman RA, Bilaniuk LT, Gennarelli T, et al: Cranial computed tomography in diagnosis & management of acute head trauma. Am J Roentgenol 131:27–34, 1978
9. Zimmerman RA, Bilaniuk LT: Radiology of pediatric craniocerebral trauma, in Shapiro K (Ed): Head Trauma, New

York, Futura Publishing Company, 1983, pp 69–142,

10. Zimmerman RA, Bilaniuk LT: Computed tomographic staging of traumatic epidural bleeding. Radiology 144:809–812, 1982
11. Zimmerman RA, Bilaniuk LT, Bruce D, et al: Computed tomography of craniocerebral injury in the abused child. Radiology 130:687–690, 1979
12. Zimmerman RA, Bilaniuk LT, Dolinskas C, et al: Computed tomography of acute intracerebral hemorrhagic contusion. Comp Axial Tomogr 1:271–280, 1977
13. Zimmerman RA, Bilaniuk LT, Gennarelli T: Computed tomography of shearing injuries of the cerebral white matter. Radiology 127:393–396, 1978
14. Zimmerman RA, Bilaniuk LT, Bruce D, et al: Computed tomography of pediatric head trauma: Acute cerebral swelling. Radiology 126:403–408, 1978

*Raul Bejar*
*Ronald Coen*

# 12

# Neonatal Intracranial Pathology and Ultrasonography

Real-time echoencephalography (RTE) is an ideal diagnostic tool for timing the onset and following the evolution of major brain lesions in preterm infants. Intraventricular–subependymal hemorrhages (IVH//SEHs), intraparenchymal bleeds (IPH), subarachnoid hemorrhages (SAH), cerebellar hemorrhages, multifocal necrosis of the white matter, ventriculitis, cerebral abscess, brain atrophy, and most of the malformations of the brain can be evaluated. Computed tomography (CT) preferentially is used to diagnose more superficial lesions, such as subdural hemorrhages.[15]

## HEMORRHAGIC PATHOLOGY

### Intraventricular–Subependymal Hemorrhages

These are the most common brain lesion in premature infants less than 34 weeks of gestation. These hemorrhages, which occur in 40–70 percent of the population at risk, originate from pockets of germinal matrix in the region of the caudate nucleus.[2,5,11,18] The bleeding may remain localized in the germinal matrix, the so called subependymal hemorrhage (SEH). If the hemorrhaging continues, the SEH enlarges and eventually ruptures into the ventricular cavity [intraventricular hemorrhage (IVH)]. In full-term infants IVHs originate mainly in the choroid plexus.[2,5,8,11,18]

These hemorrhages are detected easily with RTE because blood has a higher acoustic impedance than the brain and the cerebrospinal fluid (CSF). Thus intracranial hemorrhages are more echogenic than the surrounding

BRAIN INSULTS IN INFANTS AND CHILDREN
0-8089-1723-4

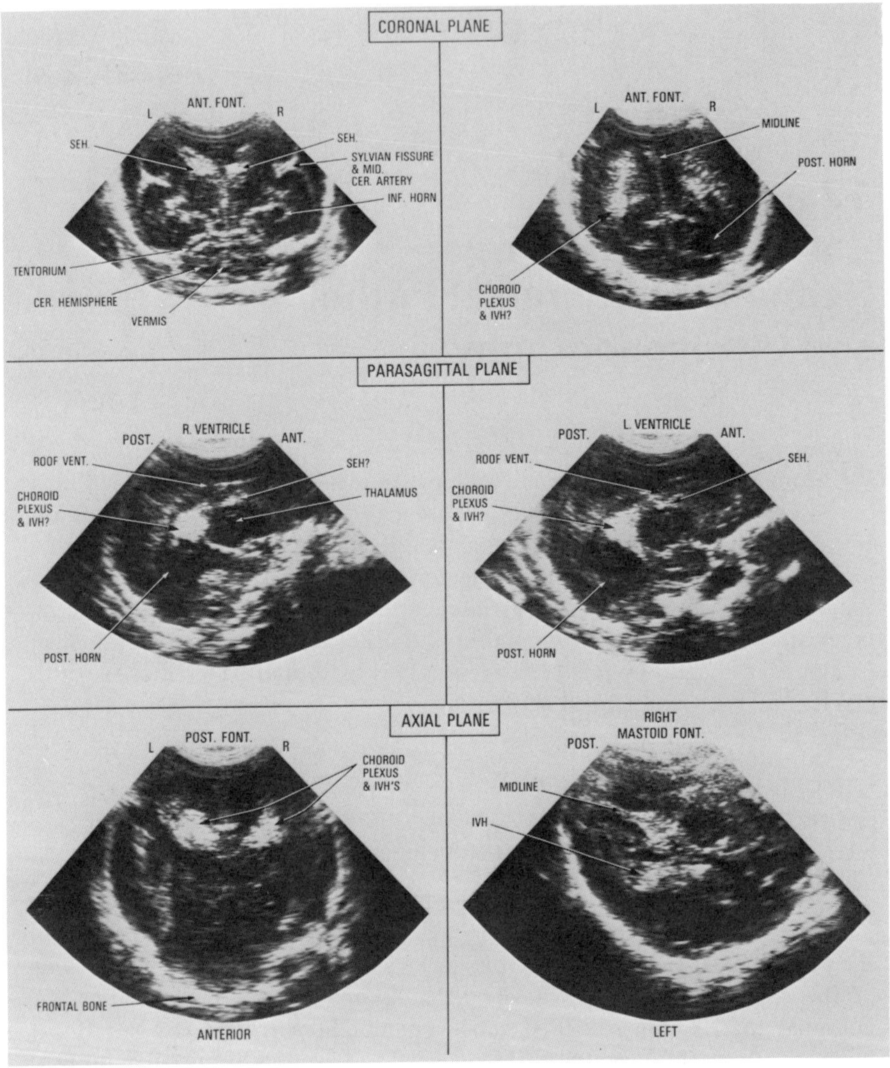


**Figs. 12-1 and 12-2.** Postmortem ultrasound studies (**Fig. 12-1**) and pathological studies (**Fig. 12-2**) in a premature infant with small SEH/IVHs. The ventricular cavities are partially obstructed by SEH. The small SEH (2 mm) in the right caudate nucleus is seen in the coronal and sagittal planes. The studies of the axial plane through the posterior and mastoid fontanel showed IVHs. These hemorrhages were not clearly visualized in the modified coronal and sagittal studies from the anterior fontanel.

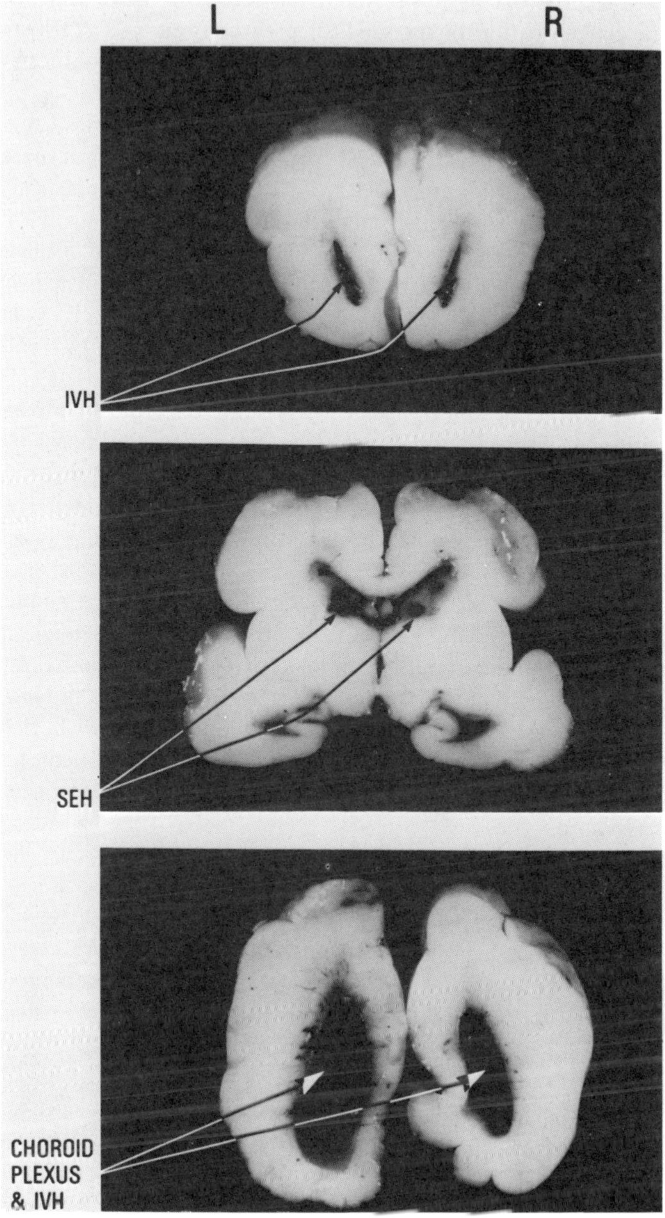


(**Fig. 12-2.** Continued)

tissues. Overall, RTE is a more sensitive technique for detecting intracranial hemorrhages than is CT. The threshold for detecting an IVH with CT is a hemoglobin concentration in the CSF of greater than 5–6 g/100 ml. Real-time echoencephalography can detect fluid blood with an hematocrit of about 5 percent.[2,15]

Small and large IVH/SEHs and their sequential changes are shown in Figures 12-1–12-5. Very small (2 mm) SEHs and their changes (extension or resolution) are shown in Figures 12-1 and 12-2. The SEHs appear as areas of increased echogenicity inside the caudate nucleus, pushing up the floor and external wall of the ventricular cavity with partial obliteration of the ventricle. Large IVH/SEHs appear as extensive echodense structures inside the ventricles (ventricular cast), enlarging the ventricular cavity (Figs. 12-1–12-4).

Studies from the anterior fontanel may not detect small IVHs. Intraventricular blood tends to sediment in the posterior horn. Small IVHs can be diagnosed when the occipital horns are visualized from the posterior or mastoid fontanels. These fontanels are closer to the occipital horns than is the anterior fontanel. The occipital horns will be in the focal distance of the transducer, and a greater amount of ultrasonic energy will reach the sedimented red blood cells, thus increasing the sensitivity and precision of the technique.

Intraventricular–subependymal hemorrhages are not a sudden event. They usually expand slowly (Figs. 12-3, and 12-4). This phenomenon is probably secondary to the high fibrinolitic activity of the germinal matrix.[7] In some infants the hemorrhages may extend very rapidly. The sudden flooding and distension of the ventricles by blood is associated with the clinical symptoms of shock, convulsions, hypoxemia, and decreased hematocrit. If a small SEH/IVH progresses to a large SEH/IVH in several days, the bleeding is usually asymptomatic.

On the basis of changes produced in ventricular size, we classify IVH/SEH's in four grades:

| | |
|---|---|
| Grade 1 | IVH or SEH without ventricular dilatation |
| Grade 2 | IVH or SEH with minimal ventricular enlargement |
| Grade 3 | IVH or SEH with large ventricular dilatation |
| Grade 4 | Intraparenchymal hemorrhage |

Only dilatation produced directly by blood is considered. The ventricular size is measured in the sagittal (body of the ventricle at midthalamus) and axial planes (atrium at the level of the choroid plexus). Ventricular dilatation is classified as follows:

| | |
|---|---|
| Mild dilatation | ventricles 7–10 mm |
| Moderate dilatation | ventricles between 11–15 mm |
| Large dilatation | ventricles >15 mm in any of the planes |

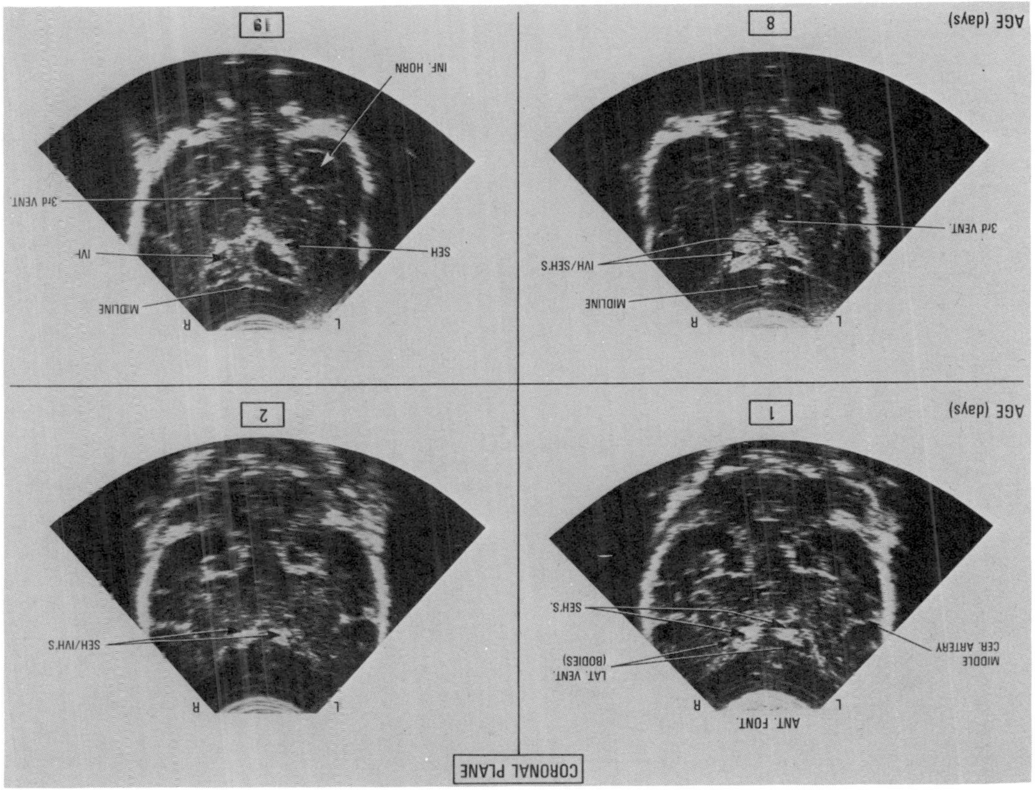


**Fig. 12-3.** Sequential studies, coronal plane, showing the slow extension of a small SEH/IVH. The infant had small SEH/IVH bilaterally that progressed to large SEH/IVHs. Note the dilation of the ventricles by the intraventricular clots, the cystic transformation of the intraventricular casts with the choroid plexus inside, and the initiation of posthemorrhagic ventricular enlargement by CSF.

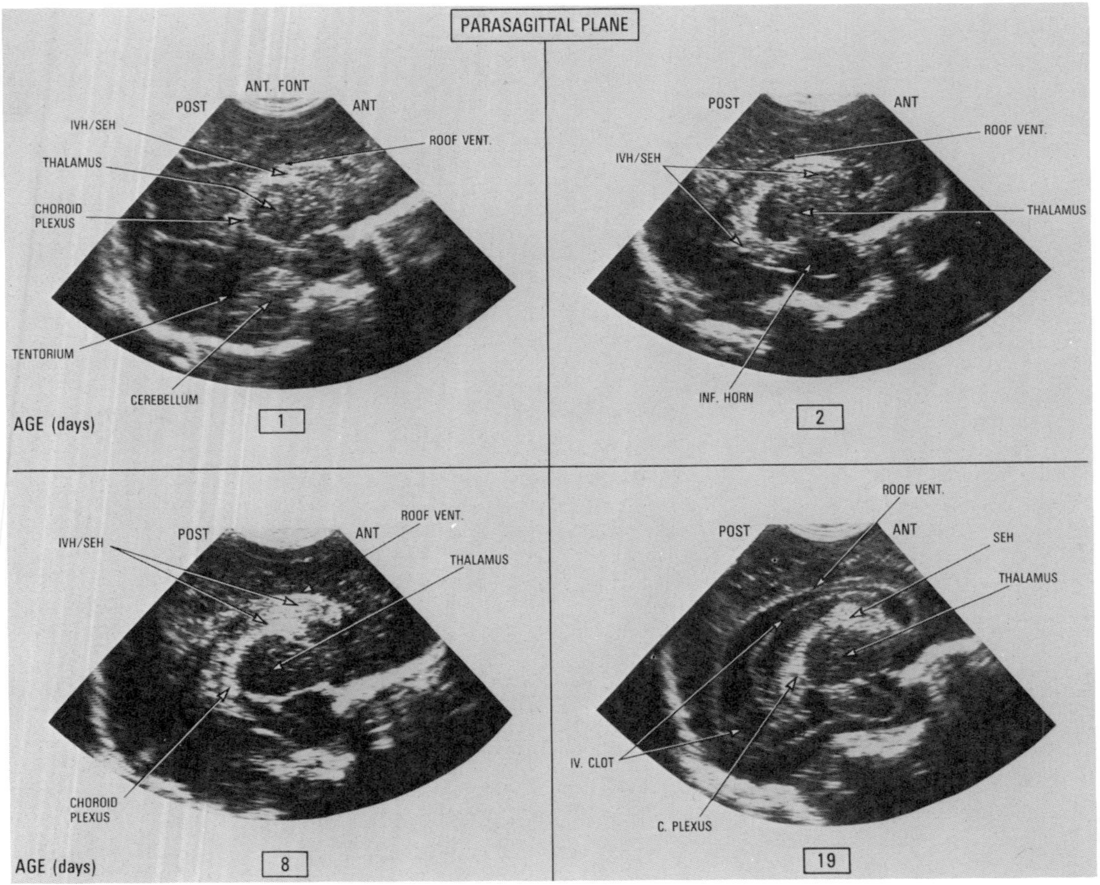


**Fig. 12-4.** Sequential studies, parasagittal plane, of patient in **Fig. 12-3**, showing the slow extension of a small SEH/IVH. The infant had small SEH/IVH bilaterally that progressed to large SEH/IVHs.

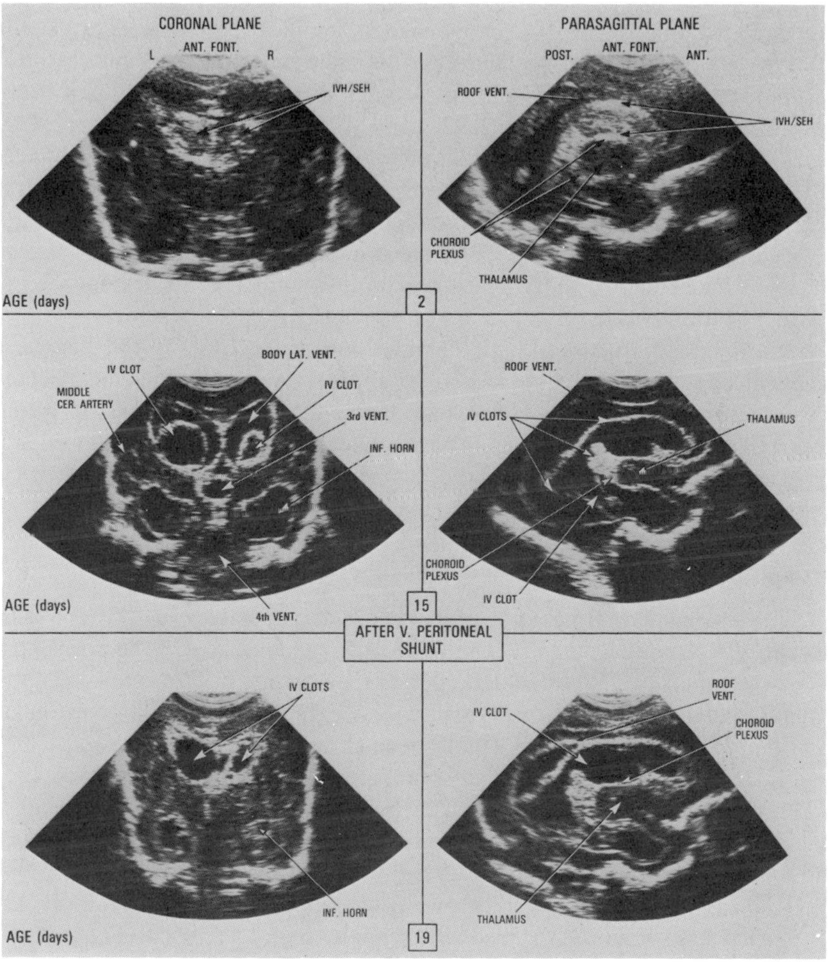


**Fig. 12-5.** Large IVH/SEH, posthemorrhagic hydrocephalus, and changes in the size of the ventricles produced by a VPS. The ventricles are filled with very echogenic material (blood) and distended by blood clots. Two weeks later the clots are cystic and posthemorrhagic hydrocephalus has developed. Note that the ventricular cast appears "anchored" to the choroid plexus and the caudate nucleus. A VPS reduced significantly the size of the ventricular cavities draining practically all of the CSF; however, the ventricles remained enlarged by the intraventricular clots.

Intraventricular–subependymal hemorrhages can produce obstruction of the CSF pathways or decreased absorption of CSF with the consequent ventricular dilatation. Whatever the size of the bleed, the ventricles usually enlarge. In most cases the dilatation is mild to moderate and resolves spontaneously. Posthemorrhagic hydrocephalus develops in 30–40 percent of the infants with large IVHs (Figs. 12-4 and 12-5). Real-time echoencephalography is the most appropriate technique for diagnosing and following changes in the ventricular size and correct evaluation of the therapeutic procedures (Fig. 12-5). Intraventricular–subependymal hemorrhages resolve in several weeks, depending on the size of the bleed and the individual patient. Large intraventricular clots usually persist for 3 or 4 months. Clots are not seen in CT scans after 2 weeks.[2,5,18]

Clots undergo characteristic changes with time. Initially they are very echogenic, and then low echogenic areas appear. Eventually the clots become cystic and the choroid plexus visualizes inside the cystic clot (Figs. 12-4 and 12-5). Large intraventricular clots may cause the ventricles to remain dilated for a time beyond correction of the posthemorrhagic hydrocephalus with a ventricular–peritoneal shunt (VPS) (Fig. 12-5).

#### Intraparenchymal Hemorrhages and Porencephaly

Intraparenchymal hemorrhages (IPH) are associated with IVH/SEHs. Recent reports suggest that IPH's are secondary to necrosis of the periventricular white matter.[19] When liquefaction of the necrotic tissue occurs, the IVH extends into the brain parenchyma. A clot extending from the ventricular cavity into the white matter is usually seen (Figs. 12-6–12-9).

Intraparenchymal hemorrhages are a serious complication since they indicate destruction of the brain parenchyma. Eventually the intraparenchymal clots will follow the same evolution as the IV clots, and then become cystic and are reabsorbed completely in several weeks. A cavity [porencephalic cyst (POR)] communicating with the ventricle appears. IPH's and POR are commonly associated with posthemorrhagic hydrocephalus (Figs. 12-6–12-9).

In porencephaly associated with hydrocephalus, the increased intraventricular pressure is transmitted to the cyst. The pressure is applied directly to the white matter. Posthemorrhagic hydrocephalus associated with POR is an indication for early derivation of the CSF. Ventricular–peritoneal shunt can reduce the size of the lateral ventricles and the porencephalic cyst, minimizing the deleterious effects of compression and ischemia of the brain parenchyma (Figs. 12-6–12-9).[3]

#### Subarachnoid Hemorrhage (SAH)

The etiology of SAH in premature infants is unknown. Asphyxia and birth trauma are considered the most common causes.[18] In our experience

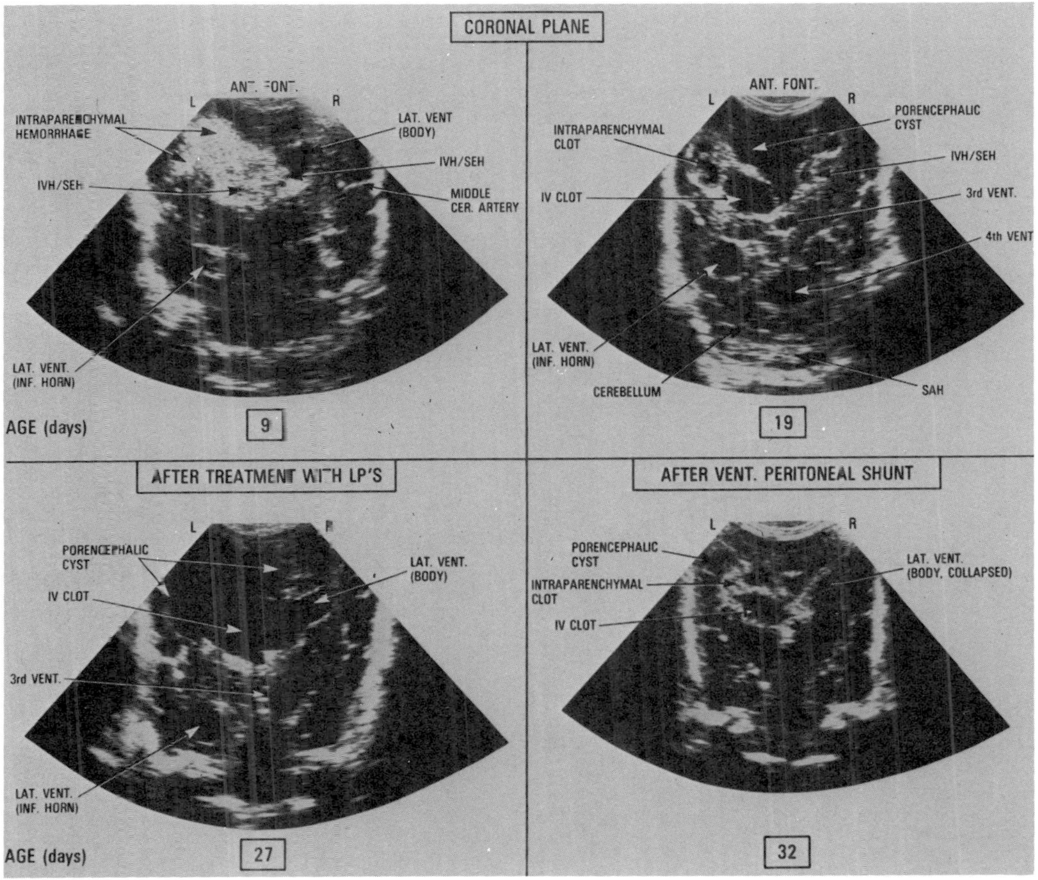


**Fig. 12-6.** Coronal sagittal studies in a preterm infant with large IVH/SEH, extensive IPH, posthemorrhagic hydrocephalus, and porencephaly. Note the unique clot extending from the ventricle into the brain parenchyma and the changes in the intraparenchymal clot with the development of a large porencephalic cyst. The cyst communicates with the body of the left lateral ventricle secondary to the IP clot (refer to text).

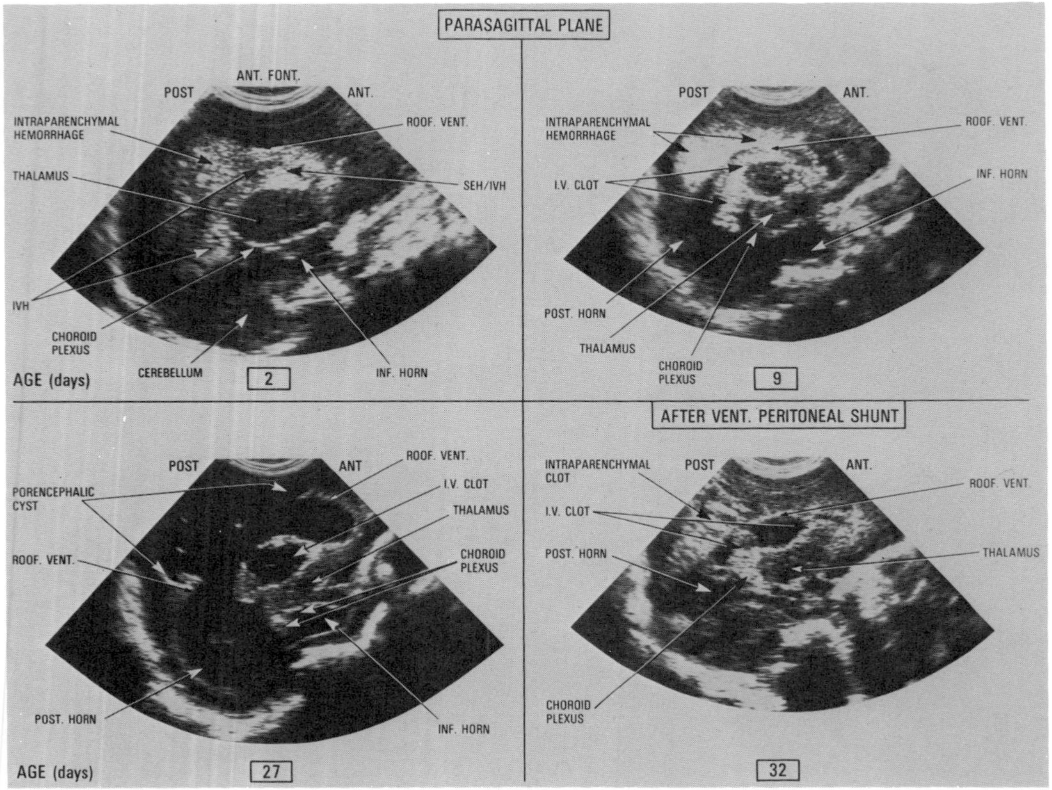


**Fig. 12-7.** Parasagittal studies of preterm infant in **Fig. 12-6**. These studies through the lateral wall of the ventricle were useful in precise delineation of the extension of the IPH and the porencephalic cyst. A VPS produced significant reduction of the ventricular size and the porencephalic cyst (refer to text).

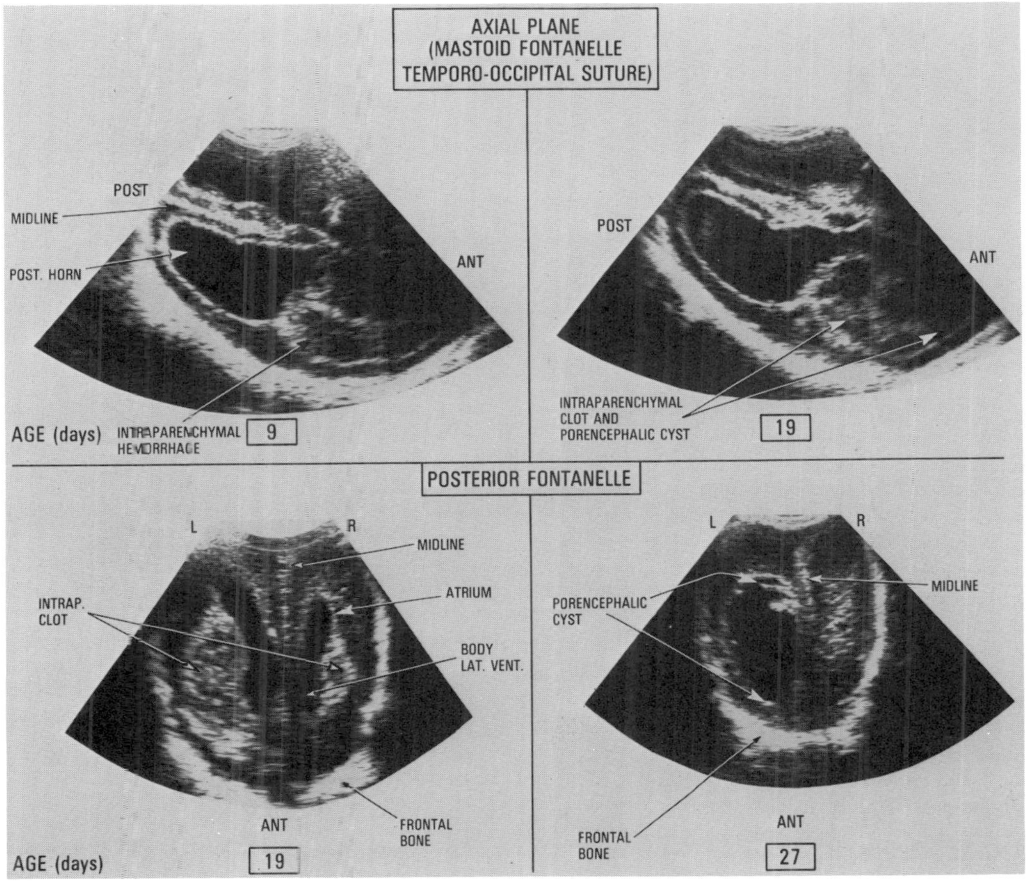


**Fig. 12-8.** Axial studies in preterm infant in **Figs. 12-6** and **12-7**. The axial views were useful in precise delineation of the extension of the IPH and the porencephalic cyst. A VPS produced significant reduction of the ventricular size and the porencephalic cyst (refer to text).

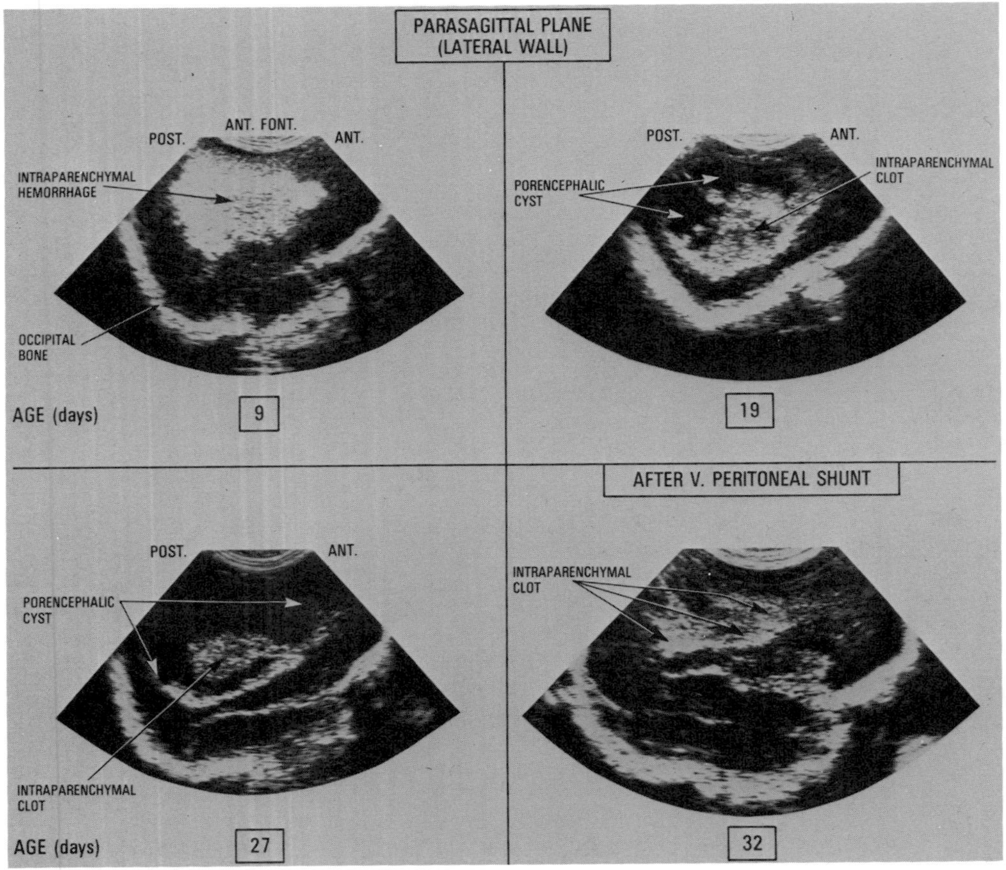


**Fig. 12-9.** Parasagittal studies in preterm infant in **Figs. 12-6, 12-7**, and **12-8**. The studies through the lateral wall of the ventricle were useful in precise delineation of the extension of the IPH and the porencephalic cyst. A VPS produced significant reduction of the ventricular size and the porencephalic cyst (refer to text).

SAHs are always associated with small or large IVHs. They occur secondary to the flow of blood from the ventricles into the subarachnoid space. Whatever the etiology, these hemorrhages must be diagnosed since they may block the passage of CSF in the basal cisterns or in the arachnoid villi and produce posthemorrhagic hydrocephalus.

Subarachnoid hemorrhages have been difficult to diagnose precisely with CT or RTE. Increased echogenicity in the Sylvian fissure was considered diagnostic of SAH. This criterion is associated with high incidence of false positive and negative diagnosis. The cisterna magna and the supracerebellar cistern are the areas to be scanned with RTE for diagnosis of these hemorrhages.[1,17] Subarachnoid hemorrhages are characterized by echoes in the anechoic cisterns (Figs. 12-10 and 12-11). Scanning of the posterior fossa in the modified coronal, sagittal, and coronal planes (see Chapter 10) provides unequivocal diagnosis of SAH. These studies are useful in determining if hydrocephalus associated with SAH is produced by obstruction of the CSF flow, and also for evaluation of the effectiveness of therapeutic maneuvers employed to control the ventricular enlargement (Figs. 12-10 and 12-11).

### Intracerebellar Hemorrhages (ICEH)

Intracerebellar hemorrhages are diagnosed unequivocally when the posterior fossa is visualized in the sagittal, parasagittal, modified coronal, and coronal planes (see Chapter 10). Sagittal studies show only the highly echogenic vermis, which should not be confused with an intracerebellar hemorrhage. The parasagittal, modified coronal, and coronal planes are most useful in diagnosing cerebellar hemorrhages. Intracerebellar hemorrhages are characterized by areas of increased echogenicity in the normally low-echogenic cerebellar hemispheres. (Figs. 12-12 and 12-13).[16]

Intracerebellar hemorrhage may associate with large SAH impairing the visualization of intracerebellar bleed. Coronal studies from the mastoid fontanels and sutures through the cerebellar hemispheres help to differentiate the ICEHs from the SAHs (Figs. 12-12 and 12-13). Sequential studies show that ICEHs become cystic with time. This finding is also useful for making a positive diagnosis (Figs. 12-12 and 12-13).

### Epidural Hemorrhages and Subdural Collections

These lesions are better diagnosed with CT. When the epidural hemorrhages and subdural collection are in the area visualized by the sector scanner, they can be diagnosed with RTE. Subdural collections appear as nonechogenic spaces between the calvarium and the cortex, displacing the

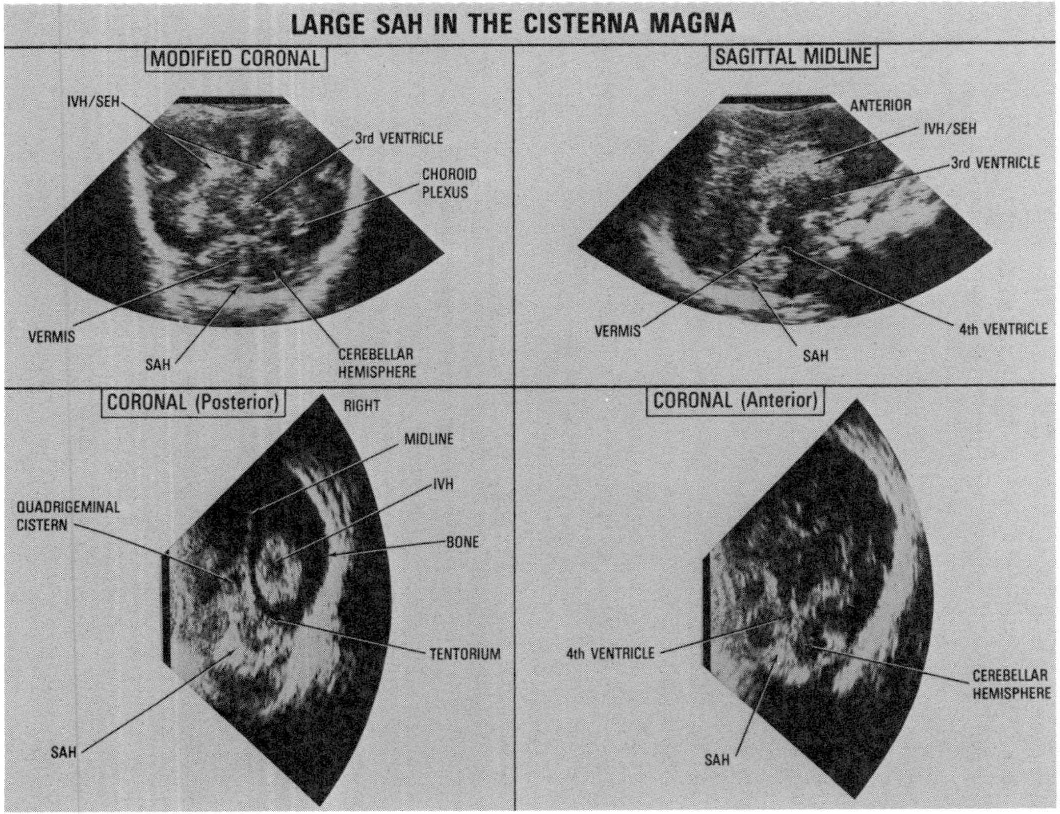


**Fig. 12-10.** Large SAHs in the posterior fossa in a premature infant with IVH/SEHs. The coronal studies of the posterior fossa through the mastoid fontanel were useful for diagnosis of SAH. Note the increased echogenicity in the cisterna magna and supracerebellar cistern.

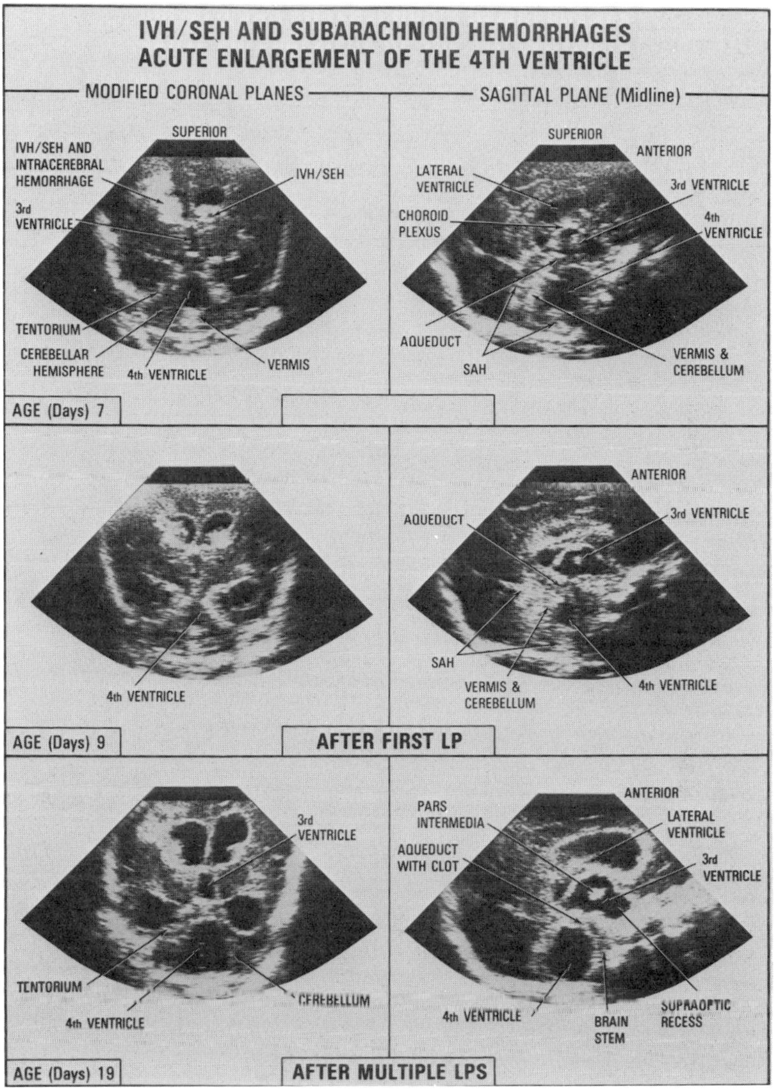


**Fig. 12-11.** Large SAHs in the posterior fossa in a premature infant with IVH/SEHs. The fourth ventricle enlarged acutely. Lumbar punctures transiently decompressed the fourth ventricle without significant change in the size of the lateral ventricles. By 19 days the fourth ventricle was gigantic, displacing the brain stem anteriorly. A VPS corrected the hydrocephalus but failed to reduce the size of the fourth ventricle, indicating bicompartmental hydrocephalus.

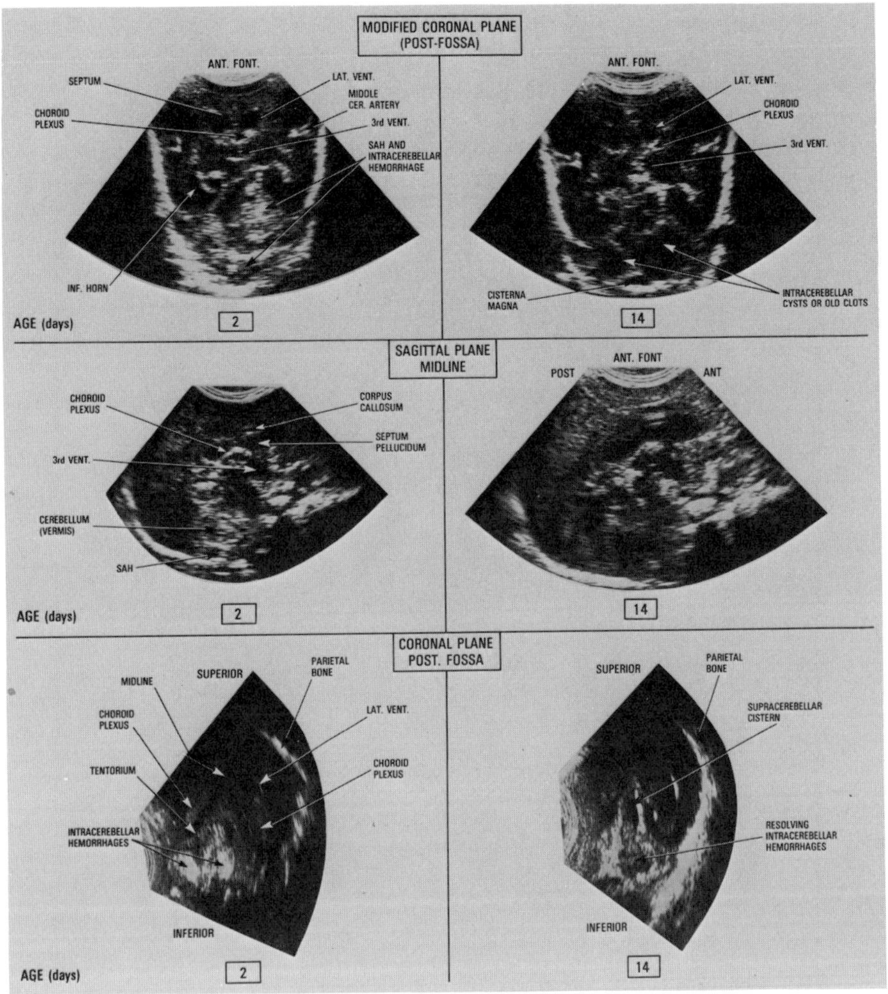


**Fig. 12-12.** Postmortem ultrasound studies in a premature infant with large SAH in the posterior fossa and extensive intracerebellar hemorrhages (hemorrhagic infarctions). The modified coronal and sagittal studies revealed an enlarged posterior fossa occupied by very echogenic material. Simultaneous studies in the coronal plane from the mastoid fontanel through the cerebellar hemispheres revealed intracerebellar hemorrhages. Note the changes in the echogenicity of the intracerebellar hemorrhages with time.

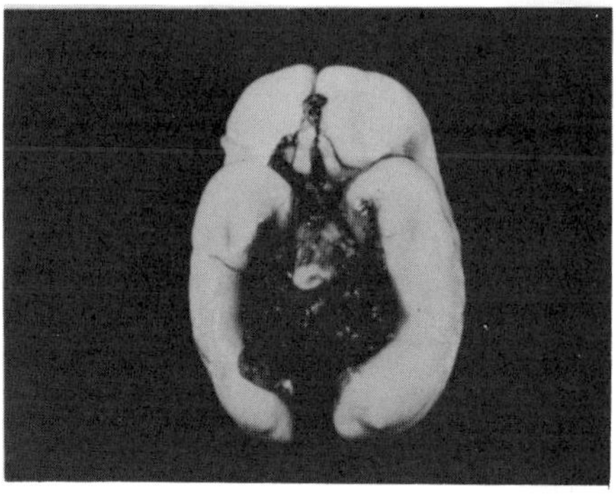

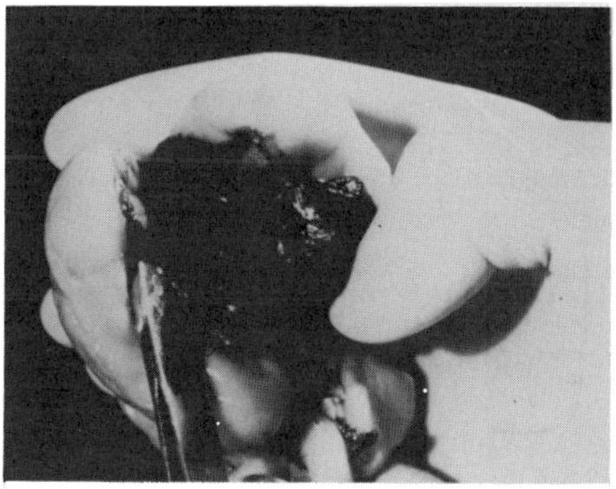

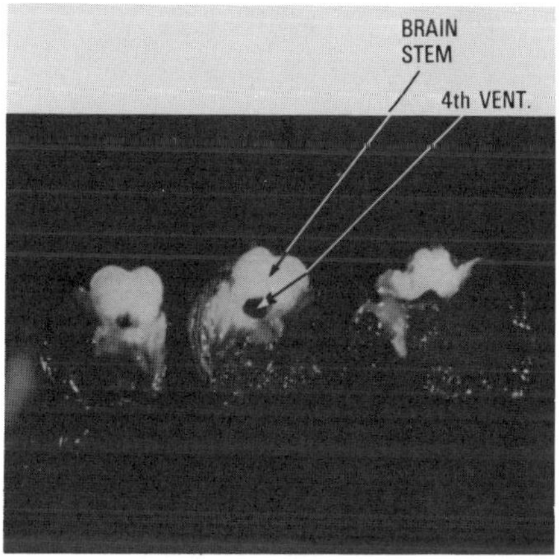


**Fig. 12-13.** Pathological studies of patient of **Fig. 12-12** (see text).

brain parenchyma toward the midline. The epidural hemorrhages are very echogenic areas immediately underneath the skull (Fig. 12-14).

## MULTIFOCAL NECROSIS OF THE WHITE MATTER (PERIVENTRICULAR LEUKOMALACIA)

Multifocal necrosis of the white matter (MFNWM) is a severe lesion associated with abnormal neurological and intellectual development. This complication is characterized pathologically by multiple foci of coagulation necrosis in the white matter adjacent to the lateral walls of the ventricles. The necrotic zones liquefy and cavitation develops. Eventually the cysts disappear by collapse or organization by glial cells.[4,12–14,18]

Multifocal necrosis of the white matter is considered a consequence of cerebral ischemia. The precise etiology, incidence, and natural evolution are

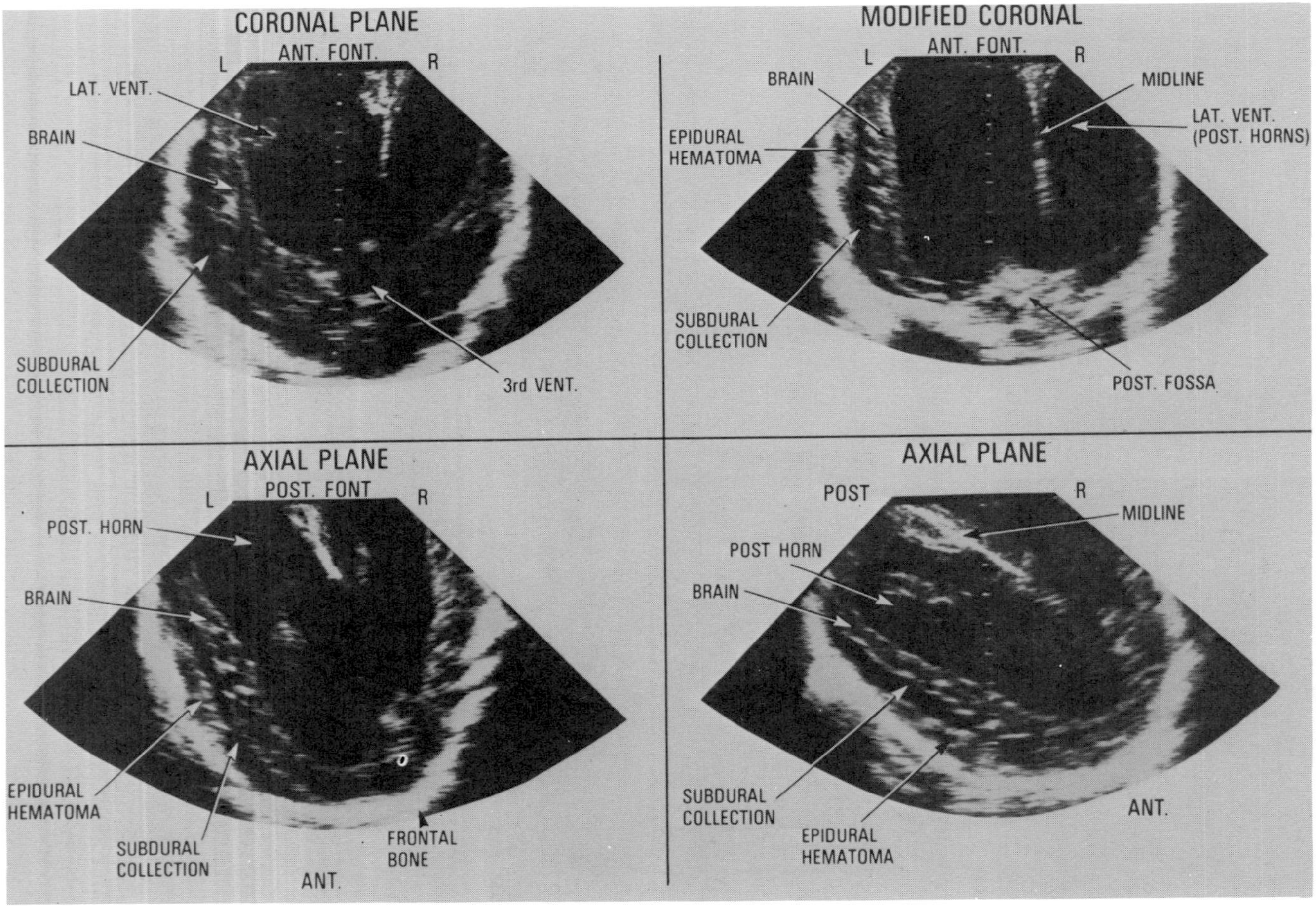
CORONAL PLANE
ANT. FONT.
L
R
LAT. VENT.
BRAIN
SUBDURAL COLLECTION
3rd VENT.
MODIFIED CORONAL
ANT. FONT.
L
R
BRAIN
EPIDURAL HEMATOMA
MIDLINE
LAT. VENT. (POST. HORNS)
SUBDURAL COLLECTION
POST. FOSSA
AXIAL PLANE
POST. FONT
L
R
POST. HORN
BRAIN
EPIDURAL HEMATOMA
SUBDURAL COLLECTION
FRONTAL BONE
ANT.
AXIAL PLANE
POST
R
MIDLINE
POST HORN
BRAIN
SUBDURAL COLLECTION
EPIDURAL HEMATOMA
ANT.

unknown since the diagnosis has been made, until recently, by direct examination of the brain. Hypoxia, asphyxia, birth trauma, infection, and endotoxemia have been associated with MFN.[4,12–14,18]

Real-time echoencephalography is useful in diagnosing this lesion. Echodense and cystic white matter lesions are considered diagnostic of MFN.[4,12–14] Multifocal necrosis of the white matter appears to have different ultrasonic stages. Initially, the white matter is very echogenic at the lateral walls and roof of the ventricles in the frontal areas, posterior horns, and atria. Increased echodensity of the white matter is a common finding in preterm infants. The majority of the patients may not have necrosis, and the echodensity in the white matter resolves in several weeks. In patients with necrosis multiple cysts develop in the highly echogenic areas. The cavitations usually vanish by three or four months.[4]

Studies of the parasagittal planes through the lateral walls of the ventricles and the modified coronal planes through the roof of the atria and posterior horns are very useful in diagnosing and following cavitation of the white matter (Figs. 12-15–12-19).

In postmortem studies the present authors found that the echodense white matter is associated with congestion, microhemorrhages, and petechial and perivascular hemorrhages. Ischemic necrosis may or may not be present. Consequently, highly echogenic white matter is nonspecific for the diagnosis. An unequivocal diagnosis of MFNWM may be made only when cavitation appears in the white matter.[4]

Using this criteria, the present authors have found that 17 percent of the preterm infants less than 34 weeks of gestation admitted to our unit have this lesion. Approximately half of them showed cavitation at birth or during the first week indicating that the infant's brain was damaged prenatally. Cavitation usually develops 10–15 days after significant insult to the immature brain. The patient shown in Figure 12-19 is a typical example of very early cavitation and intrauterine brain injury. This infant did not have respiratory distress syndrome, patent ductus arteriosus, or asphyxia. He was never ventilated and required only 30 percent oxygen for a few hours.

The highly echogenic parenchyma is associated with nonspecific low attenuation of the periventricular white matter in simultaneous CT studies. Computed tomography does not show the cysts, congestion or microhemorrhages of the white matter. When cavitation develops, prominent low attenuation may appear in CT (Figs. 12-15–12-18). These abnormalities will vanish by the fourth month. "Normal" CT or RTE studies several months after birth

**Fig. 12-14.** Subdural collection and epidural hemorrhage in a premature infant with congenital hydrocephalus (day 1). The epidural hemorrhage is characterized by an area of increased echogenicity immediately underneath the skull. The subdural collection has the same echogenicity as the CSF.

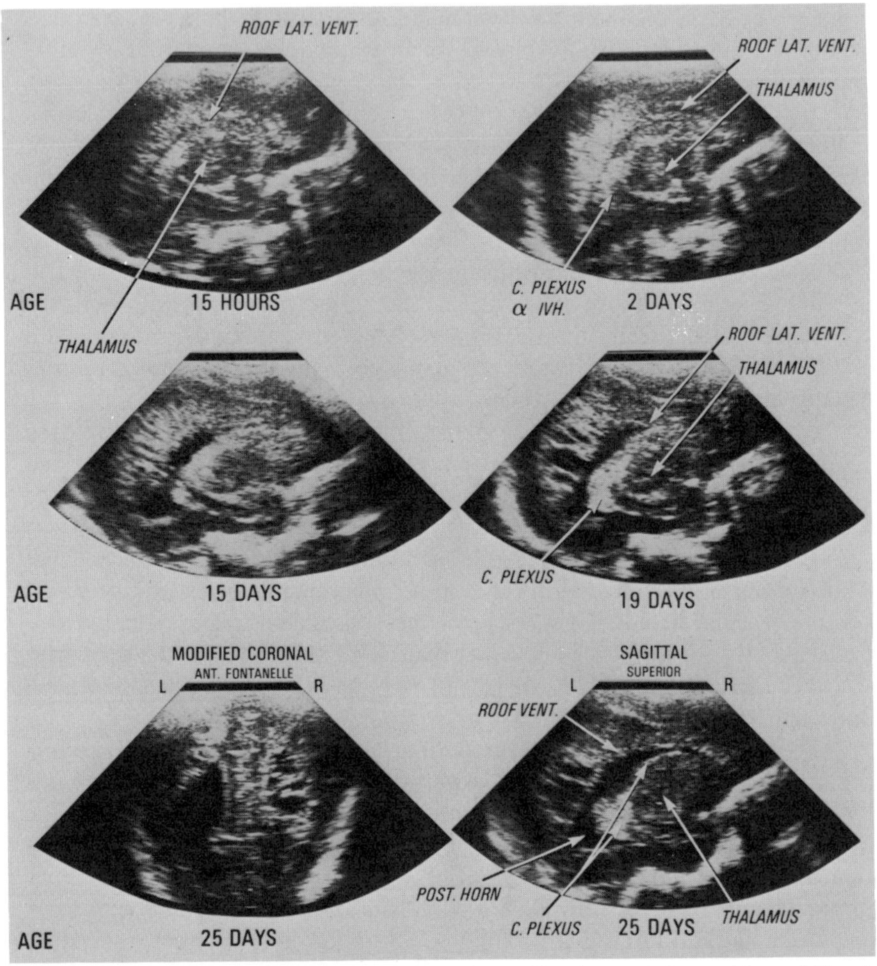


**Fig. 12-15.** Real-time echoencephalographic studies in an infant with multifocal necrosis of the white matter. The white matter was highly echogenic on day 1. The echodensity increased and extended by day 2. Cavitation developed on day 15.

do not rule out severe perinatal insult and significant damage of the immature brain.[4]

## BRAIN INFECTIONS

### Ventriculitis

Ventriculitis is a common complication of purulent meningitis in newborn infants. Ventriculitis probably occurs as the result of hematogeneous

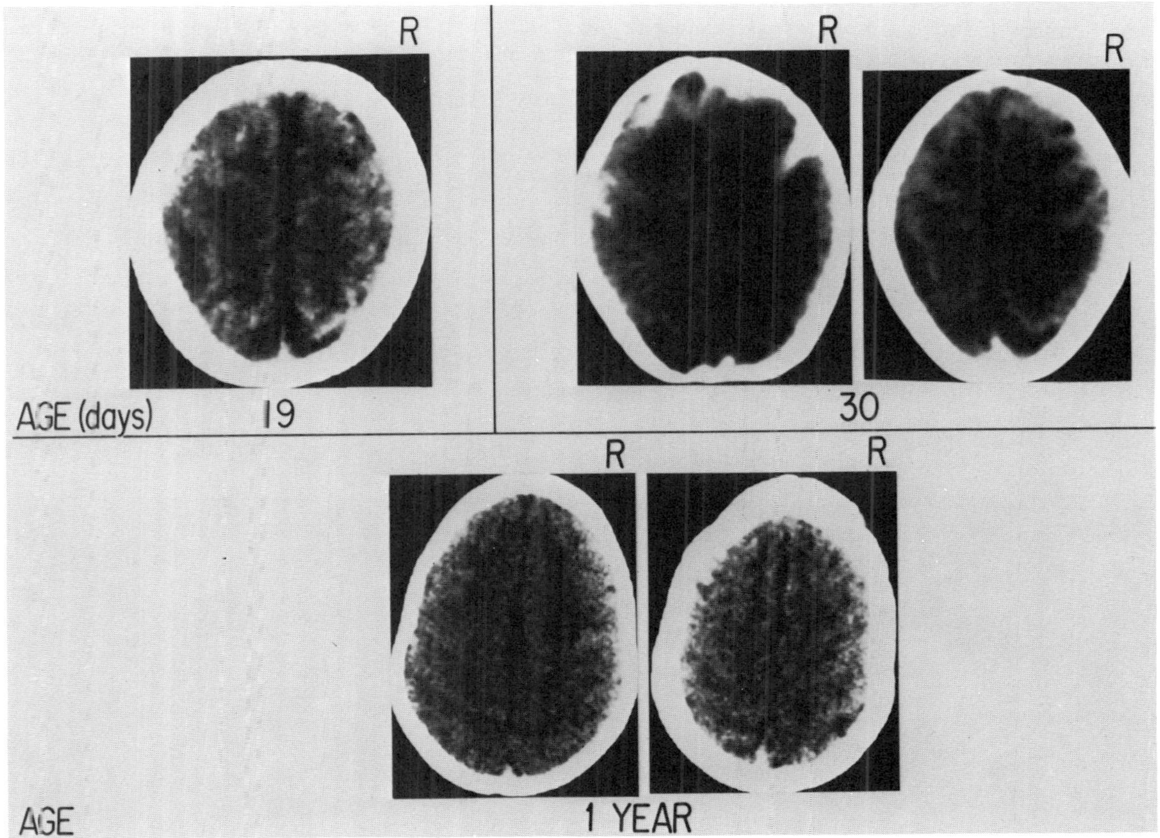


**Fig. 12-16.** CT studies of patient of **Fig. 12-15**. Focal low attenuation as present in CT studies on days 19 and 30. By 1 year the low attenuation had disappeared.

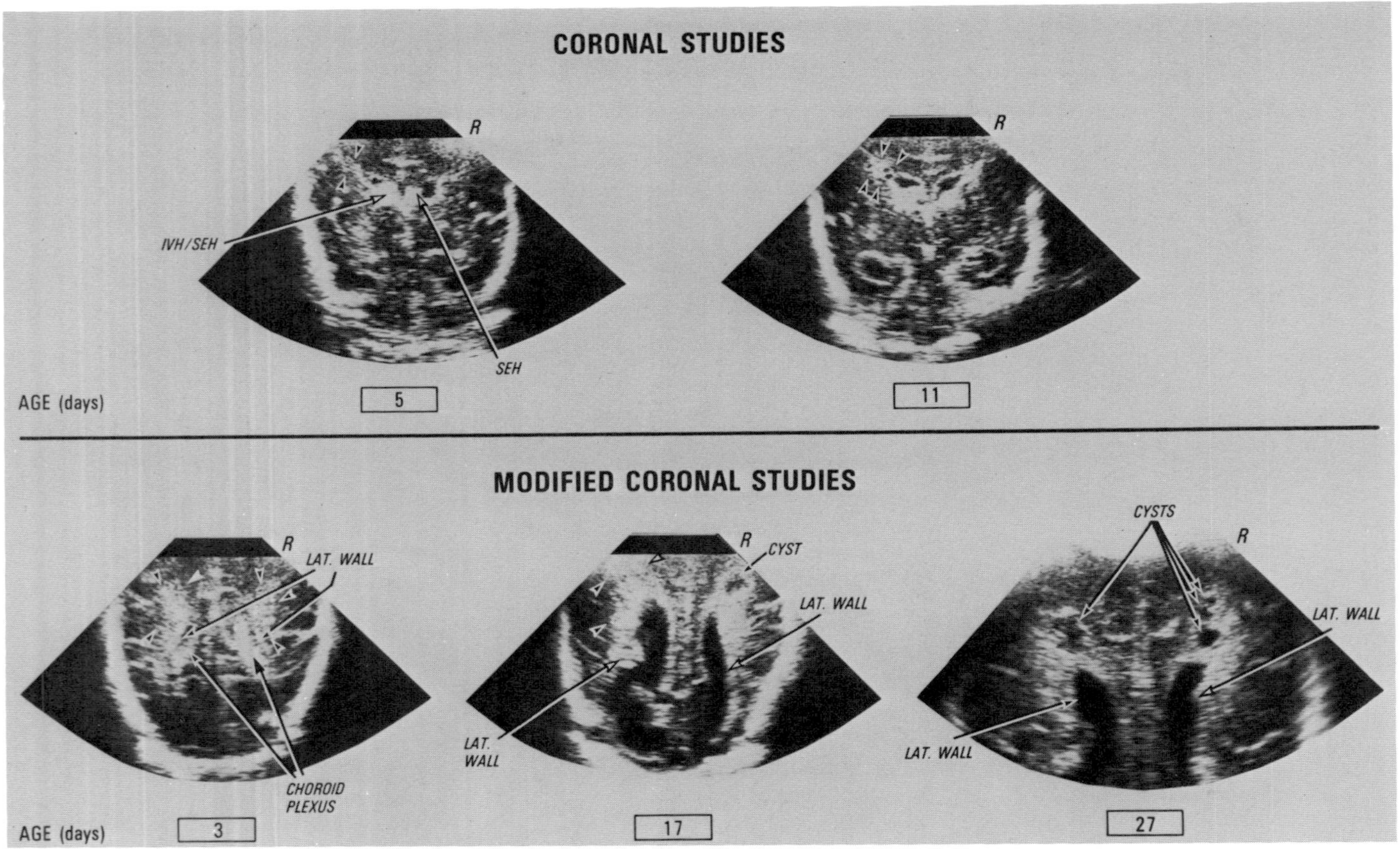


**Fig. 12-17.** Real-time echoencephalographic studies in an infant with multifocal necrosis of the white matter. Cysts developed by day 11 in the external angles of the anterior horns and by day 17 on the roof and lateral walls of the atria. The parasagittal studies were useful in determination of the size and extension of the cysts.

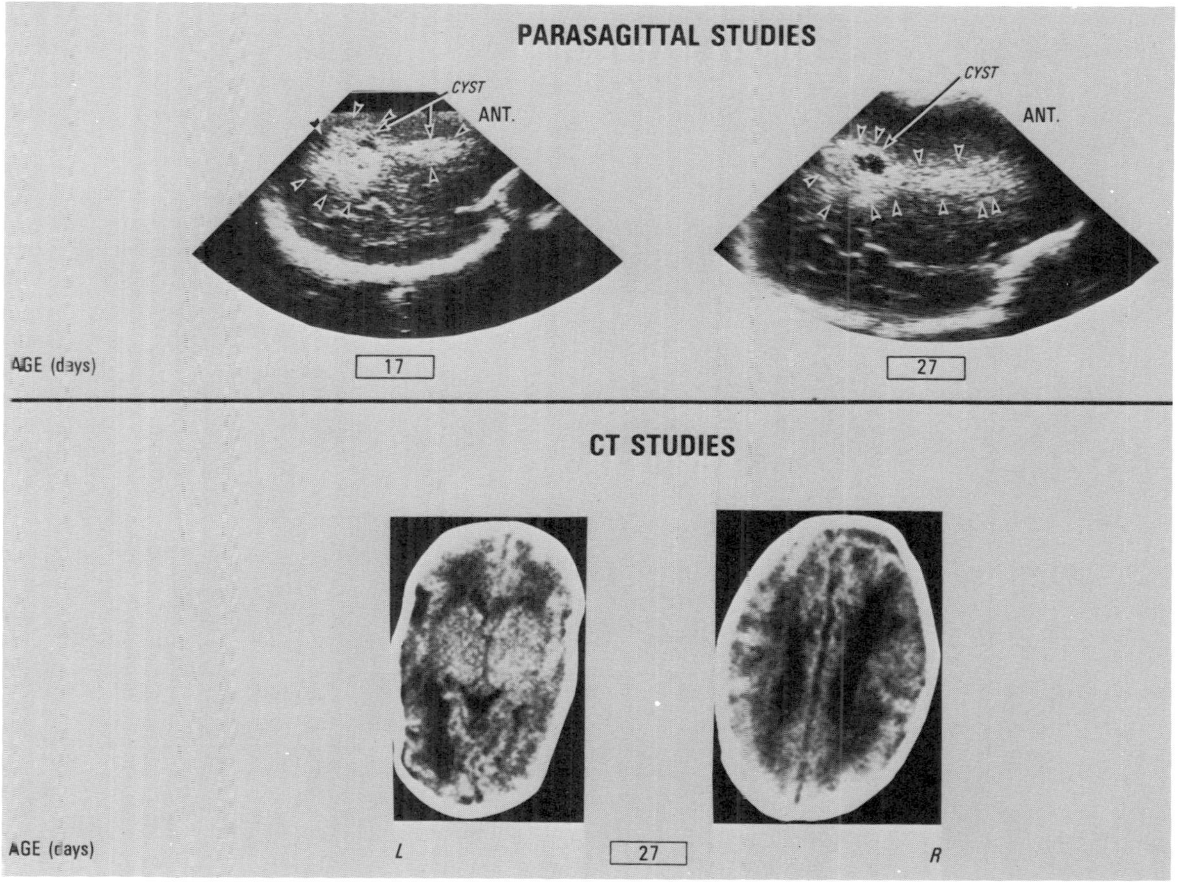


**Fig. 12-18.** A CT study done of patient in **Fig. 12-17** when cavitation was present showed only minimal low attentuation of the white matter compatible with incomplete myelinization of the brain.

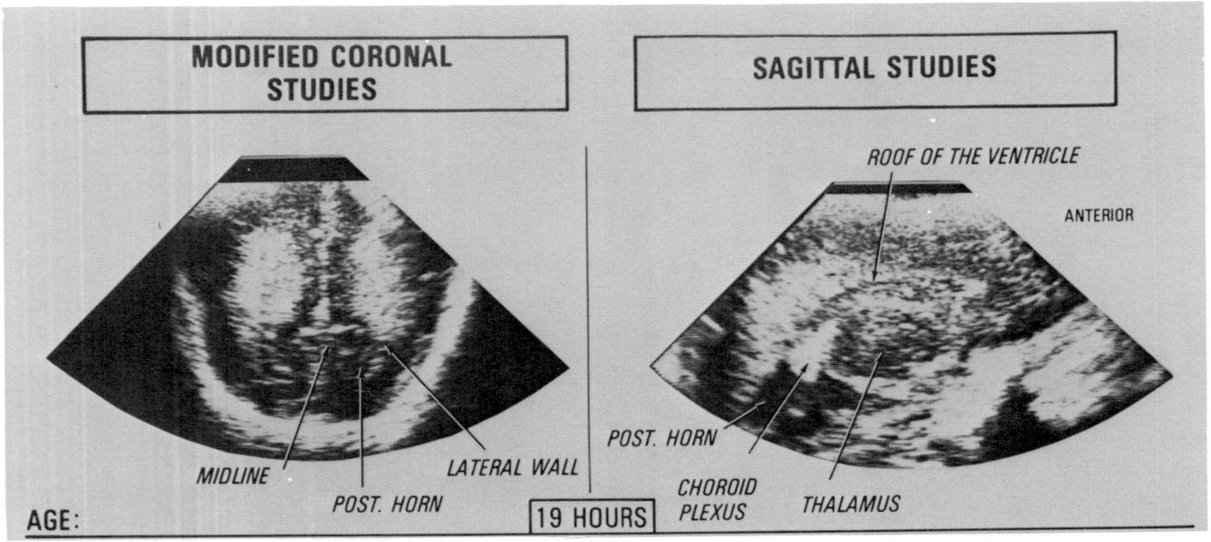


**Fig. 12-19.** Real-time echoencephalographic studies in a preterm infant who developed cavitation on day 4, indicating that the brain was damaged prenatally.

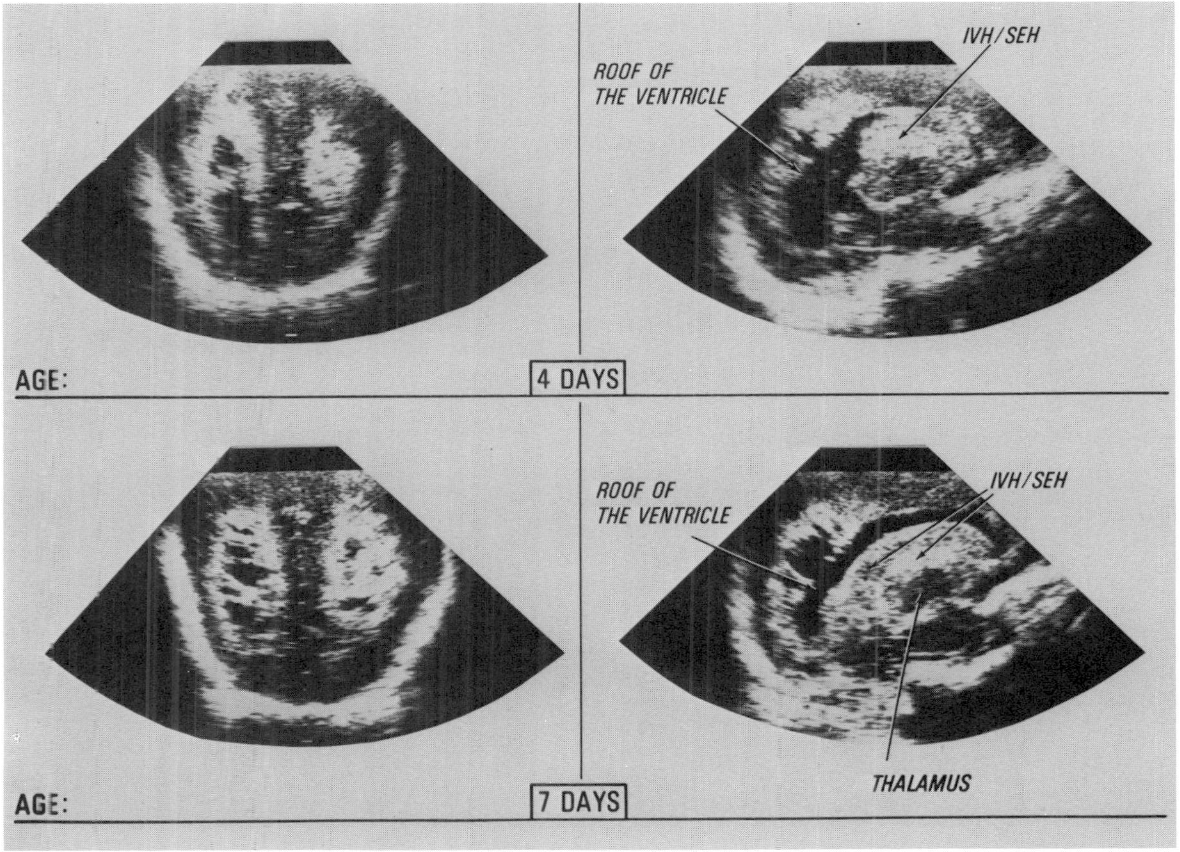


(**Fig. 12-19.** Continued)

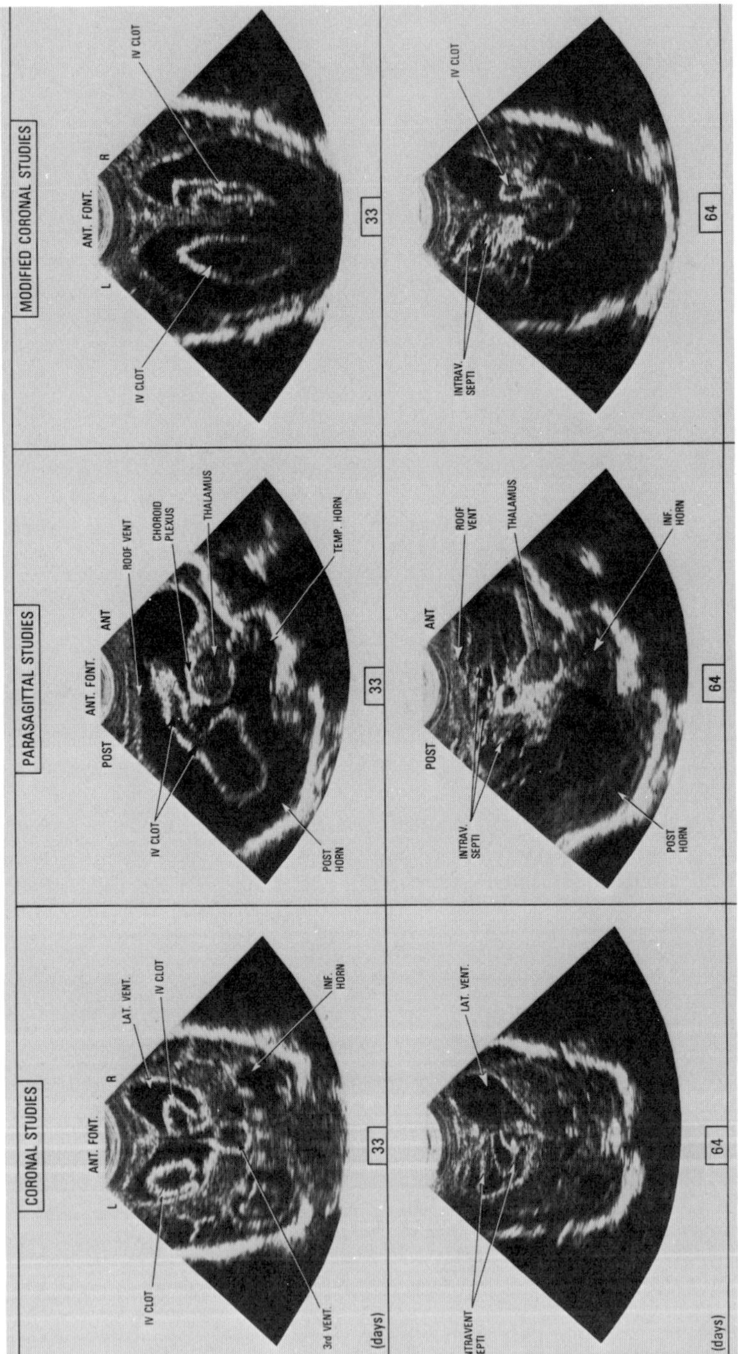
CORONAL STUDIES
PARASAGITTAL STUDIES
MODIFIED CORONAL STUDIES
AGE (days)
L
ANT. FONT.
R
LAT. VENT.
IV CLOT
INF. HORN
IV CLOT
3rd VENT.
33
POST
ANT. FONT.
ANT
ROOF VENT
CHOROID PLEXUS
THALAMUS
TEMP. HORN
IV CLOT
POST HORN
33
L
ANT. FONT.
R
IV CLOT
IV CLOT
33
AGE (days)
LAT. VENT.
INTRAVENT SEPTI
64
POST
ANT
ROOF VENT
THALAMUS
INF. HORN
INTRAV. SEPTI
POST HORN
64
IV CLOT
INTRAV. SEPTI
64

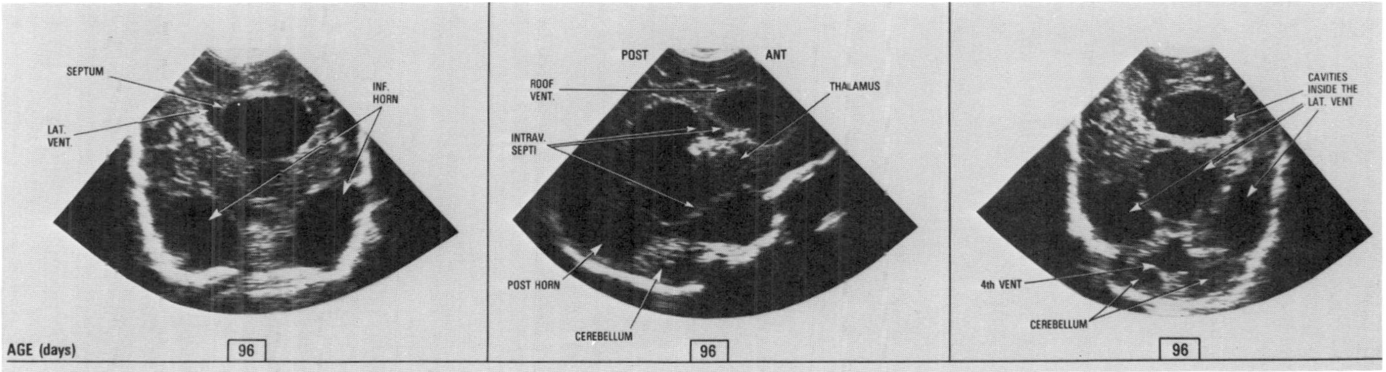


**Fig. 12-20.** RTE studies in a preterm infant with ventriculitis after placement of a VPS. Note the septations extending from one wall to the other and the eventual thickening of the septa with the formation of a multiloculated hydrocephalus and total disruption of the brain anatomy.

spread of the infection to the choroid plexus. The presence of a foreign body in the ventricular cavity such as a catheter from a VPS may provide a site for persistent infection of the ventricular cavities.[18]

Ventriculitis leads to compartmentalization of the ventricular cavity by inflammatory adherences extending from wall to wall.[10] The first stage is characterized by very thin septations that are clearly visualized with RTE (Fig. 12-20).

The septa become thicker and lead to multilocular hydrocephalus and total disorganization of the brain anatomy (Fig. 12-20). Sequential RTE studies in patients with meningitis usually provide an early diagnosis of this severe complications (Fig. 12-20).

## CONGENITAL MALFORMATION

### Dandy-Walker Malformation

This malformation is characterized by hydrocephalus, hypoplasia of the cerebellar vermis, and cystic changes involving the fourth ventricle, the so-called Dandy-Walker cyst.[9]

The hydrocephalus and cyst are visualized by application of RTE in the modified coronal plane. Hypoplasia of the vermis and the extension of the cyst are visualized easily in the sagittal and coronal studies of the posterior fossa. Coronal views show the enlarged fourth ventricle, the absence of the vermis, and the wide communication between the fourth ventricle and the cyst (Fig. 12-21).

### Arnold-Chiari Malformation

This disorder is present in infants with meningomyeloceles. In the Arnold-Chiari type II malformation there is downward displacement of the medulla and cerebellum through the foramen magnum into the canal of the cervical vertebrae. This obstructive lesion is associated with hydrocephalus, dilatation of the third ventricle and absence of the septum pellucidum.[9]

The diagnosis is suspected when a myelomeningocele is present at birth and confirmed easily with RTE, using the sagittal plane. Real-time echoencephalographic studies show a small cerebellum, low position of the fourth ventricle, absence of the cisterna magna, and displacement of the cerebellum through the foramen. Supratentorial studies show the hydrocephalus, the absence of the septum pellucidum, and the enlargement of the third ventricle (Fig. 12-21).

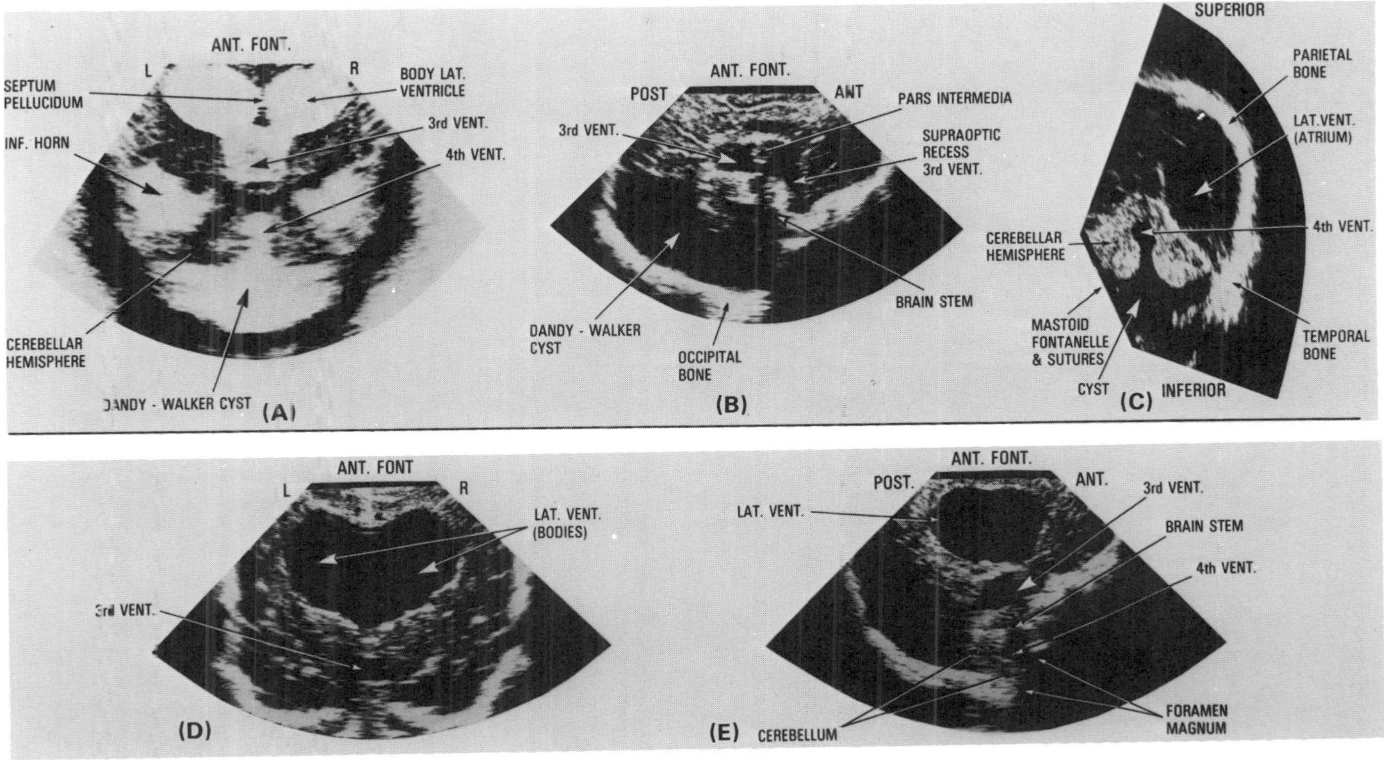


**Fig. 12-21.** Real-time echoencephalographic studies: (**A**) Dandy-Walker malformation, modified coronal plane; (**B**) Dandy-Walker malformation, sagittal plane (midline); (**C**) Dandy-Walker malformation, coronal plane (posterior fossa); (**D**) study in an infant with congenital hydrocephalus and Arnold Chiari malformation, coronal plane; (**E**) same infant as in (**D**), sagittal plane (midline). In (**A**)–(**C**) note the posterior fossa cyst in the modified coronal and sagittal planes. The coronal studies showed that the vermis was absent and that there was an open communication between the fourth ventricle and the cyst. In (**D**) and (**E**) note the low position of the fourth ventricle, the absence of the cisterna magna, and the extension of the inferior part of the cerebellum into the foramen magnum.

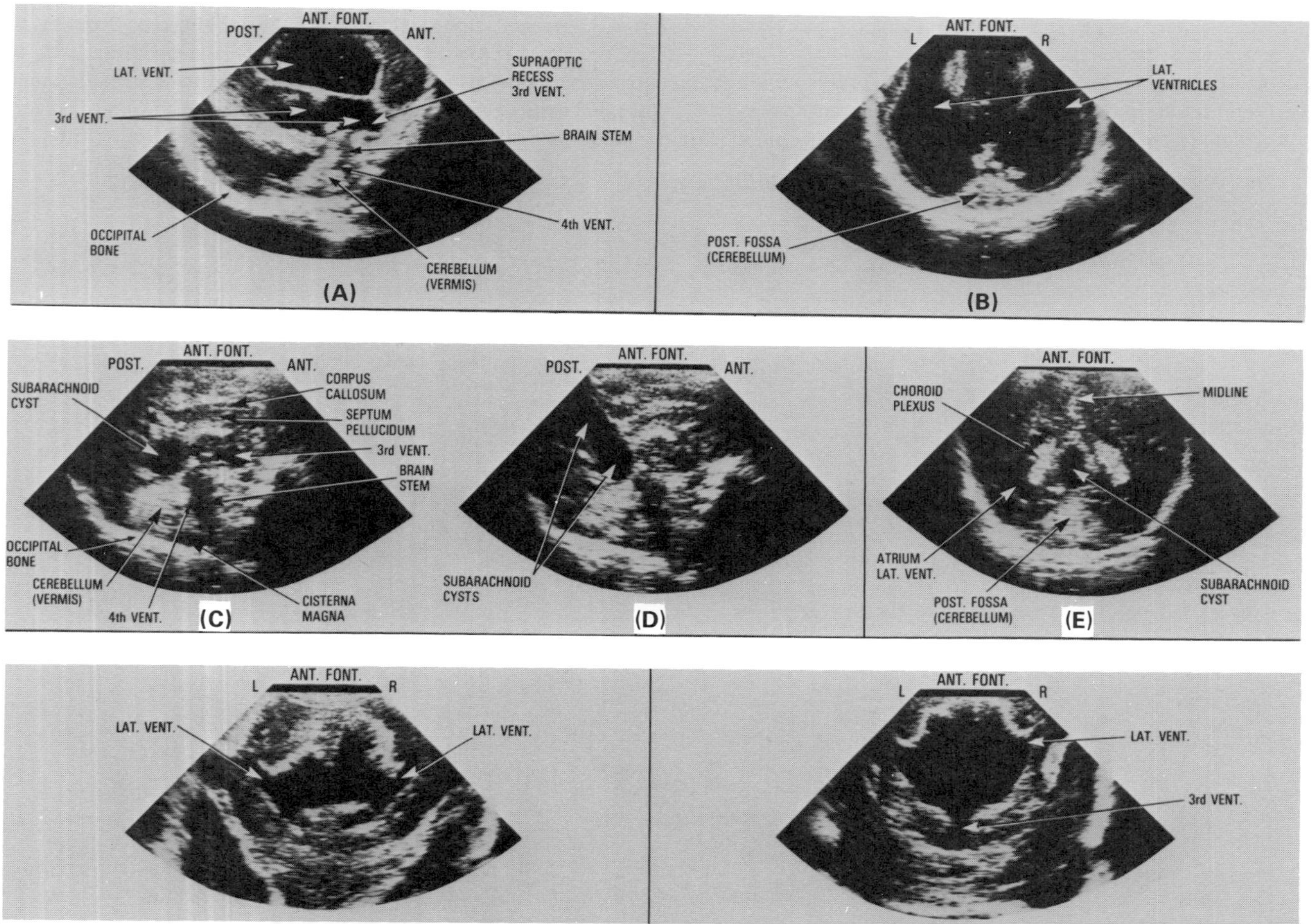
POST.
ANT. FONT.
ANT.
LAT. VENT.
3rd VENT.
SUPRAOPTIC RECESS 3rd VENT.
BRAIN STEM
4th VENT.
OCCIPITAL BONE
CEREBELLUM (VERMIS)
(A)
ANT. FONT.
L
R
LAT. VENTRICLES
POST. FOSSA (CEREBELLUM)
(B)
POST.
ANT. FONT.
ANT.
SUBARACHNOID CYST
CORPUS CALLOSUM
SEPTUM PELLUCIDUM
3rd VENT.
BRAIN STEM
OCCIPITAL BONE
CEREBELLUM (VERMIS)
4th VENT.
CISTERNA MAGNA
(C)
POST.
ANT. FONT.
ANT.
SUBARACHNOID CYSTS
(D)
ANT. FONT.
CHOROID PLEXUS
MIDLINE
ATRIUM LAT. VENT.
POST. FOSSA (CEREBELLUM)
SUBARACHNOID CYST
(E)
ANT. FONT.
L
R
LAT. VENT.
LAT. VENT.
ANT. FONT.
L
R
LAT. VENT.
3rd VENT.

### Congenital Hydrocephalus

Anatomically, congenital hydrocephalus may be divided into communicating and noncommunicating types. The latter is the most frequent form and is the consequence of a blockage within the ventricular system. Sylvian aqueductal stenosis and Arnold-Chiari malformation are the most common causes of obstructive hydrocephalus.[9]

Aqueductal obstruction is characterized in RTE by large dilatation of the lateral ventricles and enlargement of the third ventricle with a normal-sized fourth ventricle. If the hydrocephalus is very large, the posterior fossa is smaller than usual and the cerebellum is displaced toward the occipital bone with disappearance of the cisternal magna. However, the cerebellum is never dislodged into the foramen magum, differentiating aqueductal obstruction from type II Arnold-Chiari malformation (Fig. 12-22).

### Absence of the Corpus Callosum

The corpus callosum is a great commissure connecting the hemispheres of the brain. Absence of the corpus callosum may be partial or complete and is secondary to a defect of development or is acquired as a result of vascular lesions or intrauterine encephalomalacia. Porencephaly, hydrocephalus, mycrogyria and fusion of the hemispheres are defects associated with this malformation.[9]

With RTE, this lesion is characterized by narrow frontal horns and marked separation of the anterior horns and bodies of the lateral ventricles. There is dilatation of the posterior horns and third ventricle, dorsal displacement of the third ventricle, and ventricular cavities with the appearance of "vampire wings" (Fig. 12-22).

### Subarachnoid Cysts

These are true cysts lined by layers of cells from the arachnoid and filled with CSF. Three major etiologies are postulated: localized entrapment of fluid during embriogenesis, residual subdural hematoma, and fluid extravasation

---

**Fig. 12-22.** Real-time echoencephalographic studies: (**A**) stenosis of the aqueduct, sagittal plane (midline); (**B**) stenosis of the aqueduct, modified coronal plane; (**C, D**) subarachnoid cyst, sagittal plane (midline); (**E**) subarachnoid cyst, modified coronal plane; (**F, G**) agenesis corpus callosum. In the patient with congenital hydrocephalus secondary to aqueductal stenosis (**A, B**), the third ventricle is gigantic but the fourth ventricle is of normal size. In (**C**)–(**E**) a large subarachnoid cyst is shown emerging from the quadrigeminal plate and extending to the cortex. In (**F**) and (**G**) ultrasound scans reveal agenesis of the corpus callosum secondary to intrauterine infarction of the brain.

secondary to leptomeningeal tear or ventricular rupture. The cysts may develop in the posterior fossa or in the supratentorial compartment.[9] In the posterior fossa they may be differentiated from the Dandy-Walker malformation by the presence of vermis and normal fourth ventricle. In the supratentorial compartment the cysts are most commonly located in the middle cranial fossa and arise from the suprasellar cistern or the quadrigeminal plate cistern. These cysts may occur anywhere in the subarachnoid space but often are observed in the vicinity of the cerebral convexities, the suprasellar region, and the interhemispheric fissure.

The cysts may be asymptomatic or produce symptoms through compression of the brain and hydrocephalus. An asymptomatic cyst extending from the quadrigeminal plate to the cortex through the interhemispheric fissure is shown in Fig. 12-22.

## CONCLUSION

Real-time echoencephalography through the fontanels and sutures has changed the neuroradiological evaluation of intracranial pathology in newborn infants. With this technique the most common pathology in the supratentorial and infratentorial compartments may be diagnosed and followed sequentially. Our knowledge of the etiology, incidence, and natural evolution of these lesions has improved as a result of the use of RTE.

## REFERENCES

1. Babcock D: Cranial Ultrasonography of infants. Williams & Wilkins, Baltimore, 1981
2. Bejar R, Curbelo V, Coen R, et al: Diagnosis and follow-up intraventricular and intracerebral hemorrhages by ultrasound studies of infant's brain through the fontanelles and sutures. Pediatrics 66:661, 1980
3. Bejar R, Saugstad O, Gluck L: Increased hypoxanthine concentrations in cerebrospinal fluid of infants with hydrocephalus. J Pediatr 103:41, 1983
4. Bejar R, Coen R, Merritt TA, et al: Periventricular necrosis in preterm infants: Sonographic observations. Pediatr Res, (in press)
5. Dykes FD, Lazzara A, Ahmann P, et al: Intraventricular hemorrhage: A prospective evaluation of ethiopathogenesis. Pediatrics 66:42, 1980
6. Enzmann D, Britt R, Lyons B, et al: High resolution ultrasound of experimental brain abscess evolution: Comparison with computed tomography and neuropathology. Radiology 142:95, 1982
7. Gilles F, Price R, Kevy S, et al: Fibrinolitic activity in the ganglionic eminence of the premature human brain. Biol Neonate 18:426, 1971
8. Hambleton G, Wigglesworth J: Origin of intraventricular hemorrhage in the preterm infant. Arch Dis Childh 51:651, 1976
9. Icenogle D, Kaplan A: A review of congenital neurologic malformations. Clin Pediatr 20:565, 1981
10. Kalsbeck J, De Sousa A, Kleiman M, et

al: Compartmentalization of the cerebral ventricles as a sequela of neonatal meningitis. J Neurosurg 52:547, 1980
11. Lebed M, Schifrin B, Waffran F, et al: Real-time B scanning in the diagnosis of neonatal intracranial hemorrhage. Am J Obstet Gynecol 142:851, 1982
12. Levene MI, Wigglesworth JS, Dubovitz V: Hemorrhagic periventricular leukomalacia in the neonate: A real-time ultrasound study. Pediatrics. 71:794, 1983
13. Levinton A, Gilles F: Acquired perinatal leukoencephalopathy. Ann Neurol 16:1, 1984
14. Manger M, Feldman R, Brown J, et al: Intracranial ultrasound diagnosis of neonatal periventricular leukomalacia. J Ultrasound 3:59, 1984
15. Norman D: Computed tomography in intracranial hemorrhage, in Norman D, Korokbin M, Newton T (Eds): Computed Tomography. St. Louis, Mosby, 1977, p 279
16. Perlman J, Nelson J, McAlister W, et al: Intracerebellar hemorrhage in a premature newborn: Diagnosis by real-time ultrasound and correlation with autopsy findings. Pediatrics 71:159, 1983
17. Schneider M: Neonatal cranial ultrasound. Pediat Ann 12:133, 1983
18. Volpe JJ: Neurology of the Newborn. Company, Saunders Co., Philadelphia, 1981.
19. Volpe J, Hercosvitch P, Perlman J, et al: Extensive impairment of regional cerebral blood flow with intraventricular hemorrhage and hemorrhagic intracerebral involvement. Pediatrics 72:589, 1983

*Thomas G. Luerssen*

# 13

# Magnetic Resonance Imaging

Magnetic resonance imaging (MR) is a recent development in neurodiagnostic imaging that is now becoming available for expanded clinical use. As this clinical experience accumulates, it is likely that the impact of MR on patient management will approach another landmark in neurodiagnosis, computed tomography (CT). Although MR provides information presented in a format quite similar to that of high-resolution CT, the physical principles underlying the acquisition of MR and CT data are completely different. Magnetic resonance imaging not only provides anatomical information, but is capable of providing physiological and biochemical information. Magnetic resonance is currently being used in the clinical setting along with standard neuroradiographic techniques, and this work has demonstrated that MR can augment the standard neurodiagnostic studies and supplant certain invasive or complex neurodiagnostic studies without sacrificing any diagnostic accuracy. In some instances MR has been clearly superior to any other neurodiagnostic technique.

## PRINCIPLES OF IMAGING

Although it is not necessary to understand the complex physical principles underlying MR, it is important to comprehend the basic mechanisms underlying the acquisition of the data so that one can appreciate the unique character of the information MR provides. Several detailed descriptions of the physics of magnetic resonance are available.[2,6]

The essential elements of MR involve the interaction of atomic nuclei with an externally applied uniform magnetic field and an oscillating electro-

BRAIN INSULTS IN INFANTS AND CHILDREN
0-8089-1723-4

magnetic field applied at a predetermined frequency. Atomic nuclei are composed of protons and neutrons (except for the hydrogen nucleus, which consists only of a single proton). These nucleons possess an intrinsic spin, and when they are grouped together within the atomic nucleus, their spins become additive, resulting in a net nuclear spin. In general, those nuclei with an even number of protons and neutrons will have a zero net spin and are not useful for MR imaging. Odd-numbered nuclei, however, do have a net spin and are useful for imaging. Nuclei available for study by MR are $^{1}H$,* $^{13}C$, $^{15}N$, $^{19}F$, $^{23}Na$, $^{29}Si$, and $^{31}P$.

Spinning nuclei are much like spinning bar magnets in that they will generate tiny magnetic fields around them. Under normal circumstances, these "spinning magnets" are randomly oriented, but if they are placed into a strong uniform magnetic field, they will align themselves within this field, oriented along the magnetic lines of force. At this point, the spinning nuclei come to behave in much the same way as a child's spinning top aligned in the earth's magnetic field. That is, if they happen to be tipped over slightly, they will begin to wobble rhythmically around the lines of force, a motion that physicists call *precession.* The frequency at which a nucleus precesses depends on the strength of the magnetic field and the particular nucleus involved, a situation that has been related mathematically and is thus predictable. This means that a particular nuclear species within a heterogeneous population of nuclei (such as a biological tissue) can be studied by "tuning in" to its frequency and then analyzing its distribution by causing changes in the tilt and phase of spin of the isolated nuclear species. These changes are induced by the application of radiofrequency waves, which causes the external oscillating magnetic field mentioned previously.

The application of radiofrequency pulses causes a particular population of nuclei to resonate, which means it induces corresponding spins and corresponding tilt away from the lines of force of the static magnetic field. By manipulating the radiofrequency pulse, one can control the amount of tilt and the phase of spins of a certain group of nuclei. Furthermore, by applying this external force, one adds energy to the system. When the radiofrequency pulse is "turned off," the system "relaxes" and gives off the energy that was previously applied. During relaxation, two things happen: the nuclei drift back to become realigned with the static magnetic field, and these spins drift back out of phase. It is the energy given off during relaxation that is detected, usually by the same coils that applied the radiofrequency energy, and is subsequently processed into images.

Both of the relaxing states can be measured. The relaxation component along the lines of force of the static field is called $T_1$ (longitudinal or

---

*The proton is currently the most widely used nucleus for imaging purposes.

spin–lattice relaxation) and describes the interaction of the nucleus with its total environment. Naturally, this depends on the nature of the tissue in which the nucleus resides. The relaxation component of the spin drifting out of phase is called $T_2$ (transverse or spin–spin relaxation) and describes the interaction between neighboring nuclei. This is another means of distinguishing among tissues. Following the detection of this energy, the signals are processed by the computer and displayed on a screen or photographed. The advantage of MR is that the data can be further refined by altering the way the nuclei are perturbed and measuring their various responses.

As far as the patient is concerned, undergoing a study by MR is quite similar to undergoing a CT Scan. The length of time required for a MR study varies with the number of planes to be studied and what parameters of observation are selected by the radiologist. On the average, a MRI study lasts about 20 minutes.

## MAGNETIC RESONANCE IMAGING AND PEDIATRICS

Magnetic resonance imaging provides several specific advantages that directly apply to the pediatric patient:

1. Noninvasive.
2. Absence of ionizing radiation.
3. High degree of gray–white discrimination.
4. Nonreconstructed multiplanar images.
5. No bone artifact.
6. Very sensitive for study of hemorrhage, CSF abnormalities and brain water.

Of primary importance is that MR is a remarkably sensitive means of delineating CNS anatomy that does not expose a child to any ionizing radiation. This means that MR may have a significant impact on the long-term follow-up of pediatric head injuries and neoplasms (Fig. 13-1), as well as congenital malformations (Fig. 13-2).

Calcium is not imaged by proton MR. This allows one to view anatomy that is occasionally obscured by bone. The absence of bone artifact with MR allows extremely sensitive studies of the posterior fossa and craniocervical junction. A significant proportion of pediatric CNS pathology occurs in the posterior fossa and the diagnostic accuracy of MR for the diseases and anomalies in this region is excellent.[3]

Because of the difference in water content between gray and white matter, the proton relaxation characteristics of these two tissues is different. Magnetic resonance imaging can discriminate gray and white matter very

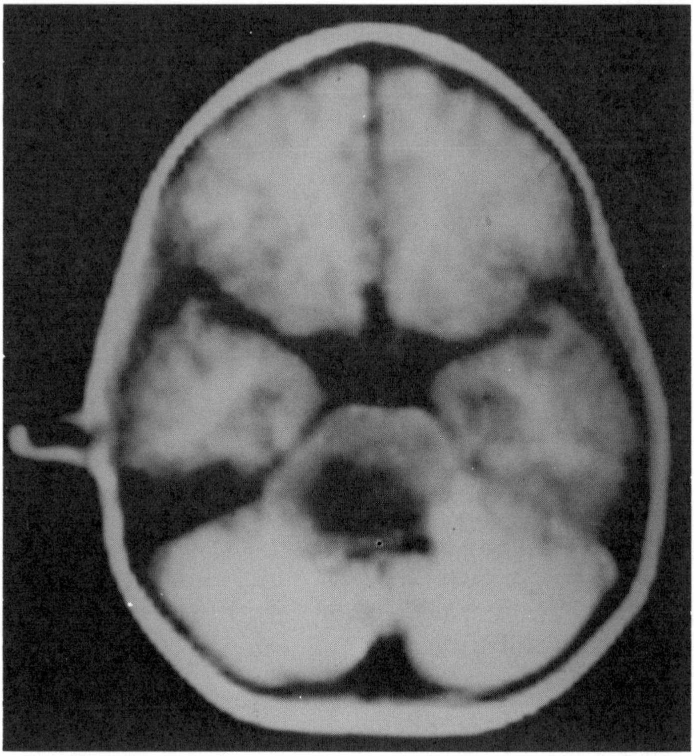

**Fig. 13-1.** $T_1$, partial saturation image in the axial plane demonstrating the presence of a brainstem glioma. Note the sensitivity of MR for demonstrating the asymmetry of the tumor and its relationship to anatomic landmarks. This may be useful for guiding a surgical approach or for planning therapy.

well, thereby making it useful for the study of multiple sclerosis, the leukodystropies, and certain congenital malformations (Fig. 13-3).[1]

Magnetic resonance imaging has been shown to be extremely sensitive for the detection of blood. Furthermore, the relaxation characteristics of blood apparently change with time, and MR may be useful not only for detecting hemorrhage, but also for determining the age of the hemorrhage.[5]

Finally, MR is very sensitive for the study of cerebrospinal fluid (CSF) and brain water and for the abnormalities of each that occurs in hydrocephalus and as a reaction to tumors or trauma. In general, it appears that MR may be superior to almost all other neuroradiographic techniques for the study of the aforementioned problems. What is more important, however, is that the increasing clinical experience with MR is likely to result in the discovery of even more advantages that can be directly applied to the pediatric setting.

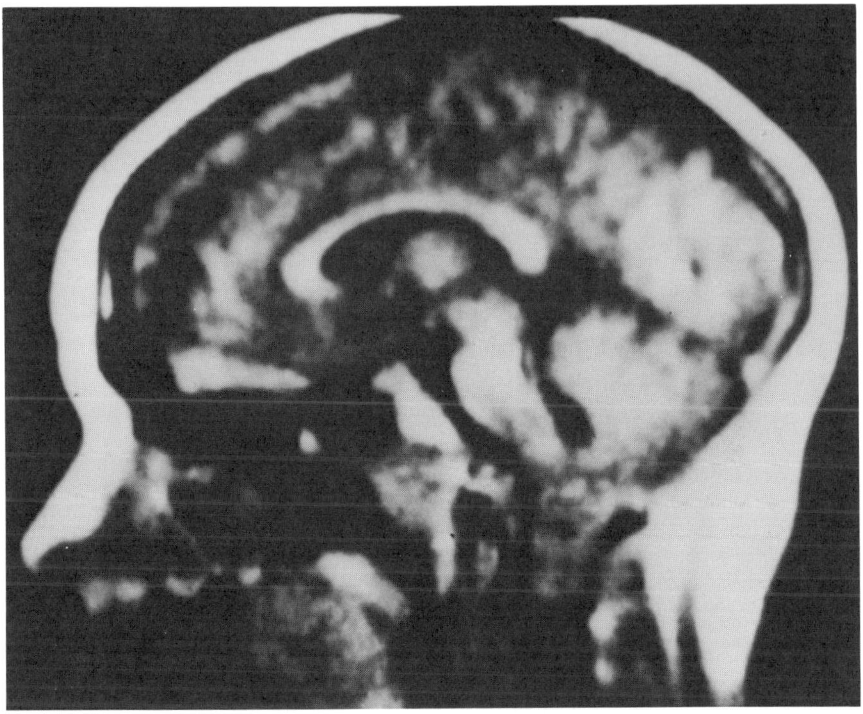

**Fig. 13-2.** $T_1$, partial saturation image in the midsagittal plane demonstrating the characteristic anatomic findings of the Chiari I malformation. Note the low-lying cerebellar tonsils extending into the cervical spinal canal.

There are some disadvantages to MR, some of which have already been alluded to:

1. Relatively long scan times.
2. No calcium imaging.
3. Ferromagnetic interference.
4. Extrinsic radiowave interference.
5. Possible biologic risk.

Scanning times may be relatively long compared to state-of-the-art CT and may be quite long if multiple planes and relaxation parameters are required. Because calcium is not imaged with MR, abnormal calcifications of brain parenchyma or tumors or secondary bony changes of the cranium or spine are not seen. Magnetic resonance images are degraded to varying degrees by the presence of some external or implanted metallic devices and by extrinsic sources of radiowaves. The availability of MR will subsequently affect the clinician's choice of such things as surgical clips, shunts, and cranial

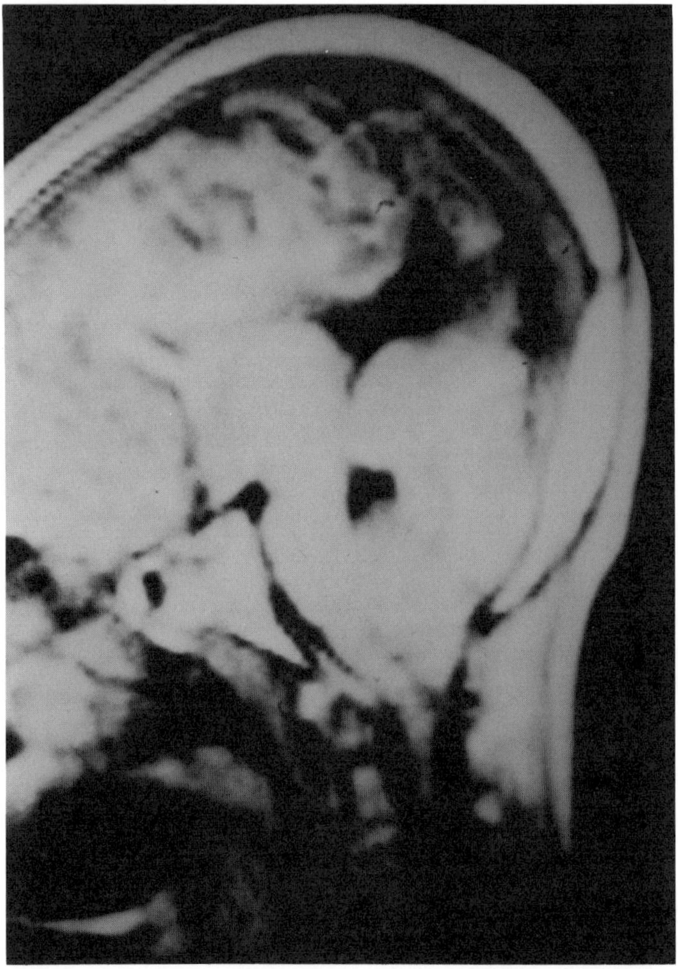

**Fig. 13-3.** $T_1$, partial saturation image in the parasagittal plane demonstrating partial agenesis of the posterior portion of the corpus callosum and an associated hindbrain malformation.

prostheses. Furthermore, these problems with ferromagnetic interference tend to complicate (but not exclude) the performance of MR studies under general anesthesia.

Although there are concerns about the biologic risks of MR, the effects of static and variable magnetic fields and the effects of exposure to radiofrequency energy have been studied and have been found to be safe within certain guidelines and ranges.[4] A large number of people (adults and children) have undergone studies by MR, and no ill effects have been reported.

Magnetic resonance imaging seems to offer a wide range of potential applications in clinical medicine and laboratory investigation. Although the current advantage of MR is its exquisite sensitivity for structural detail, MR is much more than merely an anatomic imaging technique. As more experience with this new imaging modality is obtained, it is likely that there will be a corresponding advance in the radiologist's ability to accurately identify pathological tissues, perhaps to the point of identifying disease processes as early as the time of local chemical or physiological alterations.

Other complex metabolic and physiological parameters are susceptible to MR analysis. Cerebral blood flow has been measured. The application of magnetic resonance phenomena to other nuclei such as sodium, phosphorous, fluorine, and carbon, as well as the use of paramagnetic compounds, may allow extensive studies of metabolism and normal or pathological physiology.

Despite all the extensive research and the expected applications, it is unlikely that MR will become a diagnostic panacea. However, it does seem to offer a unique versatility that can be extensively exploited for the investigation of biologic systems. Magnetic resonance imaging will definitely have its own intrinsic strengths and limitations and a specific place in the care of pediatric patients.

### Acknowledgments

The author is grateful to Dr. Robert A. Zimmerman, Division of Radiology, Hospital of the University of Pennsylvania, for his advice and assistance and to Drs. Luis Schut, Derek A. Bruce, and Leslie N. Sutton, Division of Neurosurgery, The Children's Hospital of Philadelphia, for allowing the ongoing study of some of the patients.

The author is also grateful to Ms. Kathryn M. Swan for her secretarial assistance.

### REFERENCES

1. Johnson, MA, Pennock, JM, Bydder, GM, et al.: Clinical NMR imaging of the brain in children. AJNR 4:1013–1026, 1983
2. Pykett, IL, Newhouse, JH, Buonanno, FS, et al.: Principles of nuclear magnetic resonance imaging. Radiology 143:157–168, 1982
3. Randall, CP, Collins, AG, Young, IR, et al.: Nuclear magnetic resonance imaging of posterior fossa tumors. AJNR 4:1027–1034, 1983
4. Saunders, RD, Orr, JS: Biologic effects of NMR, In Partain, CC, James, AE, Rollo FD, et al (Eds): Nuclear Magnetic Resonance Imaging, Philadelphia, Saunders, 1983, pp 383–395
5. Sipponen, JT, Sepponen, RE, Sivula, A: Nuclear magnetic resonance imaging of intracerebral hemorrhage in the acute and resolving phases. J Comp Assist Tomogr 7:954–959, 1983
6. Zermeno, A: The nuclear magnetic resonance phenomenon: An introduction, in Hickey, RC (Ed): Current Problems in Cancer, vol VII, no 3, Chicago, Year Book Medical Publishers, 1982, pp 4–19

# PART IV

# The Comatose Child

*Hector E. James*

# 14

# Therapy-Directed Diagnosis in Coma

Coma is considered as a disturbance of consciousness in which the child cannot respond to the environmental stimuli and thus cannot give an arousal response. We will therefore, employ this term for children who are unable to open their eyes, give verbal responses, or follow commands.

The term "coma" signifies a preterminal state of brain function in many diseases; thus coma should be considered as a life-threatening state by the medical personnel initially in contact with the child.

## THERAPY-DIRECTED DIAGNOSIS

The therapeutic attempts during the first few minutes often determine whether the child will survive, irreversible brain damage or severe intellectual damage will ensue, or the child will be intellectually normal.[2]

### Airway Control

It is most important that the examiner determine the degree of ventilatory embarrassment and assume airway control on initial contact with a child with consciousness impairment. A practical rule is that in children who are unable to open their eyes, follow commands, or verbalize, intubation be strongly considered. This is the only way that adequate ventilation can be assured. It is of particular importance in the patient with recurrent seizures. The technique to be employed for airway control is discussed in detail in Chapter 17.

BRAIN INSULTS IN INFANTS AND CHILDREN
0-8089-1723-4

**Systemic Assessment and Support**

Almost simultaneously determination of the blood pressure and pulse and placement of intravenous (IV) lines should be performed. Blood samples for complete blood count (CBC), arterial blood gases, calcium, electrolytes, blood urea nitrogen (BUN), blood ammonia should be taken; toxicology screening should be done; and if the patient was on anticonvulsant therapy, the levels of that particular drug(s) in the blood should be measured. Immediately following this, 0.5–1.0 g/kg of a solution of G/W 50 percent should be given and the response assessed. This is for the possibility of coma due to hypoglycemia. Intravenous fluid replacement should be performed preferably with colloid or with judicious use of crystalloid. The physician should always refrain from liberalizing IV crystalloid since a rapid shift of water into the brain by the altered blood–brain barrier mechanics can magnify intracranial hypertension.

An indwelling bladder catheter is essential in a child in coma, not only for urine analysis or drug screening, but because marked distention due to urinary retention can account for combativeness, systemic hypertension, and poor assessment of fluid balance. At this time a more thorough assessment of the patient's systemic and neurological examination is performed, and further history is obtained from the family. The history of drug ingestion, seizures, anticonvulsant therapy, and febrile illnesses should be sought. Such information will rapidly guide the physician to more definitive diagnosis and therapy. The absence of a history of trauma does not mean that "silent" trauma did not occur, such as that associated with child abuse. This should always be considered in the presence of bruising or preretinal hemorrhages.

Inasmuch as the physician obtains a prompt chest x-ray in a child with acute lung disease, the similar concept of a definitive diagnostic examination should lead to a cranial CT in a comatose child. If a mass lesion such as as intracranial hematoma is found, prompt surgical decompression can follow.

Infants may lapse into coma from meningitis without classical meningeal

**Table 14-1** *Intoxications and Pupillary Examination in Coma*

| Mydriasis | Miosis |
|---|---|
| Amphetamines | Barbiturates |
| Antihistamines | Opiates |
| Atropine | Propoxyphene |
| Cocaine | Meperidine |
| Ephedrine | Methadone |
| Ethyl Alcohol | Carbon Monoxide |
| Glutethimide | Organophosphates |
| | Thallium |

signs such as nuchal rigidity, which can be seen in older children. Meningitis is always a diagnostic concern in a comatose child. When coma is present, a prompt CT scan is necessary in order to reveal the presence or absence of an intracranial mass lesion. Following this, if no mass lesion is present, a lumbar puncture should be done to study the cerebrospinal fluid (CSF). If infection is suspected, broad-spectrum IV antibiotic therapy should be instituted pending the result of the CSF studies.

Acute intoxication may be very difficult to diagnose. Pupillary examination may be of assistance in arousing the suspicion of the physician to the etiologic agent. The changes brought about the different agents is seen in Table 14-1. The physician should be made aware that there is individual variation in the pupillary response and the possibility of an ingestion of a combination of intoxicants. Pupillary inequality may be present in ingestion, as has been seen with barbiturate overdose.[3]

An outline of the initial phase of management of the child in coma is seen in Figure 14-1.

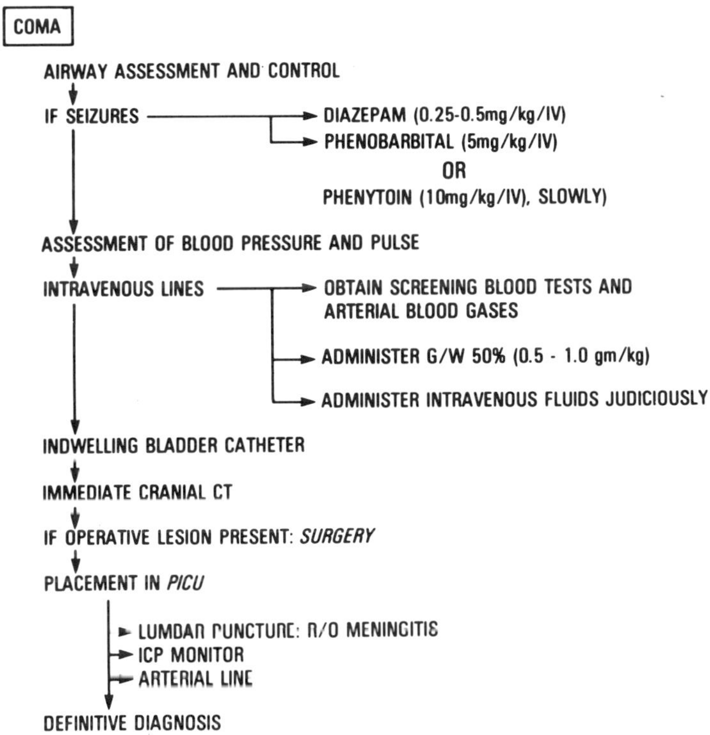


**Fig. 14-1.** Therapy-directed diagnosis in nontraumatic coma (PICU = pediatric intensive care unit).

## DEFINITIVE DIAGNOSIS

With the patient now in the pediatric intensive care setting, the results of the initial studies can be analyzed and further testing performed. The clinical course will determine the need of further therapy, such as placement of arterial lines and an intracranial pressure monitor[1] or, if the patient is improving, withdrawal of therapy.

The different causes coma (see Chapter 15) should now be considered if the preliminary screening studies are nondiagnostic

## REFERENCES

1. Bruce DA, Berman WA, Schut L: Cerebrospinal fluid pressure monitoring in children: Physiology, pathology, and clinical usefulness, in Advances in Pediatrics, vol 24, New York, New York Medical Publishers, 1977, pp 223–290
2. James HE: Coma in Infants, Children and Adolescents, in Nussbaum M (Ed): Pediatric Intensive Care, Mount Kisco, New York, Futura Publishing Co., 1984, pp 35–54
3. Mathew H: Acute poisoning: Some myths and misconceptions. Br Med J 1:519–522, 1971

*Doris A. Trauner*
*Hector E. James*

# 15

# Evaluation of Coma

Acute presentation of coma in any age group is a medical emergency. Intensive supportive care must be instituted immediately, the etiology determined so that specific treatment can be instituted, and neurologic evaluations be precise so that the course of the disease can be followed carefully with early detection of deterioration in status. Staging of coma is extremely useful in determining initial severity of the problem and in following the effectiveness of the treatment regimen.

The term "coma" is used to indicate a level of unconsciousness that is unresponsive to external stimuli, that is, in which verbal, tactile, or painful stimuli do not evoke a response. Any disturbance in the normal level of consciousness is alarming and should be defined and treated where necessary. The term "lethargy" implies that the the person is sleepy but awake and follows verbal commands when stimulated. The term "stupor" suggests that the child falls asleep when left alone but can be aroused by verbal or painful stimuli. The term "obtundation" denotes that the patient is unconscious but responds to some stimuli, such as crying out or moaning in response to pain. At times coma is subclassified into "light" and "deep," with light being synonymous with obtundation, or is used to describe the patient who postures nonpurposefully in response to pain. It is evident that these terms are somewhat imprecise and do not necessarily imply the same state to different observers. For this reason, a more precise staging system to describe alterations in consciousness is very helpful.[4]

BRAIN INSULTS IN INFANTS AND CHILDREN
0-8089-1723-4

## STAGING OF THE COMATOSE PATIENT

Methods of evaluating the level of coma, or staging, have been described for a variety of clinical situations, particularly for head trauma, Reye's syndrome, and hepatic encephalopathy (see chapter 20). Each system has merit for the particular clinical problem it is meant to address but may not be applicable to all causes of coma. The Glasgow Coma Score (GCS),[2] which was developed for use in head trauma, however, may have more general applications to all causes of impaired consciousness in that it is a uniform, numerical rating system that can be reproduced by any one examining the patient. It is thus helpful in both the initial and longitudinal follow-up evaluations of the comatose patient. This scale is discussed in Chapter 16.

## CAUSES OF COMA

Many diverse problems can result in an alteration in consciousness. Although the etiologies are multiple, they may result in one clinical presentation, that of a comatose child. A clear differential diagnosis and orderly approach to this medical emergency are necessary to prevent undue delays in treatment (see Chapter 14).

### Trauma

Both accidental and nonaccidental trauma should be strongly considered in a child who presents with acute loss of consciousness, even if there is no clear history of injury. Closed head trauma can produce loss of consciousness secondary to a subdural, epidural, or intracerebral hemorrhage; diffuse brain swelling; or cerebral contusion. Internal abdominal injury may cause bleeding, shock, and loss of consciousness secondary to cerebral ischemia.

### Metabolic Encephalopathy

Coma may ensue because of acute metabolic abnormalities, even in a seemingly healthy child. Unsuspected renal or hepatic disease, hypertension, and diabetes mellitus are all relatively common causes of metabolic encephalopathy.[5] Reye's syndrome usually follows a viral infection and is associated with evidence of liver dysfunction. Dehydration, especially when accompanied by hypo- or hypernatremia, may cause lethargy or coma. For an approach to the metabolic causes of coma, see the following list:*

1. Alterations of pH (acidosis, alkalosis)
2. Organ or system failure (hepatic, renal, etc.)

---

*For further analysis of this classification, see James.[1]

3. Alterations of water balance (dehydration, overhydration, etc.)
4. Electrolyte alterations
5. Vitamin deficiency and dependence status

### Seizures

Sustained or frequently recurring seizure activity can result in prolonged alteration in consciousness. Even when the clinical signs of seizure activity have abated, electrographic seizures may persist and account for continued unconsciousness. In addition, after the seizures stop, the patient may enter a prolonged postictal state that resembles a deep sleep from which full arousal is not possible. There are several types of status epilepticus. Generalized major motor status is the result of prolonged convulsive activity. Petit mal status occurs when the petit mal, or absence, seizures are so frequent that the child cannot awaken between spells. Psychomotor or partial complex status is the result of recurrent psychomotor seizure activity, which may render the patient confused, disoriented, or amnestic even though that patient can be aroused and may even have some confused conversational abilities. The latter two categories of status may be difficult to diagnose unless the patient has a clear history of a prior seizure disorder; even then, it may not be obvious that the problem is related to seizure activity. An EEG is extremely useful in diagnosing this disorder.[3]

### Toxins

A multitude of potentially toxic substances are available for children to ingest, from medications such as salicylates to leaves and berries of poisonous plants such as holly. Toxin ingestion must be considered in any child with unexplained coma, even if the parents are certain that an ingestion could not have occurred. A toxicology screen on urine and blood is essential in this situation.[5] Intoxication resulting from the following agents may produce coma:

1. Heavy metals (organic mercury, lead, etc.)
2. Pharmocological agents (anticonvulsants, antidepressants, etc.)
3. Alcohol
4. Venoms (snake bites, tick paralysis, etc.)
5. Miscellaneous (botulism, carbon monoxide, etc.)

### Infections

Viral, bacterial, and fungal diseases can produce alterations in consciousness either as a result of direct invasion of the nervous system (meningitis, encephalitis, or brain abscess) or by releasing toxins systemically which affect

**Table 15-1** *Infectious Agents that Can Produce Alterations in Consciousness*

| |
|---|
| Active Infection |
| Bacterial |
| Fungal |
| Protozoan |
| Rickettsial |
| Viral |
| Postinfection and Parainfectious |
| Acute Hemorrhagic Leukoencephalopathy |
| Encephalomyelitis |
| Reye's Syndrome |
| Overwhelming Systemic Infection |

the nervous system (Table 15-1). In regard to the former situation, lethargy or coma may be the presenting symptom of a CNS infection, especially in infants and young children. In particular the bacterial meningitides and herpes simplex encephalitis are prone to cause rapid impairment in consciousness. In the latter situation, diseases such as pertussis and typhoid fever can produce a toxic encephalopathy without direct involvement of the nervous system by the infectious agent.

### Anoxia

Lack of oxygen to the brain, as from shock, drowning, pulmonary insufficiency, suffocation, or strangulation, will result in numerous metabolic derangements in the brain sufficient to produce coma. Once the precipitating event is over, it may be difficult to establish the etiology of the resulting comatose state. Arterial blood gas determinations may be helpful in this situation, as well as a careful examination for evidence of strangulation or suffocation.

### Management of the Comatose Child

Since a comatose child is a medical emergency, a preplanned, logical approach is essential in preventing unnecessary delays in diagnosis and treatment as discussed in Chapter 14.

After the patient has been stabilized and an examination completed, other diagnostic tests may be required. If the child has a fever and stiff neck, a lumbar puncture is necessary to determine whether CNS infection is present, and antibiotics are administered promptly by the IV route. If there is suspicion of head trauma or mass lesion, computed tomography (CT) of the head is indicated as soon as possible. An electroencephalogram (EEG) is essential in diagnosing electrographic status epileticus.

If an immediately treatable cause of the problem (e.g., hypoglycemia, uremia, meningitis, hypertension) is not detected, or if the cause is known and is likely to produce brain damage, supportive therapy should be instituted immediately as further evaluation continues along the criteria listed for the possible etiologic categories previously enumerated in this chapter. If the child is paralyzed and cannot be evaluated clinically, continuous EEG monitoring is extremely useful in detecting seizure activity and evidence of deterioration or improvement in brain electrical activity.

Finally, it is important to be aware that children in coma may change rapidly, and that it is thus imperative that continuous assessment of blood pressure, respiratory and cardiac status, and fluid intake and output be made and that frequent examinations of the child be performed by someone familiar with coma management. It is seldom possible to predict outcome initially, since many children will eventually return to normal function even after prolonged coma. If agressive management is undertaken rapidly and complications such as shock and hypoxia corrected and prevented subsequently, the potential for a favorable outcome will be optimized.

## REFERENCES

1. James HE: Coma in infants, children, and adolescents, in Nussbaum M (Ed): Pediatric Intensive Care, 1983, pp 35–53, Mount Kisco, New York, Futura Publishing Co.
2. Jennett B, Bond M: Assessment of outcome after severe head injury: A practical scale. Lancet 1:480, 1975
3. Lockman LA: Coma, in Swaiman KF, Wright FS (Eds): The Practice of Pediatric Neurology. St. Louis, Mosby, 1982, pp 148–160
4. Plum F, Posner JB: Diagnosis of Stupor and Coma, ed 3. Philadelphia, FA Davis, 1980
5. Trauner DA: Toxic and Metabolic Encephalopathies, in Wiederholt WC (Ed): Neurology for Non-neurologists. New York, Academic Press, 1982, pp 225–247

*Hector E. James*
*Doris A. Trauner*

# 16

# The Glasgow Coma Scale

For many years clinicians have attempted to communicate in a uniform fashion the varying degrees of impairment of consciousness seen in patients. The common terms employed, such as coma, stupor, lethargy, and obtundation, have been discussed in Chapter 15. In clinical practice a disadvantage in the use of these terms is that they lead to differing interpretations among physicians and nurses. Misinterpretation of the patient's clinical status and the inability to compare patient populations in reference to outcome may thus result. Influence on outcome by the various treatment modalities and clinical trials are then difficult to compare because of the lack of uniform method of assessment of the patient's clinical state.

## THE GLASGOW COMA SCALE (GCS)

In an attempt to obtain a reliable prognosis as to the final outcome in a severely head injured patient within a few days from the injury, studies were made derived from combinations of predicted features in an individual patient. This was performed in such a way that the data were compiled from a data bank that accumulated the information in a cooperative study in head-injured patients. As a result of the data analysis, coma was defined by what the authors interpreted as the best predictors of outcome: the ability to open one's eyes, obey commands, and speak.[2] The GCS is thus an attempt to relate in mathematical terms eye opening in response to any stimuli, verbal behavior, or motor response (Table 16-1). The lowest score is 3 (the worst), and the highest is 15 (maximum). The authors observed that of the comatose

BRAIN INSULTS IN INFANTS AND CHILDREN
0-8089-1723-4

**Table 16-1** *Glasgow Coma Score*

| Activity | Best Response | Score |
|---|---|---|
| Eye opening | Spontaneous | 4 |
| | To verbal stimuli | 3 |
| | To pain | 2 |
| | None | 1 |
| Verbal | Oriented | 5 |
| | Confused | 4 |
| | Inappropriate words | 3 |
| | Nonspecific sounds | 2 |
| | None | 1 |
| Motor | Follows Commands | 6 |
| | Localizes pain | 5 |
| | Withdraws in response to pain | 4 |
| | Flexion in response to pain | 3 |
| | Extension in response to pain | 2 |
| | None | 1 |

Modified from reference 2.

patients who were unable to spontaneously open their eyes within 24 hours of the head injury, 64 percent were dead or vegetative at 6 months; whereas of those patients able to do so only 34 percent were vegetative.[2] This also translated into a difference in useful recovery: 54 percent of those able to open their eyes within 24 hours of head injury had a moderate to good recovery, whereas only 26 percent of those unable to open their eyes had a similar favorable recovery.[2]

It should be noted that the mean age of the patients in the data bank was 33 years[2,3]; therefore, these data should not be extrapolated freely to children. Furthermore, because of the weight of the verbal response and aspects of motor response, such extrapolation would not apply to children under 2 years. A suggested modification that could apply to infants is seen in Table 16-2.

The reader should remember that the GCS originated from a prospective study in head-injury patients. The data bank consisted exclusively of this disease, therefore, and although it is now commonly employed in other causes of coma, this was not its original purpose or design. The GCS data bank should not, therefore, be subjected to the same interpretation regarding clinical course and outcome in disorders other than head injury.

Intercurrent intoxication such as by alcohol may influence the early staging of a patient with head injury in the GCS. The same concept should be kept in mind in the postictal patient.

**Table 16-2** *Modified Coma Score for Infants*

| Activity | Best Response | Score |
|---|---|---|
| Eye Opening | Spontaneous | 4 |
| | To speech | 3 |
| | To pain | 2 |
| | None | 1 |
| Verbal | Coos, Babbles | 5 |
| | Irritable cries | 4 |
| | Cries to pain | 3 |
| | Moans to pain | 2 |
| | None | 1 |
| Motor | Normal spontaneous movements | 6 |
| | Withdraws to touch | 5 |
| | Withdraws to pain | 4 |
| | Abnormal flexion | 3 |
| | Abnormal extension | 2 |
| | None | 1 |

## PEDIATRIC ASPECTS AND THE GCS

From the previous discussion it can be understood that the outcome from the head-injury data bank applies primarily to adults. Such data should *not* be used to predict outcome from head injury or other diseases in children.

Other more recent and on going studies have addressed the problem in children and adolescents. There has not yet been a cooperative multicenter approach to the topic, but undoubtedly this will occur. In reference to outcome in head-injured children and elements of the GCS, the Children's Hospital of Philadelphia Neurosurgery service reported motor flaccidity to be the worst prognostic sign, although significant morbidity or death occurred in only 33 percent.[1] Bilateral nonreactive pupils and impaired or absent calorics yielded a 25 percent morbidity/mortality rate.[1] This differs from the Children's Memorial Hospital of Chicago where none of the children with nonreactive pupils or absent caloric responses survived.[4]

In reviewing the experience at Children's Memorial Hospital in Chicago between 1959 and 1978, the authors noted that children under 1 year of age with coma from head injury had the poorest outcome; in reference to ocular motor and verbal responses, they noted that the ocular score more consistently reflected the degree of neurological damage.[4] The most significant pathological factor associated with the poorer outcome in children under 1 year of age was the presence of subdural hematomas.[4] A neurological finding associated with a poorer outcome was the presence of hemiparesis.[4] From the reviews of their data the authors created a Children's Coma Score to better correlate outcome with mutual neurological assessment. In the ocular aspect they have modified it from assessments of eye opening to ocular responses, such as visual pursuit and pupil responsiveness. The verbal responses have been reduced to three forms: crying, absence or presence of spontaneous respirations, and apneic spells. The motor responses have been reduced to four: flexion or extension, withdrawal from pain, hypertonicity, and flaccidity. The lowest score (worst outcome) is 3, and the highest (best outcome) is 11.[4]

We feel that a more simplistic scale for an infant would be the one proposed in Table 16-2. A definite scale can be made only when a cooperative prospective study such as the GCS is undertaken employing only children.

## REFERENCES

1. Bruce DA, Schut L, Bruno L, et al: Outcome following severe head injuries in children. J Neurosurg 48:679–688, 1978
2. Jennett B, Teasdale G, Braakman R, et al: Predicting outcome in individual patients after severe head injured. Lancet 1:1031–1034, 1976
3. Jennett B, Teasdale G: Aspects of coma after severe head injury. Lancet 1:878–881, 1977
4. Raimondi AJ, Hirschauer J: Head injury in the infant and toddler. Child's Brain 11:12–35, 1984

*Nick G. Anas*

# 17

# Airway Management and Ventilation

As in any life-threatening condition, optimization of airway function is the first step in the resuscitation of the child who suffers an acute brain insult. The goal of airway support is to achieve arterial oxygenation sufficient to avoid hypoxic injury to the brain and maintain ventilation sufficient to prevent hypercapnia, which may aggravate existing intracranial or pulmonary hypertension. Efforts at brain resuscitation are in vain if inadequate pulmonary or cardiac function is responsible for secondary brain injury.

This chapter is designed to present the indications for airway intervention and the techniques for achieving that goal. This discussion is complemented by Chapter 21, which focuses on the various pulmonary disorders associated with acute brain insults and the modalities available for instituting and monitoring assisted ventilation.

## AIRWAY MANAGEMENT

The indications for airway support in the child who sustains an acute brain insult are listed in Table 17-1.

### Respiratory Rate and Rhythm

Abnormalities of respiratory rate and rhythm are common manifestations of brain injury. Plum and Posner[17] describe a variety of abnormal patterns ranging from apnea to central neurogenic hyperventilation depending on the location and the extent of the central nervous system (CNS) insult.

BRAIN INSULTS IN INFANTS AND CHILDREN
0-8089-1723-4

**Table 17-1** *Indications for Airway Management in the Child*

| |
|---|
| Abnormalities of respiratory rate and rhythm |
| Upper airway obstruction |
| Loss of pharyngeal muscle activity and tone |
| Inability to clear secretions |
| Foreign body |
| Direct trauma |
| Seizures |
| Loss of protective airway reflexes |
| Pulmonary disease |
| Failures of oxygenation |
| Failure of ventilation |
| Pulmonary hypertension |
| Respiratory muscle dysfunction |
| Fatigue |
| Shock states |
| Secondary to nerve dysfunction |
| Chest wall dysfunction |
| Intracranial hypertension |
| Prophylactic |

Automatic (metabolic) control of breathing resides in the respiratory centers of the lower pons and medulla, which are modulated by cortical centers in the awake state and perhaps during rapid-eye movement (REM) sleep. Primary disruption of the medullary respiratory centers leads to ataxic breathing, gasping, or apnea in the comatose patient. On the other hand, dysfunction of structures deep in both cerebral hemispheres or in the diencephalon may result in Cheyne-Stokes or apraxic rhythms. Regardless of the pattern observed, failure to achieve optimal arterial oxygenation or ventilation are sufficient reasons for institution of airway and ventilatory support.

### Partial or Complete Upper Airway Obstruction

This is probably the most common indication for airway support in the brain-injured child. The duration of total airway obstruction that a patient will tolerate before becoming profoundly hypoxic is a function of various factors:[7] the rates of oxygen consumption and carbon dioxide production, the blood volume and hemoglobin concentration, the lung volume, and the inspired oxygen concentration prior to obstruction. When acute total airway obstruction is experimentally produced in anesthetized animals during normal tidal breathing of room air, the arterial $Po_2$ declines from 92 to 40 mmHg after 1 minute, to 10 mmHg after 3 minutes, and to 4 mmHg after 5 minutes. In addition to the hypoxic complications resulting from airway obstruction, the increase in intrathoracic pressure that occurs will exacerbate existing intracranial hypertension by diminishing the return of cerebral venous blood. In the child who sustains acute brain injury, the most common cause of airway obstruction is posterior displacement of oropharyngeal soft-tissue structures, particularly the tongue. In the awake patient, the various muscles of the upper airway are activated synchronously with the inspiratory effort to ensure a patent oropharynx. If conditions are such that the negative pharyngeal pressure created during inspiration overcomes the distending pressure exerted by the upper airway muscles, airway obstruction will occur. Clinical circumstances in which obstructive apnea is well documented include states of depressed consciousness, neuromuscular dysfunction, and seizure activity. This tendency is further promoted during REM sleep, during anesthesia, and in association with anatomic or traumatic abnormalities of the upper airway.

### Loss of Protective Airway Reflexes

The loss of protective airway reflexes (cough, gag, swallowing) commonly occurs in the child with acute brain injury in both the presence and absence of lower cranial nerve dysfunction. Either passive regurgitation or active vomiting of gastric contents may result in pulmonary aspiration.[3] The absence of cough also leaves the patient unable to mobilize mucus and debris in the peripheral pulmonary tree, resulting in vulnerability to atelectasis and pneumonia. If the patient exhibits purposeful movement in response to a painful stimulus, the protective reflexes are probably intact.[11] Close observation rather than immediate support may be indicated, bearing in mind that the patient's neurological status is dynamic.

### Pulmonary Disease

Airway support for the purpose of instituting either assisted ventilation or continuous positive airway pressure or both is often necessary in the presence of pulmonary disease: neurogenic pulmonary edema, aspiration pneumonia, the adult respiratory distress syndrome, atelectasis, and secondary bacterial pneumonias. A detailed discussion of the child with decompensating lung disease is presented in Chapter 21.

### Respiratory Muscle Fatigue

In the child who sustains head trauma or other acute insults, impaired cardiac or pulmonary function commonly interferes with brain resuscitation by limiting oxygen and glucose delivery. Apnea as a result of respiratory muscles fatigue will occur if substrate delivery to the respiratory muscles does not match energy demands. It has been shown in a dog model that cardiogenic shock can lead to respiratory muscle dysfunction with resultant lactic acid and carbon dioxide accumulation. The increased work of breathing (acidosis leads to hyperventilation) increases the blood flow requirements of the respiratory muscles. Thus in an attempt to maintain optimal ventilation, other vital organs are deprived of their expected percentage of the cardiac output, which is already reduced. If this situation is compounded by incomplete tissue utilization of substrate, which is a characteristic of various shock states, respiratory muscle demands are further increased. The work of breathing is also increased in lung diseases by several mechanisms: interference with gas exchange, decreasing lung compliance, placing the respiratory muscle fibers at less than optimal length for maximal contractility (e.g., hyperinflation states), and depressing the cardiac output. In summary, respiratory muscle dysfunction that occurs as a result of either cardiac or pulmonary disease will interfere with brain resuscitation efforts by limiting substrate availability. Early respiratory support will often avert this complication.

### Chest Wall Instability

A stable chest wall is necessary for maintaining the optimal end expiratory lung volume (functional residual capacity) and a normal respiratory pattern. Alterations in the normal functional residual capacity (atelectasis or hyperexpansion) interfere with normal gas exchange by creating greater intrapulmonary shunting or dead-space ventilation (see Chapter 21). Chest wall stability is absent in the presence of rib fractures (flail chest), intercostal nerve or muscle damage, and often during REM sleep. Airway support may be necessary to provide continuous positive airway pressure to maintain the optimal functional residual capacity.

### Other Categories

The final categories for aggressive airway intervention in the child who sustains acute brain injury are the desire to achieve supranormal gas exchange and for "prophylaxis." Hyperventilation of the patient in order to induce an alkalotic state may be desirable as a means of increasing the tone of cerebral vascular bed in the presence of intracranial hypertension or reducing that of the pulmonary vascular bed in the presence of pulmonary hypertension. Complications of alkalosis that may prevent this maneuver are systemic hypotension, increased coronary vascular resistance, leftward shift of the oxygen dissociation curve, hypokalemia, and cardiac conduction disturbances. "Prophylactic" airway support may be desirable prior to air or land transport of the patient, for sedation for radiological procedures, or in a child with deteriorating level of consciousness.

## INSTITUTING AIRWAY SUPPORT

Airway support in the child who sustains an acute brain injury may be accomplished by several modalities: jaw and neck extension, artificial nasal and oral pharyngeal devices, endotracheal intubation, cricothyrotomy, or tracheostomy.[4] Because we most commonly employ endotracheal tube support and because regardless of the devices used the skills and principles underlying acute airway management are the same, the majority of this discussion focuses on techniques and complications of endotracheal intubation.

The most common problems encountered during endotracheal intubation are (1) difficulty with the procedure, (2) improper placement of the endotracheal tube, (3) obstruction of the airway, and (4) secondary vascular bed responses such as intracranial and systemic hypertension.

The technique of endotracheal intubation is a motor skill that is difficult to teach on the printed page and is best learned under the guidance of an experienced practitioner in a controlled environment such as the operating room. Despite this experience, problems that often sabotage the procedure of intubation include excessive oropharyngeal secretions, regurgitated gastric contents, abnormalities in airway structure, and inadequate sedation of the patient. The first two problems are avoided by vigorous airway toilet prior to and during the intubation procedure, emptying of the stomach contents by means of nasogastric suctioning (if this can be done without inducing vomiting), or the administration of atropine to decrease secretions.

Sedation or anesthetization of the child prior to intubation generally results in a less traumatic and more efficient procedure when performed by an experienced practitioner. Selection of the appropriate pharmacological agents must include knowledge of their time of onset, duration of action, and side effects, particularly with regard to cerebral flow, cerebral compliance, intracranial pressure, cerebral metabolic rate of oxygen, and systemic hemodynamic effects. For example, cerebral autoregulation is impaired by the inhalation anesthetics in a dose-related fashion. The resultant increase in intracranial pressure, in addition to an anesthetic-induced reduction in systemic blood pressure, may seriously compromise regional cerebral blood flow and cause focal or generalized ischemia. Our regimen for rapid-sequence induction[1,5] for endotracheal intubation is as follows:

1. Head tilt (extension) at 10°–15°
2. Administration of 100 percent $O_2$ for 2 minutes
3. Intravenous thiopental sodium administration at 4 mg/kg
4. Intravenous succinylcholine chloride administration at 1 mg/kg

A rise in intracranial pressure may occur following the administration of the succinylcholine (a depolarizing muscles relaxant) because of muscles fasciculation or by stimulation of the sympathetic nervous system.[6] To avoid this complication, many intensive care units employ curare (a nondepolarizing muscle relaxant) at 0.2–0.3 mg/kg and mask–bag ventilation prior to administering succinylcholine for the intubation.

Rapid-sequence intubation with the use of anesthetic or sedation agents is inappropriate in certain circumstances. There are potential difficulties with airways management and intubation in patients with cervical spine fractures (suspected or documented), cervical spine fixation, or impaired mandibular motion. Awake (blind) nasal intubation[9] with the use of topical anesthesia and minimal sedation may be successful but is difficult in the young child because of the anterior location of the larynx. The flexible fiberoptic bronchoscope is particularly useful in this situation.[14] The flexible device may be inserted into the tip of the nasal tube, which is then manipulated under visual guidance into the trachea. A rigid fiberoptic laryngoscope is also available for oral intubation.

The most common error encountered in placement of the endotracheal tube is intubation of the right main stem bronchus. This is manifest by decreased movement of the left chest wall, decreased breath sounds in the left lung field, and hypoxemia due to atelectasis and intrapulmonary shunting. The distal tip of the endotracheal tube should be positioned at least 2 cm above the carina and the position of the tube marked relative to fixed points on the patient's nose or mouth. Careful placement of the endotracheal tube under direct visualization and confirmation by airway roentgenogram are the best assurances of proper tube position.

In order to minimize damage to the airway, the cuff of the endotracheal tube is inflated to only the volume at which a "leak" is audible when applying 25–30 cm of $H_2O$ pressure. The airway of the young child is particularly vulnerable to the pressure necrosis resulting from an excessively inflated cuff,[8] although the development of high-volume, low-pressure cuffs has decreased the risk of acquired subglottic stenosis. On the other hand, a damaged cuff may require placement of another endotracheal tube, as this may result in inadequate ventilation or hypoxemia from lack of continuous positive airway pressure.

A significant problem related to endotracheal intubation is the induction of either intracranial or systemic hypertension or both. Laryngoscopy and intubation elicit a substantial hemodynamic response.[13] If the intracranial compliance is decreased or the intracranial pressure increased, the patient may be unable to withstand a marked increase in blood pressure without increase in intracranial pressure or reduction in cerebral perfusion pressure to dangerous levels. Large doses of thiopental sodium[2] (3–5 mg/kg) or low doses of fentanyl[10] (8 μg/kg) will help to blunt the intracranial response to intubation. Intravenous lidocaine will also help to control intracranial pressure by decreasing the systemic vascular response. Additionally, if difficulty is encountered with the intubation procedure, time must be taken to adequately reoxygenate and ventilate the patient by means of the mask–bag maneuver before proceeding further. Hypoxemia and acidosis are potent cerebral vasodilators that markedly increase intracranial pressure.

Systemic hypertension is a common problem in children who sustain head trauma and other acute brain insults. If this is the case, the patient must be intubated under close blood pressure monitoring, preferably with an indwelling arterial catheter and "continuous readout" of the blood pressure. Systemic hypertension may aggravate intracranial hypertension, induce secondary brain injury, or extend intracranial bleeds (particularly those associated with a ruptured intracranial aneurysm). Proper sedation may be sufficient to control the rise in blood pressure, but occasionally antihypertensive drugs must be provided prior to the intubation procedure. Again, care must be taken to avoid drugs that as a result of their systemic action also decrease cerebral vascular tone, thereby increasing intracranial pressure. In particular, sodium nitroprusside, which is a potent arterial and venous dilator, has been shown to increase intracranial pressure. Hydralazine has a similar effect in our experience. Therefore, we prefer to employ either alpha-adrenergic blocking agents (e.g., phentolamine) or beta-adrenergic blocking agents (e.g., propranolol) as antihypertensive medications.

The patient who coughs or strains because of the endotracheal tube must be monitored closely, as intracranial pressure may increase and aggravate regional cerebral perfusion deficits. In mechanically assisted patients, poor synchronization of spontaneous breathing through a ventilator may have similar effects. In these instances, sedation or perhaps neuromuscular blockade may be employed to limit patient interference with ventilation.

Although this discussion has focused on endotracheal intubation, emergency cricothyrotomy may be necessary to assure adequate oxygenation and ventilation in the following circumstances: maxillofacial or mandibular injuries, laryngeal crush injuries, suspected cervical spine injuries, and foreign body obstruction. In an emergency cricothyrotomy, a stab wound is made over the cricothyroid membrane, with no time taken for ligation of any bleeding vessels. A clamp is inserted, the cricoid and thyroid cartilages are separated, scissors are spread transversely to open the membrane, and a tracheostomy tube is immediately inserted. Complications associated with this procedure are much less common than those secondary to slash tracheostomy.

## REFERENCES


1. Barr AM, Thornley BA: Thiopentone and suxamethonium crash induction: An assessment of the potential hazards. Anesthesia 31:23–29, 1976
2. Bedford RF, Persing JA, Pobereskin L, et al: Lidocaine or thiopental for rapid control of intracranial hypertension. Anesth Analg 59(6):435–437, 1980
3. Cameron JL, Mitchell WH, Zuidema GD: Aspiration pneumonia: Clinical outcome following documented aspiration. Arch Surg 106:49–52, 1973

4. Caplan LM, Turndorf H: Airway management, in MH Worth (Ed): Principles and Practice of Trauma Care, Baltimore, Williams & Wilkins, 1982, pp 2–31
5. Cromartie RS: Rapid anesthesia induction in combat casualties with a full stomach. Anesth Analg 55:74–76, 1976
6. Joyce JT, Roizen MF, Eger EI: Effect of thiopental induction on sympathetic activity. Anesthesiology 59:19–22, 1983
7. Kennedy SK: Airway management and respiratory support, in Ropper AH, Kennedy SK, Servas NT (Eds): Neurological and Neurosurgical Intensive Care. Baltimore, University Park Press, 1983, pp 51–86
8. Klainer AS, Turndorf H, Wu WH, et al: Surface alterations due to endotracheal intubation. Am J Med 58:674–683, 1975
9. Kopman AF, Wollman SB, Ross K, et al: Awake endotracheal intubation: A review of 267 cases. Anesth Analg 54:323–327, 1975
10. Marin DG, Rosenberg H, Aukburg SJ: Low dose fentanyl blunts circulatory responses to tracheal intubation. Anesth Analg 61(8):680–684, 1982
11. Newfeld P, Cottrell JE: Neurological-Pharmacologic Considerations of Brain Protection and Resuscitation. In: Brain Failure and Resuscitation. Grenvik A, Safar P (Eds). 225–237. New York, Churchill Livingstone, 1981
12. Plum F and Posner JB: The Pathological Physiology of Signs and Symptoms of Coma. In: Diagnosis of Stupor and Coma. Plum F, Posner JB (Eds). 1–59. Philadelphia, FA Davis Co, 1972
13. Stovelting RK: Circulatory Changes During Direct Laryngoscopy and Tracheal Intubation: Influence of Duration of Laryngoscopy with or without Prior Lidocaine. Anesthesiology 47:381–383, 1977
14. Taylor PA, Towey RM: The Broncho-Fiberscope as an Aid to Endotracheal Intubation. BR J Anaesth 44:611–612, 1972

*Ronald M. Perkin*

# 18

# Pathophysiology of Childhood Shock Syndromes

The critically ill pediatric patient often presents a therapeutic challenge to the clinician, who must deal with a well-defined need to support or augment the cardiovascular response to an acute illness. In any critical care environment, the presence of hypotension identifies a patient in need of a rapid hemodynamic assessment and an equally rapid therapeutic response. This is especially true for the patient suffering from a brain insult where abnormalities in cellular oxygenation can further brain injury. Although circulatory failure is often amenable to intervention by resuscitation and support of the circulation, many patients die because of multiple organ failure. Circulatory failure is not the limiting factor for survival, therefore, as even brief periods of inadequate tissue perfusion may result in damage to several organs, and failure in one organ system may contribute to the failure of others. Central nervous system (CNS) injury often becomes the limiting factor that prevents survival.

Although shock is recognized clinically after hypotension develops, its major pathphysiological reactions occur in the period prior to the hypotensive episode.[7] It is obvious that therapy of shock states should be given promptly and adequately in early stages when it is most effective; it should be directed against underlying pathophysiological mechanisms and titrated to achieve optimal physiological goals.[7] This chapter describes the physiological natural history of the various shock syndromes in terms of their cardiovascular patterns, in order to evaluate potential underlying mechanisms. This is needed to define therapeutic goals in physiological terms so that appropriately titrated therapy will maximize survival rates and minimize complications.

BRAIN INSULTS IN INFANTS AND CHILDREN
0-8089-1723-4

## DEFINITION

Shock is an acute, complex pathophysiological state of circulatory dysfunction that results in failure to deliver sufficient amounts of oxygen and other nutrients to satisfy the requirements of the tissue beds.[6] Shock is a group of diverse, life-threatening circulatory syndromes occurring secondary to many different etiologic events including hemorrhage, trauma, sepsis, and reduced cardiac function. However, shock can rarely be ascribed to brain injury or insult.

The exact cardiorespiratory pattern manifest during shock depends on the complex interaction of host, time, and illness. The precipitating event initiates a state of cardiovascular dysfunction, and these circulatory problems are modified or augmented by complex neuroendocrine activity; products of cellular breakdown; altered metabolism; and individual host factors such as blood volume status, nutritional state, and myocardial competence. Because of the multiple factors involved, the cardiorespiratory pattern will vary considerably as the shock state evolves.[6]

## ETIOLOGY OF SHOCK SYNDROMES

### Hypovolemic Shock

The most common cause of shock in pediatric patients is acute hypovolemia, which follows a reduction in blood volume (Table 18-1).[6] Although hypovolemia does not occur secondary to closed head injuries in adults, infants with open cranial sutures may lose a significant proportion of circulating blood volume intracranially, especially if decompression into the scalp occurs. In addition, children with a functioning cerebral fluid shunt and intracranial hemorrhage may become hypovolemic. In general, however, hypovolemia in children and adults with head injuries is due to other causes.[6]

Loss of circulating blood volume is followed by a series of cardiac and peripheral homeostatic adjustments that attempt to restore the systemic arterial blood pressure and perfusion pressure in critical organs such as the heart and the brain.[11] This occurs at the expense of blood flow to the renal, mesenteric, and cutaneous circulations.[11] Whether these adjustments are adequate to maintain cardiovascular homeostasis is determined by the patient's preexisting status and the amount and rate of blood volume loss.

Compensated phases of hypovolemic shock are characterized by decreases in central venous pressure, stroke volume, and urine output, and by increases in heart rate, systemic vascular resistance, and myocardial contractility. Systemic arterial blood pressure is frequently normal as a the result of increased systemic vascular resistance.[6,7] With continued loss of blood volume

**Table 18-1** *Common Causes of Hypovolemia in Children*

Whole-Blood Loss
- Hemorrhage
  - External
  - Internal (e.g., gastrointestinal bleeding, hepatic or splenic rupture, fractures, major vessel injury, intracranial bleeding)
- Relative Loss
  - Pharmacological (e.g., barbiturates, vasodilators)
  - Positive-pressure ventilation
  - Spinal cord injury
  - Sepsis or Anaphylaxis

Plasma Loss
- Burns
- Capillary leak syndromes (e.g., inflammation, sepsis, anaphylaxis)
- Protein losing syndromes (e.g., nephrosis, intestinal obstruction)

Fluid and Electrolytic Loss
- Vomiting
- Diarrhea
- Renal
  - Altered intrinsic renal function
  - Excessive diuretic use
  - Endocrine causes (e.g., adrenal insufficiency, diabetes insipidus)

or delayed or inadequate replacement, the intravascular fluid losses surpass the compensatory abilities and decompensated phases appear. The pronounced systemic vasoconstriction and hypovolemia result in damage to blood vessels, kidneys, liver, pancreas, and bowel. The patients become hypotensive, acidotic, lethargic, and oliguric.

It is important to emphasize that arterial pressure falls only after compensations are exhausted, which may occur long after the precipitating event and after severe reduction in cardiac output.[7] Cerebral blood flow may be more dependent on cardiac output than systemic arterial pressure when intravascular volume is decreased. Systemic arterial pressure is a relatively crude guide to cardiac performance.

### Spinal Shock

The presence of hypotension secondary to spinal cord injury is frequently overlooked in the multiply injured patient. It occurs as a result of massive vasodilation and is relatively easy to differentiate from hypovolemic shock. The pulse is normal or decreased, the skin is dry and warm, and the urine output is normal. Because of the loss of sympathetic control to the heart and peripheral circulation, cardiovascular control and regulation is poor. In the face of a circulating volume deficit, constriction of the venous capacitance vessels does not occur to maintain cardiac filling pressures. In the presence of overtransfusion because of the lack of sympathetic-induced tachycardia and increased contractility, pulmonary edema may develop. For those reasons, hypotension should not be treated unless there is evidence of inadequate tissue perfusion. Treatment involves careful fluid infusion and vasoactive drugs.

### Cardiogenic Shock

Cardiogenic shock is the state in which an abnormality of cardiac function is responsible for the failure of the cardiovascular system to meet metabolic needs. The common denominator is depressed cardiac output and, in most instances, is the result of decreased myocardial contractility.[4,6] The possible etiologies of cardiogenic shock in children are:

1. Congenital heart disease
2. Dysrhythmias
3. Drugs
4. Hypoxemia and ischemia
5. Acidosis
6. Hypothermia
7. Metabolic disorders (hypoglycemia and hypocalcemia)
8. Myocardial contusion
9. Extrinsic inflow or outflow obstruction (tension pneumothorax or pneumopericardium, pericardial effusion)
10. Increases in systemic or pulmonary vascular resistances
11. Late stages of shock of any eitology

Compensatory mechanisms for the decreased stroke volume in cardiogenic shock can further depress cardiac function.[6] Transient compensatory increases in myocardial contractility may occur but eventually give way to deterioration of myocardial function from progression of the underlying disease or the failure of compensations. For these reasons, frequently only one cardiorespiratory pattern, in varying degrees of severity, is observed in cardiogenic shock. The patients are tachycardic, hypotensive, oliguric, and acidotic. Cardiac output is depressed and elevations of central venous pressure, pulmonary wedge pressure, and systemic vascular resistance are observed.

**Septic Shock**

Septic shock occurs frequently and is associated with high mortality rates in children as well as adults.[1,5,8] Sepsis is a systemic disease caused by microorganisms or their products in the blood. When sepsis leads to circulatory insufficiency and inadequate tissue perfusion, shock is present. Septic shock remains a major cause of death in critically ill patients. Despite careful use of antibiotics, adequate hemodynamic monitoring and aggressive surgery, mortality occurs in 60–70 percent of these patients.

Recent innovations in medical practice have increased the likelihood of sepsis and subsequent shock. Aggressive resuscitation protocols may employ corticosteroids, antibiotics, and the use of invasive medical devices, all of which contribute to an increase in blood stream invasion with microorganisms. Although the most common offending organisms are gram-negative bacteria, septic shock may occur following infections with gram-positive bacteria, fungi, rickettsiae, and viruses.[10] Regardless of the offending organisms, similar cardiorespiratory responses appear to be host dependent.[10]

In comparison to other forms of shock the pathophysiology of septic shock is markedly different. The precise mechanisms causing circulatory dysfunction in septic shock are not clear. This appears to be the result of many interrelated factors, including direct effect of the organism or its by-products on the cardiovascular system; cardiovascular effects of secondary products, including the products of activated protein cascade systems (complement, coagulation, kallikrein) and toxic myocardial factors; liberation of other vasoactive agents (serotonin, endorphins, prostaglandins, histamine); derangement of intermediary metabolism failure of oxygen extraction at the cellular level; host compensatory mechanisms; and underlying host factors such as preexisting cardiovascular, nutritional, and immunologic status.[6]

It is impossible to predict the effect of these factors at the microcirculatory level. Recent evidence suggests that metabolic and cardiorespiratory changes are intimately related as part of a common process and that survival patterns in critically ill septic patients are determined long before hypotension is recognized.[1,8]

The clinical pattern and presentation of septic shock may vary a great deal, depending on the dynamic interplay of the invading organism, elapsing time, and the host status (Table 18-2).[6] Abnormal hemodynamic responses comprise a primary hallmark of septic shock. In early stages, it is characterized by a high cardiac output, a low peripheral resistance, and a normal or increased oxygen uptake, all of which constitute a compensated hyperdynamic state. The immediate hemodynamic burden of survival in septic shock is dependent on adequate myocardial function and effective blood volume; thus an initial hypodynamic phase may occur. Survival has been related to the ability to establish a hyperdynamic state. The significance of ventricular

**Table 18-2** *Stages of Septic Shock*

| Compensated Hyperdynamic* | Uncompensated Hyperdynamic | Cardiogenic |
|---|---|---|
| ↑ CI | ↑ CI | ↓ CI |
| ↓ SVR | ↓↓ SVR | ↑ SVR |
| nl BP | ↓ BP | ↓ BP |
| nl $Vo_2$ | ↓ $Vo_2$ | ↓ $Vo_2$ |
| nl or ↑ pH | ↓ pH | ↓ pH |
| nl A − $Vo_2$ | ↓A − $Vo_2$ | ↑ A − $Vo_2$ |

*Abbreviations: CI = cardiac index; SVR = systemic vascular resistance; BP = systemic blood pressure; nl = normal; $Vo_2$ Consumption; A − $Vo_2$ = arteriovenous oxygen content difference.

failure and the inability to maintain an adequate cardiac output have been stressed by numerous investigators, suggesting that there is an initial strong correlation between cardiac index and survival.[6,9]

If sepsis is unchecked and uncorrelated, there is steady deterioration in cardiovascular performance. In early stages of decompensation a hyperdynamic cardiovascular state, reflected by increased cardiac output, appears to fail to supply peripheral metabolic needs, resulting in metabolic acidosis. Hypotension presents inspite of an increased cardiac output; the peripheral vascular resistance is inappropriately low for the level of cardiac output.[6] Many patients die of refractory hypotension as a result of a very low systemic vascular resistance.[5]

Deterioration of the septic process characteristically shows a fall in oxygen consumption during a period when cardiovascular function and oxygen availability remain increased. The reduction in oxygen consumption reflects a very severe impairment of oxidative metabolism at a time of major metabolic and physiological stress.[8] This decrease in oxygen consumption is the earliest predictor of an increased chance of physiological decompensation and death.

In some patients, with further progression of septic shock, increasing evidence of myocardial failure becomes evident and is associated with a progressive multisystem organ failure.[6] This late or cardiogenic stage is manifest by a hypodynamic cardiovascular picture that is indistinguishable from late shock of any etiology. All aspects of cardiac performance rapidly deteriorate, even with agressive support.

### Traumatic Shock

Acute injury results in increased automonic neural activity, which in turn stimulates the central cardiac and respiratory centers to increase heart rate, myocardial contractility, and alveolar ventilation. Unless limited by hypovolemia or impaired myocardial function, the early cardiorespiratory pattern consists of increased cardiac output, central blood volume, and oxygen delivery. Such a sympathetic nervous hyperactivity has been documented in head injury. In some patients with severe head injury the intensity of the hyperdynamic state exceeds levels reported in other types of trauma.[3]

There is evidence that the hyperdynamic response, if extreme, may damage the myocardium. The finding of subendocardial hemorrhages in 50 percent of autopsied patients with severe head injury suggests myocardial damage from the hyperdynamic state.[3] In addition, the hyperdynamic state may result in increased cerebral blood flow and intracranial pressure.

## MONITORING

Adequate monitoring generates information, allowing definition of the patient's exact cardiorespiratory pattern, which is helpful in diagnosis, prognosis, and treatment.[2,6] Occasionally, in patients with clearly definable causes of shock, which are rapidly corrected, the only requirements for effective patient monitoring include the accurate measurement and recording of vital signs, including heart rate, respiratory rate, temperature, and systemic arterial blood pressure (by cuff), together with observation of the patient's color, activity, and peripheral perfusion.

More agressive monitoring is required for critically ill children with shock and multisystem dysfunction that is more complex, does not respond rapidly to initial therapeutic measures, or is likely to place the patient at risk for many hours or days. Many invasive and noninvasive bedside monitoring devices are now available and are complemented by an ever-widening range of laboratory measurements.[2] In addition to obtaining a detailed history and receiving thorough and repeated physical examinations, critically ill patients should have continuous electrocardiographic display and heart rate monitoring, skin or core temperature (or both) recordings, continuous intra-arterial systemic blood pressure and pulse wave form display, careful fluid intake and output measurements, and an initial chest roentgenogram that is either repeated daily or when the patient's condition deteriorates.

Patients who have elevated systemic vascular resistance, pulmonary edema, or pulmonary hypertension or who require IV inotropic or vasoactive agents for therapy should receive measurement of central venous filling pressures, pulmonary artery pressure, and cardiac output with the use of a pulmonary artery thermodilution catheter. Measurement of these variables will allow the physician to make accurate diagnoses; choose the proper therapeutic agents; and rapidly, repeatedly, and objectively assess the results of therapy. Hemodynamic therapy of critically ill patients in shock is impossible without measurement of preload, arterial blood pressure, and cardiac index, along with calculation of pulmonary and systemic vascular resistance.

## REFERENCES


1. Abraham E, Shoemaker WC, Bland RD, et al: Sequential cardiorespiratory patterns in septic shock. Crit Care Med 11:799, 1983
2. Bachbindiner N, Ganz W: Hemodynamic monitoring: Invasive techniques. Anesthesiology 45:146, 1976
3. Clifton GL, Robertson CS, Kyper K, et al: Cardiovascular response to severe head injury. J Neurosurg 59:447, 1983
4. Lappas DB, Powell WMJ, Daggett WM: Cardiac dysfunction in the perioperative period: Pathophysiology, diagnosis, and treatment. Anesthesiology 47:117, 1977
5. Parker MM, Shelhamer JH, Bacharach SL, et al: Profound but reversible myocardial depression in patients with septic shock. Ann Intern Med 100:483, 1984
6. Perkin RM, Levin DL: Shock in the pediatric patient. Part I. J Pediatr 101:163, 1982
7. Shoemaker WC: Pathophysiology and therapy of shock and syndromes, in Shoemaker WC, Tompson WL, Holbrook PR (Eds): Textbook of Critical Care. Philadelphia, Saunders, 1984, pp 52–72
8. Seigal JH, Cerra FB, Coleman B, et al: Physiological and metabolic correlations in human sepsis. Surgery 86:163, 1979
9. Weil MH, Nishijima H: Cardiac output in bacterial shock. Am J Med 64:920, 1978
10. Wiles JB, Cerra FB, Seigal JH, et al: The systemic septic response: Does the organism matter? Crit Care Med 8:55, 1980
11. Zeifach BW, Bronek A: The interplay of central and peripheral factors in irreversible hemorrhagic shock. Prog Cardiovasc Dis 18:147, 1975

# PART V

# Therapy for Impending Brain Insults

*Ronald M. Perkin*

# 19

# Management of the Child in Shock

Since circulatory shock is a clinical syndrome reflecting inadequate tissue oxygenation, therapeutic efforts—in addition to treatment of the primary underlining process—involve optimization of cardiac output and arterial oxygen content. Improvement of cardiac output involves manipulation of the four major determinants of ventricular performance: heart rate, preload, afterload, and contractility.[13]

## HEART RATE AND RHYTHM

Dysrhythmias affect cardiac performance chiefly by their effect on heart rate.[13] Bradydysrhythmias often result in a decreased cardiac output, although there may be an initial compensatory increase in stroke volume. Tachydysrhythmias result in depressed cardiac output as a result of impaired diastolic filling time and may decrease perfusion of the myocardium, particularly the subendocardium. Standard therapy to optimize heart rate and rhythm should be used in addition to a search for factors that predispose to dysrhythmias (e.g., electrolyte imbalance, hypoxemia, alteration in systemic pH, abnormal core temperature, drugs). Electrocardiographic (ECG) abnormalities and myocardial damage are known to occur in patients with severe brain insults, particularly intracerebral hemorrhage of traumatic or spontaneous origin.[6,15] The most frequent ECG abnormalities are changes suggestive of ischemic myocardial injury and are probably the result of sympathetic nervous hyperactivity.[15] Fatal dysrhythmias have been reported in otherwise healthy head-injured patients.[6] The high frequency and potential seriousness

BRAIN INSULTS IN INFANTS AND CHILDREN
0-8089-1723-4

of this problem suggest that ECG changes should be looked for in all infants and children with neurological insults.

## PRELOAD

Preload establishes the end-diastolic ventricular volumes, which are clinically assessed by measurement of right and left artrial pressures.[13] Changes in preload greatly alter cardiac output. Reduction of preload, leading to decreased cardiac output, is most commonly a result of hypovolemia but may also result from displacement of blood from the thorax (e.g., positive-pressure ventilation) or cardiac compression (e.g., tamponade).[13] An absolute or relative blood volume deficit is often the primary component of the shock syndromes.[17] Regardless of the etiology of shock, therefore, the possibility of hypovolemia must be considered and efforts made to restore an effective circulating blood volume. It is emphasized that fluid resuscitation should not be withheld in patients with associated central nervous system (CNS) dysfunction. Frequently, restoration of adequate circulating blood volume will reverse some neurological manifestations and prevent irreversible ischemic injury from lack of perfusion. However, overhydration in patients with potential or actual cerebral edema should be avoided.[13]

Restoration of lost blood volume by fluid infusion is the principal goal in shock states, but considerable controversy exists in regard to administration of the appropriate fluid.[7,9,18] Volume restoration includes the use of either crystalloid or colloid solutions (or both) in addition to blood when indicated for whole blood loss or anemia. Crystalloids are electrolyts containing solutions that are distributed among the body compartments depending on chemical composition and tonicity.[7,18] The two most common crystalloid fluids used for resuscitation are 0.9 percent sodium chloride (normal saline) and lactated Ringer's solution. The disadvantage of these solutions is that they are distributed rapidly throughout the extracellular fluid volume. Since 25 percent of the extracellular fluid volume is located in the plasma volume and 75 percent in the interstitium, most of the administered fluid leaves the vascular system almost immediately and goes into the tissue to increase interstitial fluid and lymph and to cause edema.[7] Large infusion of crystalloid solutions may result in cerebral edema. Because 5 percent dextrose in water does not contain electrolytes, it moves freely in and out of extracellular and intracellular spaces without significantly increasing plasma volume. Hypotonic fluids are thus seldom used for fluid resuscitation, especially in patients with neurological injury.

The colloids used in the treatment of shock include plasma, prepared plasma fractions, and synthetic plasma substitutes. These solutions contain large molecules that are restricted primarily to the intravascular space, where they exert an oncotic effect.[7] Therefore, Isooncotic solutions such as 5 percent albumin or fresh-frozen plasma produce a relatively greater plasma expansion than isotonic crystalloid solutions for the same volume of fluid infused.

Proper selection of resuscitation fluid can be accomplished only after the patient is assessed and the following questions answered: What type of fluid has been lost? What are the specific underlying physiological problems? What are the specific physiological actions of each type of fluid? Changes in red cell volume, colloid osmotic pressure, and serum sodium content should be taken into account in selection of initial resuscitation fluids.[9]

The amount of fluid necessary to restore effective circulating blood volume depends on the fluid deficit and the rate of on going loss. The total amount of fluid required often exceeds the total volume lost because of expanded capacity of the vascular space and dysfunction of cellular membranes.[9] In cases of hypovolemic shock uncomplicated by myocardial dysfunction, the fluid resuscitation should proceed as outlined in Figure 19-1. If no improvement occurs as manifest by a rise in systemic arterial pressure,

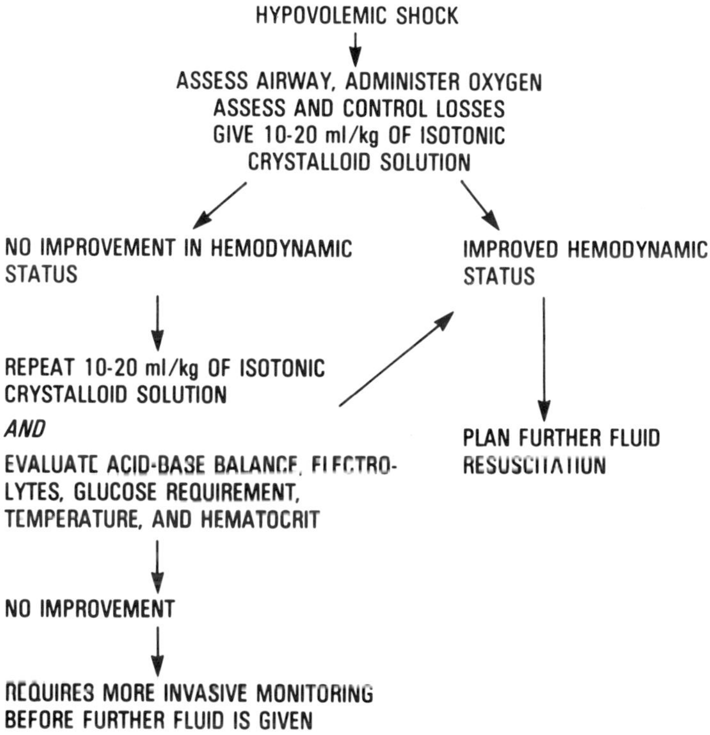


**Fig. 19-1.** Initial approach to fluid management in a child with uncomplicated hypovolemic shock.

improved peripheral perfusion, adequate urine output, and decreased metabolic acidosis after two infusions of isotonic crystalloid solution at 10–20 ml/kg, no further fluid should be given without more accurate monitoring.[13] In patients with cardiogenic or septic shock, efforts to improve cardiac output and tissue perfusion by volume loading must be careful monitored from the onset.[12] Cardiac filling pressures (preload) must be raised to a point where cardiac output becomes adequate and then carefully adjusted for optimal levels.[12] Cardiac output may be judged by the mixed venous $Po_2$, with the aim of achieving a $Po_2$ of greater than 30 mmHg or by actual measurement of cardiac output. Oxygen-carrying capacity is evaluated by measurement of the hematocrit, which should be at least 30–35 percent.

It is emphasized that if cerebrovascular autoregulation is altered, the response to large fluid infusion and rapid change in arterial pressure may be acute brain swelling. For this reason, the brain-injured patient in shock should have an intracranial pressure monitor inserted to observe the intracranial pressure response to fluid infusion and other resuscitation therapies.

## CONTRACTILITY, VASCULAR TONE, AND AFTERLOAD

In some severely ill patients, adequate oxygen delivery may not be possible even after efforts are made to optimize preload, afterload, heart rate, and arterial oxygen content. In these situations depression of myocardial contractility likely exists as a result of either the presence of myocardial disease or damage, continuing hypoxemia and acidosis, or the presence of a circulating myocardial depressant factor.[13] Therapy must focus on enhancing contractility of the myocardium. The following factors influence myocardial contractility:

- Arterial oxygen content
- Myocardial blood flow
- Acid–base balance
- Glucose
- Electrolyte and mineral imbalances
- Thyroid and adrenal function
- Temperature
- Drugs

Therapeutic measures to improve myocardial contractility include improvement in myocardial oxygen delivery, reduction of myocardial oxygen demands, correction of extramyocardial factors, appropriate utilization of inotropic drugs, and avoidance of cardiac-depressant drugs. Barbiturates, particularly phenobarbital and thiopental sodium, have been used effectly in brain-injured patients with increased intracranial pressure (ICP) that is refractory to corticosteroids, mannitol, and hyperventilation; however, this treatment may be complicated by hypotension with an adverse impact on survival.[19]

Myocardial oxygen delivery is contingent on the maintenance of coronary blood flow and adequate oxygen content of the coronary perfusate. In many cases of heart failure and circulatory shock, coronary blood flow becomes dependent on aortic diastolic pressure, ventricular end-diastolic pressure, and diastolic time. Any compromise of coronary blood flow leads to subendocardial ischemia, which results in a self-perpetuating process that eventually leads to terminal heart failure.[13] Therapeutic measures designed to increase coronary perfusion pressure (aortic diastolic pressure minus ventricular end-diastolic pressure) or optimize heart rate may improve subendocardial perfusion, correct the imbalance of energy supply and demand, and thus improve myocardial contractility. Occasionally the judicious use of vasopressor such as norepinephrine is required in order to increase aortic diastolic pressure and improve coronary blood flow. In some patients, naloxone may act as a vasopressor while reversing some of the pathophysiological changes seen in shock.

Measures to increase the arterial oxygen content should be instituted as hypoxemia is a common accompaniment of circulatory shock. In approaching the problem of hypoxemia, one must consider all factors that determine the partial pressure of oxygen in arterial blood ($Pa{O_2}$). These determinants include ventilatory, circulatory, and metabolic factors as well as the quantity and quality of hemoglobin present. Therapeutic intervention that changes circulatory (e.g., cardiac output) and metabolic (e.g., oxygen consumption) determinants of the $Pa{O_2}$ may result in dramatic change in $Pa{O_2}$ without altering underlying lung function. Sudden changes in $Pa{O_2}$ are usually circulatory or metabolic in origin if gross ventilatory changes have been excluded (e.g., pneumothorax, malpositioned or obstructed endotracheal tube). For further discussion of the ventilatory factors, the reader is referred to Chapters 17 and 21.

Acid–base and electrolyte disorders accompanying many major physiological disturbances may contribute to myocardial dysfunction. An appropriate cellular millieu must exist before the administration of on inotropic drugs is considered.[13] Correction of acidosis may restore cardiac output and eliminate the need for more aggressive therapy. Correction with sodium bicarbonate is indicated when marked metabolic acidosis exists (arterial blood pH $<7.20$). Electrolyte abnormalities, metabolic alkalosis, fluid overload, and hypertonicity are recognized complications of bicarbonate therapy.[14]

Abnormalities in electrolyte and mineral concentrations may adversely affect myocardial contractility.[14] Hypocalcemia, hypophosphatemia, and hypomagnesemia all impair myocardial function and should be corrected.[14]

Glucose is a necessary energy substrate for metabolism in the myocardium. Severe hypoglycemia may result in myocardial depression and circulatory failure. Because myocardial glycogen stores are limited, glucose must be provided to preserve the myocardium and enhance its performance. Insulin and potassium may be added to facilitate muscle uptake of glucose and to prevent hypokalemia. Administration of solutions consisting of glucose, insulin, and potassium (GIK) have been used in patients with circulatory failure of multiple etiologies, and it is well documented that GIK administration improves cardiac performance in these patients.[5] Such infusions improve contractility, restore cell membrane potentials, and lower the concentration of plasma free fatty acids.[5]

Hypothermia, defined as a core temperature of 35°C or less, is relatively common in trauma patients. A number of disease states predispose to hypothermia: diabetic ketoacidosis, sepsis, hypoglycemia, cerebral trauma, spinal cord injuries, burns, and malnutrition. Hypothermia has profound neurological, cardiovascular, and respiratory manifestations. As core body temperature decreases, mentation deteriorates. Below 30°C, loss of consciousness with unreactive dilated pupils, apnea, and absence of deep tendon reflexes is seen. Hypothermia also causes a progressive depression of cardiac output.[13] This decrease in cardiac output is related to depressed contractility, increased afterload, and alteration in heart rate. The initial heart rate response to cold is tachycardia, but blow 32°C bradycardia is noted. When the core temperature drops blow 28°C, ventricular fibrillation or asystole can occur, and these rhythms are seldom responsive to atropine, pacing, or countershock. Hypothermia increases the viscosity of blood, resulting in decreased conductance through the coronary vessels and other vascular beds, followed by decreased effective cardiac output and oxygen transport. The initial goal in the treatment of hypothermia is to rapidly attain a core temperature of 30°C to prevent cardiac dysrhythmias. Vital signs, cardiograms, arterial pH and blood gases, blood glucose, and electrolytes must be closely monitored.

Although volume expansion and correction of extracardiac abnormalities may enhance cardiac function, occasionally treatment relies on the use of drugs with the ability to restore or augment myocardial contractility or improve cardiac output and bring about a restoration and maintenance of blood flow.[8] In acute situations, it is most desirable to use drugs that are short-acting and administered by continuous IV infusion because the hemodynamic situation may rapidly change.

Catecholamine drugs are frequently used in the various shock syndromes (Table 19-1).[8] The catecholamines are the most potent possible inotropic agents available; however, their effects are not limited to inotropy. They also possess chronotropic effects and complex effects on the vascular beds of the various organs of the body.[2,10] Their use may, therefore, in some instances be complicated by undesirable vascular actions or toxic effects on the myocardium.[10]

Vasodilating drugs are often advocated in the management of shock because of improvement of ventricular function by reducing afterload. "Afterload" is a term utilized to express the total force opposing ejection from the ventricle. The force is composed of resistive, compliant, viscous, and inertial components. The vascular resistance is probably the largest single component.

In some patients with circulatory failure, an afterload mismatch is present.[16] A mismatch occurs when the level of afterload is excessive for the inotropic state and there is inadequate compensation by an accompanying change in preload.[16] In this situation, afterload becomes the critical factor determining cardiac output and the two are inversely related.[3] In some patients a reduction in afterload may improve cardiac output, which thus forms the rationale for use of vasodilators (Table 19-2).

The mechanism and the site of action differ considerably among the various vasodilators.[3,11] Before therapy is initiated, therefore, an exact hemodynamic profile should be obtained and the mechanisms causing elevated vascular resistance determined. The use of vasodilators in shock is generally limited to those situations in which cardiac dysfunction exists and is associated with elevated ventricular filling pressure, elevated systemic vascular resistance, and normal or elevated systemic arterial blood pressure.[13] Use of vasodilators in hypertensive patients with cardiovascular dysfunction and CNS injury is often a dilemma. The high pressure may be viewed as a contributor to increased intracranial pressure or as a risk factor for intercerebral bleeding. Alternatively, the high pressure may represent a response that is necessary to produce adequate cerebral perfusion. In addition, many vasodilators decrease cerebrovascular resistance, thereby increasing cerebral blood flow and perhaps intracranial pressure. For these reasons, vasodilators should not be used in patients with neurological disease unless monitoring of intracranial pressure or cerebral blood flow (CBF) (or both) is available. Other causes of elevated systemic vascular resistance and pressure, such as pain, anxiety, hypervolemia, hypoxia, hypothermia, and drug effect, must be considered and treated prior to use of vasodilators.

## OTHER ASPECTS OF THERAPY

Stress ulceration and erosive gastritis may occur acutely in patients who are critically ill. Acute ulcerations of the stomach and duodenum commonly occur in the victims of severe trauma, hemorrhage, shock, sepsis, burns, and intracranial disease. Bleeding or perforation can almost always be prevented

**Table 19-1** *Catecholamines*

| Drug | Recommended Dose | Comment |
|---|---|---|
| Norepinephrine | 0.05–1.0 μg/kg/min (alpha, beta) | Predominant alpha-adrenergic stimulation overshadows the $beta_1$ effects on the myocardium; used only in situations in which arterial pressure has decreased to levels that acutely jeopardize coronary and cerebral perfusion; may cause hypocalcemia, hypoglycemia, ischemic dysrhythmias, and ischemia of renal and splanchnic beds |
| Epinephrine | 0.005–0.02 μg/kg/min (beta)<br>0.02–1.0 μg/kg/min (alpha, beta) | Vasodilation of splanchnic bed and skeletal muscle at low doses; major metabolic effects: increases free fatty acids, and increases glucose; higher doses may lead to renal and mesenteric ischemia; reserved for situation where the failing myocardium is unresponsive to other inotropic drugs |
| Isoproterenol | 0.01–0.5 μg/kg/min (beta) | Synthetic catecholamine that acts almost exclusively on beta-adrenergic receptor as an agonist; positive inotropic and chronotropic effects while decreasing systemic and pulmonary vascular resistances; seldom useful in shock because it increases cutaneous and muscular |

**Table 19-1** *(continued)*

| Drug | Recommended Dose | Comment |
|---|---|---|
| | | vasodilation, thus redistributing blood to nonessential areas; indicated in therapy of cardiac failure complicated by bradycardia or asthma and perhaps pulmonary hypertension |
| Dopamine | 0.02–2.0 μg/kg/min (dopaminergic)<br>2.0–10.0 μg/kg/min (beta, dopaminergic)<br>10.0–20.0 μg/kg/min (alpha, beta)<br>>20.0 μg/kg/min (alpha) | Stimulates cardiac beta receptors by direct and indirect mechanisms; has unique vasodilating effects on certain vascular beds, especially renal vasculature, but also on mesenteric coronary and intracerebral vascular beds; the specific peripheral effects of dopamine make this catecholamine particularly useful when low-dose infusions can restore cardiovascular stability and also augment renal function |
| Dobutamine | 1.0–10.0 μg/kg/min (alpha, beta) | Relatively new synthetic catecholamine with a biochemical structure similar to that of isoproterenol; racemic mixture—overall activity is due to the sum of the activation of individual stereoisomers; positive inotropic effect with minimal chronotropic or peripheral vascular effects |

**Table 19-2** *Vasodilators*

| Drug | Recommended Dose | Comment |
| --- | --- | --- |
| Phentolamine | 2–20 μg/kg/min | Nonspecific alpha-adrenergic blocker; reduces peripheral vascular resistance with progressive increase in cardiac output; coronary and cerebral beds not influenced unless intravascular volume is inadequate |
| Sodium nitroprusside | 0.5–8.0 μg/kg/min | Nonspecific vascular smooth-muscle relaxant affecting both arteriolar resistance and venous capacitance bed; dilates the cerebral circulation and may result in increased cerebral blood flow and increased intracranial pressure |
| Trimethaphan camsylate | Begin at 2–3 μg/kg/min | Blocks sympathetic motor reflexes; dilates venous and arterial beds; negative inotropic effect—cardiac output may decrease; no cerebral vascular dilation—cerebral blood flow may decrease; causes histamine release; exact dose requirements vary |
| Hydralazine | 0.1–0.5 mg/kg every 3–6 h or 1.0–5.0 μg/kg/min | Smooth-muscle relaxant active primarily on the arteriolar resistance bed; long-acting; dilates cerebral vascular bed; may produce undesirable tachycardia |

by titrating gastric acidity every hour or two to a pH of 4.0 or greater with antiacids.

Disseminated intravascular coagulation (DIC) occurs to some extent in all shock patients and represents an inappropriate activation of the clotting process. Clotting disorders have been described after a variety of cerebral insults, particularly head injury. Brain has the highest level of thromboplastin of any body tissue, and disruption of the blood–brain barrier can cause the release of large quantities of thromboplastin into the circulation and activation of extrinsic pathways for blood clotting. Disseminated intravascular coagulation significantly contributes to mortality, usually in the form of bleeding or thrombosis. Treatment is directed at controlling infection, hypoxia, acidosis, and hypotension. Administration of vitamin K, platelets, and fresh frozen plasma should be done.[4] If the fibrinogen level is less than 100 mg/dl and does not increase with fresh-frozen plasma, cryoprecipitate should be given.[4] The use of heparin is controversial and replacement of coagulation factors, vigorous treatment of circulatory failure and other primary defects is the major concern.[4]

Although the usually physiological response that occurs in shock is increased secretion of adrenocortical hormones, not all patients in shock have increased blood cortisol levels.[1,13] Because of the possibility of depressed adrenocortical function, all patients in shock who fail to respond to routine therapy should be provided with replacement therapy of 2–3 times normal maintenance doses of cortisol or equivalent until the status of the adrenal glands can be studied. The use of much larger doses of corticosteroids in shock remains controversial.

## REFERENCES


1. Catalona RD, Parameswaran V, Ramachandran J, et al: Mechanisms of adrenocortical depression during escherichia coli shock. Arch Surg 119:145, 1984
2. Chernow B, Rainey TG, Lake CR: Endogenous and exogenous cathecholamines in critical care medicine. Crit Care Med 10:409, 1982
3. Cohn JN: Physiologic basis of vasodilator therapy for heart failure. Am J Med 71:135, 1981
4. Colman RW, Robboy SJ, Minna JD: Disseminated intravascular coagulation: A reappraisal. Annu Rev Med 30:359, 1979
5. Denni RC, Harlow C, Cagdahl RH, et al: Enhancement of myocardial functions with glucose, insulin, and potassium. Surg Gynecol Obstet 151:185, 1980
6. Hackenberry LE, Miner M, Rea GL, et al: Biochemical evidence of myocardial injury after severe head trauma. Crit Care Med 10:641, 1982
7. Hauser CJ, Shoemaker WC: Volume therapy treatment of hypovolemia. Hosp Phys 16:38, 1980
8. Lefer AM, Spath JA: Pharmacologic basis of the treatment of circulatory shock, in Antonaccio M: Cardiovascular Pharmacology. New York. Raven Press, 1977, pp 377–428
9. Lucas CE, Ledgerwood AM: The fluid problem in the critically ill. Surg Clin North Am 63:439, 1983

10. Lucchesi BR: Inotropic agents and drugs used to support the failing heart, in Antonacio M, (Ed): Cardiovascular Pharmacology. New York, Raven Press, 1977, pp 337–376
11. Miller RR, Fennell WH, Young JB, et al: Differential systemic arterial and venous actions and consequent cardiac effects of vasodilator drugs. Progr Cardiovasc Dis 24:353, 1982
12. Packman, MI, Rackow EC: Optimum left heart filling pressure during fluid resuscitation of patients with hypovolemic and septic shock. Crit Care Med 11:165, 1983
13. Perkin RM, Levin DL: Shock in the pediatric patient. Part II. J Pediatr 101:319, 1982
14. Perkin RM, Levin DL: Common fluid and electrolyte problems in the pediatric intensive care unit. Pediatr Clin North Am 27:567, 1980
15. Rogers MC, Zakha KG, Nugent SK, et al: Electrocardiographic abnormalities in infants and children with neurologic injury. Crit Care Med 8:213, 1980
16. Ross J: The failing heart and the circulation. Hosp Pract 19:151, 1983
17. Shoemaker WC: Pathophysiology and therapy of shock syndromes, in Shoemaker WC, Thompson WL, Holbrook PR (Eds): Textbook of Critical Care. Philadelphia, Saunders, 1984, pp 52–72
18. Shoemaker WC, Hauser CJ: Critique of crystalloid versus colloid therapy in shock and shock lung. Crit Care Med 7:117, 1979
19. Traeger SM, Henning RJ, Dobkin W, et al: Hemodynamic effects of phenobarbital therapy for intracranial hypertension. Crit Care Med 11:697, 1983

*Doris A. Trauner*

# 20

# Management of Reye's Syndrome

## CLINICOPATHOLOGICAL FEATURES

Reye's syndrome[7] is an acute metabolic encephalopathy involving liver and brain, which primarily effects children, although adult cases are now recognized. This disorder is associated with viral infections but is not the result of direct infection of the nervous system. Viruses most commonly associated with this disease are influenza B and varicella.

There is a typical biphasic course to the illness. The initial phase is a viral illness, usually resembling influenza or upper respiratory infection. The child is typically recovering from this viral ailment when there is sudden onset of vomiting, followed rapidly by lethargy, hyperexcitability, obtundation, and coma, all within 24–48 hours after the onset of vomiting. Seizures may occur at any time. Hyperventilation is a prominent finding. Abnormalities of liver function are almost always present, and the liver may be enlarged on examination. Increased intracranial pressure is a common complication and may be difficult to control. There is a 40 percent mortality rate.

The disorder is more subtle in infants under 1 year of age, and the diagnosis is often missed.[3,10] These patients may have little or no vomiting, and the first indication of Reye's syndrome may be sudden respiratory disturbances, including apnea. Mortality and morbidity are high in this age group.

Numerous metabolic abnormalities have been described in this disorder. Most are associated with hepatic involvement and include elevated serum transaminases, hyperammonemia, hypoglycemia (more common in children under the age of 4 years[2]), lactic acidemia, hyperaminoacidemia, short-chain fatty acidemia, and elevations of creatinine phosphokinase and uric acid.

BRAIN INSULTS IN INFANTS AND CHILDREN
0-8089-1723-4

Whether any of these abnormalities accounts for the clinical manifestations is unclear. In experimental animals, the major features of Reye's syndrome can be reproduced by infusion of short-chain fatty acids.[11] Hyperammonemia is known to produce coma as well. Other diseases that are clinically similar to Reye's syndrome (Jamaican vomiting sickness, Udorn encephalopathy) are known to be caused by exogenous plant toxins. Although several potential environmental toxins have been suggested as potential precipitating or causal factors in Reye's syndrome, there is no clear evidence that this disorder is caused by exogenous toxin. The strongest circumstantial evidence for a possible exogenous factor is found in salicylates. A high percentage of children with Reye's syndrome have received aspirin for their antecedent illnesses, and in one study it was concluded that children who are treated with aspirin are more likely to develop Reye's syndrome than children who are given acetaminophen for the same viral illness.[9] Recent recommendations from the American Academy of Pediatrics and other support groups are that children with varicella and flulike illnesses should not be given aspirin for symptomatic relief.

Several pathological changes have been observed in cases of Reye's syndrome.[4,6] The most striking abnormalities are found in the liver, which is often enlarged and pale yellow. Microscopic examination reveals diffuse microvesicular fatty accumulation within hepatocytes, with no evidence of inflammation or necrosis. Fatty changes may also been seen in kidney, heart, and skeletal muscle. Histochemical stains of liver tissue demonstrate reduction in activity of succinic acid dehydrogenase. Ultrastructural changes are found primarily in mitochondria, which are swollen and pleiomorphic, with disruption of cristae and absence of mitochondrial dense bodies. Similar mitochondrial abnormalities have been observed in brain and muscle, and these findings have led to the hypothesis that this is primarily a mitochondrial disorder. In view of these findings, bedside needle biopsies of liver are often diagnostic.

Reye's syndrome was first recognized as a clinical entity in 1963.[7] Since that time, various treatment regimens have been proposed and utilized. Because the etiology remains unclear, no specific therapy is available. Intensive supportive care has been the mainstay of treatment. In recent years recognition of the need to monitor and control intracranial pressure has increased.[8,12] In addition, attempts to reverse the numerous metabolic abnormalities associated with Reye's syndrome are utilized.[13] The remainder of the discussion in this chapter details the current approaches to treatment.

## STAGING OF REYE'S SYNDROME

Patients with severe forms of Reye's syndrome require intensive monitoring, and aggressive treatment regimens are usually employed. For this reason, it is important to define the severity of illness prior to initiating treatment and to follow the course of the disease in a systematic way. Several systems for "staging" the severity of the disease have been suggested, but the National Institute of Health Consensus Development Conference on the Diagnosis and Treatment of Reye's Syndrome recommended that a uniform staging system be used throughout the country so that various therapeutic approaches could be compared among centers treating the disease. The system has five stages:

*Stage I.* The patient is lethargic but follows verbal commands and has purposeful response to pain. Pupillary reactions are brisk and oculocephalic reflexes present.

*Stage II.* The patient is combative or stuporous, verbalizes inappropriately, and has purposeful or nonpurposeful reaction to pain. Pupillary reactions are sluggish, and there may be conjugate deviation of the eyes.

*Stage III.* The patient is comatose with decorticate posturing spontaneously and in response to painful stimuli. Pupillary responses are sluggish, and eyes have conjugate deviation on "doll's eyes" maneuvers.

*Stage IV.* The patient is comatose with decerebrate posturing spontaneously and in response to painful stimuli. Pupils are sluggishly reactive, and there are inconsistent or absent oculocephalic reflexes.

*Stage V.* The patient is comatose with flaccid posture; there is no response to painful stimuli and no pupillary response to light, and oculocephalic reflexes are absent.

## TREATMENT

Patients with Reye's syndrome have a number of problems that complicate their management. They are prone to sudden respiratory problems, including apnea. Hyperthermia, even in the absence of infection, is a common problem. These patients are subject to developing thick mucus plugs that may obstruct bronchioles and further complicate intracranial pressure problems by increasing intrathoracic pressure.

Supportive care must take into account all of these potential problems. Any patient with suspected Reye's syndrome should be treated in a pediatric intensive care unit even in the mild stages, since sudden deterioration is common. For patients in Stages I or II, correction of electrolyte imbalances, control of temperature and blood pressure, and IV administration of 10 percent glucose are recommended treatment approaches. There is some evidence that treatment of children in the mild stages with hypertonic glucose solutions decreases the likelihood that the disease will progress to more severe levels.

Any child who is unresponsive to verbal commands (i.e., stages III–V) should be intubated and mechanically ventilated, using neuromuscular blockade with an agent such as pancuronium bromide if necessary to reduce resistance from coughing or muscle tension. Under the circumstances, continuous EEG monitoring is needed. Careful cardiovascular monitoring of such patients necessitates the use of arterial and central venous pressure catheters or a Swan-Ganz catheter. Strict fluid control should be maintained. Chest physiotherapy is used in removing mucus plugs and minimizing intrathoracic resistance.

Since intracranial pressure elevations are common in this disorder, it is useful to continuously monitor ICP. Intracranial pressure should be maintained below 20 torr, provided mean arterial blood pressure (MABP) is 70 or greater. In order to prevent cerebral ischemia, cerebral perfusion pressure (CPP = MAPB − ICP) must be 50 or greater. Thus a "safe" ICP must be calculated by use of CPP rather than a standard value for ICP alone. For further discussion on intracranial volume and pressure, the reader is referred to Chapter 2.

Control of ICP may be accomplished in any of several ways. Muscular paralysis and assisted, controlled hyperventilation may be sufficient in some cases. If necessary, diuretics such as mannitol, may be employed. We have found that doses as low as 0.25 g/kg IV are effective in controlling ICP in Reye's patients.[12] The limiting factor in the use of this agent is hyperosmolality, which may cause mannitol to be ineffective and may also compromise renal function. If serum osmolality is kept below 310 by manipulation of IV fluids, mannitol can be effective without renal impairment. For further discussion on the use of diuretics, the reader is referred to Chapter 26.

The use of high-dose barbiturate therapy in the treatment of Reye's syndrome is controversial. Although this approach will lead to control of ICP, there is no clear evidence that this improves survival.[5] In addition, barbiturate therapy is accompanied by a number of complications and may actually prolong the course of the acute illness.[1] This form of treatment should thus be reserved for the most severe and intractable ICP problems in the most seriously ill patients (see Chapter 27).

Other modes of treatment for severely ill patients include exchange transfusions to clear ammonia and other toxins and to corrected clotting abnormalities, hypertonic glucose and IV insulin administration to decrease circulating fatty acid concentrations; neomycin enemas to eliminate excess ammonia, and anticonvulsant therapy (usually phenytoin) if seizures occur.

## PROGNOSIS

Despite early recognition of the disease and more aggressive treatment in recent years, there is still a 40 percent mortality rate. When the disease is recognized in the early stages (I and II), the mortality rate is quite low, however. Thus awareness of the disease and a high index of suspicion are essential in minimizing deaths from Reye's syndrome. Survivors over the age of 1 year generally do well, returning to normal function in most instances. Infants under 1 year of age have a somewhat poorer prognosis, and many of these surivivors are permanently neurologically handicapped.

## REFERENCES

1. Brown RE, Burckart G, Thompson R: Barbiturate-associated morbidity and mortality in Reye's syndrome. J Natl Reye's Synd Found 3:29, 1982
2. Huttenlocher PR, Trauner DA: Reye's syndrome, in Vinken PJ, Bruyn GW (Eds): Handbook of Clinical Neurology, vol 29. Amsterdam, North-Holland Publishing Company, 1977, Chapter 17
3. Huttenlocher PR, Trauner DA; Reye's syndrome in infants. Pediatrics 62:84, 1978
4. Lichtenstein PK, Heubi JE, Daugherty CC, et al: Grade I Reye's syndrome: A frequent cause of vomiting and liver dysfunction. New Engl J Med 309:133, 1983
5. Miller JD: Barbiturates and raised intracranial pressure. Ann Neurol 6:189, 1979
6. Partin JC, Schubert WK, Partin JS: Mitochondrial ultrastructure in Reye's syndrome. New Engl J Med 285:1339, 1971
7. Reye RDK, Morgan G, Baral J: Encephalopathy and fatty degeneration of the viscera. Lancet 2:749, 1963
8. Shaywitz BA: Prolonged continous monitoring of intracranial pressure in severe Reye's syndrome. Pediatrics 59:595, 1977
9. Starko KM, Ray CG, Dominguez LB, et al: Reye's syndrome and salicylate use. Pediatrics 66:859, 1980
10. Sullivan-Bulyri JZ, Nelson DB, Murens DM, et al: Reye's syndrome in children less than one year old: Epidemiologic observations. Pediatrics 65:627, 1980
11. Trauner DA, Huttenlocher PR: Short chain fatty acid-induced central hyperventilation in rabbits. Neurology 28:940, 1978
12. Trauner DA, Brown F, Ganz E, et al: Treatment of elevated intracranial pressure in Reye's syndrome. Ann Neurol 4:275, 1978
13. Trauner DA: Treatment of Reye's syndrome. Ann Neurol 7:2, 1980

*Nick G. Anas*

# 21

# Acute Management of The Child With Decompensating Lung Disease

The physician managing the child with acute brain injury must appreciate the intricate relationship between the central nervous and respiratory systems. Chapter 17 emphasized the importance of airway control in order to avoid secondary hypoxic brain injury. This discussion addresses the pulmonary disorders commonly associated with brain injury, the management of respiratory failure in the brain-injured child, and the effect on the lung of the therapeutic modalities used in the treatment of brain injury.

## IDENTIFYING THE UNDERLYING DISEASE

The goal of cardiopulmonary therapy is to maximize oxygen and substrate delivery to the vital organ systems. Oxygen availability is primarily a function of the cardiac output and the arterial oxygen content, with content dependent on both hemoglobin concentration and oxygen saturation.[21] Although cardiac and pulmonary function are not independent of one another, a reduced arterial oxygen content is usually the result of either pulmonary parenchymal or vascular disease. *Hypoxemic* respiratory failure in the child with acute brain injury thus can be categorized into three groups[2,6,8,13,22]: normal end-expiratory gas volume [functional residual capacity (FRC)] but elevated pulmonary vascular resistance (e.g., neurogenic pulmonary edema, pulmonary hypertension), (2) reduced FRC but normal pulmonary vascular resistance (intrapulmonary ventilation–perfusion mismatch or shunting; e.g.,

BRAIN INSULTS IN INFANTS AND CHILDREN
0-8089-1723-4

atelectasis, pneumonia, bronchospasm[15]), (3) reduced FRC and an elevated pulmonary vascular resistance [e.g., the adult respiratory distress syndrome (ARDS)[23]]. The group of pulmonary disorders resulting primarily in inadequate alveolar ventilation (hypercapnic respiratory failure) are upper airway obstruction, nonobstructive or central apnea, and respiratory muscle fatigue. The management of these problems is presented in Chapter 17.

### Neurogenic Pulmonary Edema

Central nervous system (CNS) injuries, particularly those resulting in intracranial hypertension, manifest signs of increased sympathetic nervous system activity: tachycardia, systemic hypertension, and an elevated peripheral vascular resistance. In fact, in head-injured patients there appears to be an inverse relationship between circulating plasma norepinephrine levels and the initial Glasgow Coma Score (GCS).[4] Evidence suggests that the initial phase of "neurogenic" pulmonary edema[12,20] is also a manifestation of this centrally mediated sympathetic discharge. Alpha-adrenergic activation results in a marked increased in aortic, systemic arterial, pulmonary venous, and superior vena caval pressure. The increase in aortic pressure is accompanied by a decrease in aortic blood flow, however, indicating an increase in systemic vascular resistance (SVR). This elevation in SVR shifts blood flow from the high-resistance systemic circulation to the lower-resistance pulmonary circulation, thereby increasing pulmonary blood volume. With increasing pulmonary venous and arterial pressure, hydrostatic pulmonary edema occurs. These events of alpha-mediated systemic and pulmonary hypertension are transient and in the brain-injured child may culminate in restoration of normal vascular pressures and resolution of pulmonary edema; disruption of vascular integrity, leading to persistent pulmonary edema; or persistence of pulmonary hypertension, resulting in an increase in dead-space ventilation and a reduction in the cardiac output (increased right ventricular afterload and decreased left ventricular preload). Potential mechanisms to explain a persistent elevated pulmonary vascular resistance include humorally mediated vasoconstriction or vascular occlusion due to microembolization. The intravascular release of cerebral thromboplastin following trauma or other acute brain injury may cause the formation of fibrin microemboli or the aggregation and adhesion of platelets in the pulmonary vascular bed with the release of vasoactive substances such as thromboxanes.

### Intrapulmonary Ventilation—Perfusion Alterations

Pulmonary disorders resulting in a reduction in the FRC or an increase in airways resistance but with continued perfusion of poorly ventilated lung units are characterized by arterial hypoxemia. In the child who sustains an acute brain injury, the most common lung disorders of this type are aspiration pneumonia, atelectasis secondary to retention of secretions, and bronchospasm probably due to alteration in neurogenic control or release of smooth-muscle constricting substances such as leukotrienes or prostaglandins. Compounding these abnormalities in head-injured patients is an apparent failure of normal ventilation–perfusion regulation. Through the use of steady-state elimination of inert gases of different solubility, it has been shown that in victims of head trauma a significant percentage of the cardiac output is distributed to areas of lung with low V/Q ratios or shunt units despite normalization of the FRC.[6] This implies the loss of hypoxic regulation of pulmonary blood flow. Finally, studies of mechanical head injuries in animals have demonstrated a reduction in lung compliance that predisposes to atelectasis or alveolar hyperventilation. The data from these studies suggest that the loss of normal compliance is a function of an alteration in structure of alveolar surfactant (the substance responsible for minimizing alveolar surface tension at low lung volumes).

### Adult Respiratory Distress Syndrome

This syndrome was first defined by Petty as a pathophysiologic state characterized by severe dyspnea, hypoxemia, diffuse bilateral pulmonary infiltration, and stiff lungs following massive acute injury (to any major organ system). The functional–structural abnormalities in the ARDS patient are complex and variable but may include[1,3] (1) intrapulmonary shunting due to alveolar edema or small airways constriction, (2) permeability pulmonary edema (protein-rich fluid) due to disruption of alveolar–capillary integrity, (3) reduced pulmonary compliance due to interstitial edema or altered alveolar surfactant (surface-active agent), and (4) an increase in dead-space ventilation and/or a reduction in the cardiac output due to an increase in pulmonary vascular resistance.[18] Among the mechanisms proposed to explain the pathophysiology of ARDS, the following are most likely to occur in the child with an acute brain insult: vascular injury mediated by the cellular elements of the blood (platelets, granulocytes),[5,10] injury associated with abnormal coagulation of the blood (fibrin, thrombin), injury mediated by humoral substances (histamine, bradykinin, arachidonic acid metabolites), injury related to hypoperfusion of the lung, and (5) injury related to the loss of neurogenic regulation.

## MANAGEMENT OF RESPIRATORY FAILURE ASSOCIATED WITH BRAIN INJURY

### Monitoring

The goals of respiratory support in the head-injured patients are to maximize arterial oxygenation, maintain normal alveolar ventilation, optimize lung compliance, minimize shunt and dead-space ventilation, maintain "optimal" cardiac output, and avoid increasing intracranial pressure. In order to monitor the effectiveness of therapy (Tables 21-1 and 21-2) the following systems must be employed: continuous arterial pressure and blood gas analysis, pulmonary artery and wedge pressure monitoring with intermittent thermodilution cardiac output determination, measurement of the end-expiratory carbon dioxide concentration (to calculate dead-space ventilation), tidal volume measurement (for calculating lung compliance), and continuous intracranial pressure monitoring. To meet these goals, the equipment requirements include arterial and infrared (IR) capnograph or mass spectrometer, a portable spirometer, or pneumotachograph, and an intracranial pressure monitoring system. The calculations necessary for completing this patient information are listed in Tables 21-3 and 21-4: these should be continuously recorded at the patient's bedside.

## Therapy

### *Oxygenation*

*Positive end-expiratory pressure.* This is the most physiologically effective modality available for correcting arterial desaturation due to an increase in intrapulmonary ventilation–perfusion mismatch or shunting.[19] Positive end-expiratory pressure (PEEP) increases the functional residual capacity of the lung and thus "recruits" previously perfused but poorly ventilated or collapsed alveolar units. In pediatric patients, PEEP is most efficiently delivered by means of an endotracheal tube that is well sealed. Because all modern ventilators contain the appropriate circuits, PEEP can be delivered during either spontaneous or assisted breathing. This minimizes the time that the lung is vulnerable to airway or alveolar collapse. We institute PEEP therapy when the patient is unable to maintain an arterial $Po_2$ greater than 50 mmHg while receiving 50 percent oxygen concentration.

Positive end-expiratory pressure therapy may be counter productive if its application reduces cardiac output,[9,11] increases pulmonary vascular resistance, or reduces lung compliance. The "best PEEP" results in the maximal oxygen transport and the lowest amount of dead-space ventilation; in any patient, this number is obtained by a process of trial and error and may change with alterations in the patient's pulmonary and cardiac function. In addition, as discussed in Chapter 20, PEEP may increase intracranial pressure by inhibiting the return of cerebral blood.[16] If this effect is associated with a reduction in cardiac output, the detrimental reduction in cerebral blood flow (CBF) may outweigh the improvement in arterial oxygenation.

*Diuretics.* Administration of diuretics is most efficacious in correcting hydrostatic pulmonary edema and of less benefit in permeability pulmonary

**Table 21-1** *Respiratory Profile*

| Parameter | Normal Values (Room Air) |
|---|---|
| Arterial $PO_2$ | 95–100 mmHg |
| Arterial $PCO_2$ | 35–45 mmHg |
| Arterial pH | 7.35–7.45 |
| Arterial saturation | 98–100% |
| Arterial hemoglobin | 12–14 g% |
| Venous $PO_2$ | 35–45 mmHg |
| Alveolar $PO_2$ | 100–115 mmHg |
| Alveolar–arterial $PO_2$ | 10–15 mmHg |
| Arterial $PO_2/FIO_2$ | 400–500 |
| $V_D/V_T$* physiological | 0.33 |
| $V_D/V_T$ alveolar | 0–0.05 |
| $Q_S/Q_T$† | 0.05 |
| Static compliance | 75 ml/cm $H_2O$ |

*$V_D/V_T$ = dead-space ventilation.
†$Q_S/Q_T$ = shunt fraction.

**Table 21-2** *Hemodynamic Profile*

| Parameter | Normal Values |
|---|---|
| Blood pressure S/D<br>(mean) | 120/80 mmHg<br>80–100 mmHg |
| Heart rate | 60–90 beats/min |
| Pulmonary artery pressure (S/D)<br>(mean) | 20/10 mmHg<br>11–15 mmHg |
| Pulmonary capillary wedge (mean) | 5–12 mmHg |
| Central venous pressure (mean) | 0–9 mmHg |
| Cardiac index | 3.0–4.0 l/min/$m_2$ |
| Stroke volume index | 35–40 ml/beat/$m_2$ |
| Systemic vascular resistance index | 1700–2600 dynes-sec-cm$^{-5}$/$m_2$ |
| Pulmonary vascular resistance index | 45–225 dynes-sec-cm$^{-5}$/$m_2$ |
| Oxygen delivery | 500–700 ml/min/$m_2$ |
| Oxygen extraction | 0.20–0.25 ml/min/$m_2$ |

**Table 21-3** *Respiratory Calculations*

$$\text{Alveolar } Po_2 = (FIo_2 \times P_B - 47) - Paco_2/RQ^*$$

$$\text{Alveolar dead space } (V_D/V_T) = \frac{Paco_2 - P_E co_2 \dagger}{Paco_2}$$

$$\text{Shunt } (Q_S/Q_T) = \frac{(Cco_2 - Cao_2)\ddagger}{(Cco_2 - C\bar{v}o_2)}$$

$$\text{Static compliance} = \frac{\text{tidal volume}}{(P_{st} - \text{PEEP})}$$

$$\text{Dynamic compliance} = \frac{\text{Tidal Volume}}{(P_{max} - \text{PEEP})}$$

*$FIo_2$ = fraction of inspired oxygen; $P_B$ = barometric pressure; $RQ$ = respiratory quotient.
†$P_E co_2$ = end-tidal $CO_2$.
‡$Cco_2$ = capillary oxygen content; $Cao_2$ = arterial oxygen content; $C\bar{v}o_2$ = mixed venous oxygen contents.
§$P_{st}$ = static inspiratory pressure; $P_{max}$ = maximum inspiratory pressure.

edema. Intravenous loop diuretics (furosemide or ethacrynic acid) are utilized in our intensive care unit, as they have the advantage of augmenting the effectiveness of the osmotic agents used for intracranial hypertension. Care must be taken to avoid excessively dehydrating the patient (thereby reducing cerebral perfusion) or inducing hypokalemic metabolic alkalosis.

*Colloid fluids.* These fluids may be useful in limiting the formation of pulmonary edema fluid by increasing the serum oncotic pressure (Starling relationship). This is most likely to be beneficial by decreasing the propensity for hydrostatic pulmonary edema when the left atrial or mean arterial pressure is increased (common in head trauma) or by maintaining intravascular fluid in the presence of a damaged alveolar–capillary membrane.[14] Conflicting data exist regarding the efficacy of colloid therapy, which are considerably more expensive than crystalloid solutions. Nonetheless, we recommended the use of colloid-containing fluids for the resuscitation of the brain-injured child who has concomitant pulmonary disease.

**Table 21-4** *Hemodynamic Calculations*

Cardiac output = Blood pressure/Vascular resistance

Cardiac output = Heart rate × Stroke volume

$O_2$ delivery = Cardiac index × Arterial $O_2$ content

$O_2$ consumption = Cardiac index × (A − V) $O_2$ content

$O_2$ content = ($O_2$ Sat) (g Hb) (1.34 ml $O_2$/g Hb) + ($PO_2$) (0.003 ml $O_2$/100 ml/mmHg)

*Methylprednisolone.* Administration of methylprednisolone (30 mg/kg IV × 3 doses) has been shown to prevent the aggregation of granulocytes and subsequent complement activation in the pulmonary vascular bed, a proposed mechanism for disruption of alveolar–capillary integrity.[17] Other potential possible effects of steriods include inhibition of phospholipid (precursor of arachidonic acid) release from cell membranes, the preservation of endothelial integrity, and the inhibition of superoxide radicals (toxic oxygen byproducts). However, immune suppression as a result of high-dose steroid therapy may be a drawback in a seriously injured child. We do not routinely administer methylprednisolone to brain-injured children.

*Pulmonary vasodilators.* These are smooth-muscle relaxants or alpha-adrenergic blocking agents, which may improve arterial oxygenation in lung diseases characterized by an elevated pulmonary vascular resistance by increasing the cardiac output or decreasing dead-spacing ventilation. These drugs seldom work advantageously, however, as they are not specific for the pulmonary vascular bed. The associated reduction in the systemic vascular resistance and concomitant reduction in cardiac output offset the advantage gained in reducing the pulmonary artery pressure. In most instances pulmonary hypertension is best managed utilizing hypocapnia alkalosis (to reduce pulmonary vascular tone) and alpha-adrenergic or inotropic agents (to increase coronary blood flow).

## Ventilation

The arterial $CO_2$ content is directly proportional to the body's rate of $CO_2$ production and is inversely related to minute ventilation. Thus inadequate ventilation (hypercapnia) in the head-injured patient occurs by an excessive increase in $CO_2$ production (increased work of breathing) or by decrease in minute ventilation (decreased lung compliance, increased dead-space ventilation, apnea). We recommend the use of assisted ventilation for apnea, an arterial $P_{CO_2}$ greater than 50 mmHg, a tidal volumes less than 3 ml/kg, a vital capacity less than 15 ml/kg, dead-space ventilation greater than 50 percent, increased "work of breathing" accompanied by a reduced cardiac output, and intracranial hypertension.

In most pediatric intensive care units assisted ventilation is begun by delivering intermittent mandatory breaths (IMV) with either a volume-cycled or pressure-cycled ventilator. Delivery of IMV allows the patient to breathe spontaneously while periodically receiving a mandatory breath from the ventilator. The rate of IMV and the tidal volume (10–15 ml/kg) are preselected, and the effectiveness is determined only by analyzing arterial blood gas tensions. Although there are many techniques available for accomplishing IMV, most function with a gas reservoir that is directed into the inspiratory limb of the ventilator circuit through a one-way valve. When the patient inspires spontaneously, the valve opens, admitting gas from the reservoir. At a preselected rate, the ventilator is activated, the valve closes, and the mechanically generated tidal volume is delivered to the patient.

The choice of the type of ventilator utilized is limited by the size of the patient's airway. As a general rule, volume-cycled ventilators are preferable, as these ensure the delivery of a predetermined tidal volume regardless of changes in lung compliance. Consistent alveolar ventilation can be achieved. However, their use requires the presence of cuffed endotracheal tube to prevent air leak. Endotracheal tubes less than 5 mm in diameter are not equipped with cuffs; moreover, the young infant's airway is particularly vulnerable to pressure necrosis near the region of the cricoid cartilage. As a rule of thumb, if the patient weighs less than 10 kg, it is preferable to permit an endotracheal leak, which requires the use of a pressure-cycled ventilator.

## EFFECT OF BRAIN-INSULT-DIRECTED THERAPY ON THE LUNG

Osmotic agents such as mannitol are effective in reducing intracranial pressure by raising the serum osmolality and drawing free water from areas of the brain with an intact blood–brain barrier. Total body dehydration results, however, which adversely alters sputum viscosity (predisposing the patient to atelectasis) and reduces cardiac output. The diminution in cardiac output will result in less cerebral blood flow and, if of sufficient severity, create a lactic acidemia. Acidosis increases the work of breathing and dilates the cerebral vascular bed.

Barbiturates (thiopental and pentobarbital) are very effective in reducing intracranial pressure. However, barbiturates also reduce the cardiac output (peripheral vasodilation and direct myocardial depression) and impair pulmonary mucociliary activity (predisposing the patient to pneumonia).

Dopamine has been shown to suppress spontaneous ventilation. Elevations in the arterial $P_{CO_2}$ have been recorded in patients who were normocapnic and hypoxemic and then were administered dopamine. A resulting increase in intracranial pressure may occur in a patient with reduced cerebral compliance.

## REFERENCES

1. Bachoten M, Weibel ER: Alterations of the gas exchange apparatus in adult respiratory insufficiency associated with septicemia. Am Rev Respir Dis 116:589–615, 1977
2. Baigellman W, O'Brien JC: Pulmonary effects of head trauma. Neurosurgery 9:729–740, 1981
3. Brigham KL, Wolverton WC, Blake LH,

et al: Increased sheep lung permeability caused by pseudomonas bacteremia. J Clin Invest 54:792–904, 1975
4. Clifton GI, Ziegler MG, Grossman RG: Circulating catecholamines and sympathetic activity after head injury. Neurosurgery 8:10–13, 1981
5. Craddock PR, Fehr J, Brigham KL, et al: Complement and leukocyte mediated pulmonary dysfunction in hemodialysis. New Engl J Med 296:769–774, 1975
6. Crittenden DS, Beckman DL: Traumatic head injury and pulmonary damage. J Trauma 22:766–769, 1982
7. Deneke SM, Fanburg BL: Normobaric oxygen toxicity of the lung. New Engl J Med 303:76–86, 1980
8. Frost EAM: Respiratory problems associated with head trauma. Neurosurgery 1:300–306, 1977
9. Hemmer M, Suter PM: Treatment of cardiac and renal effects of PEEP with dopamine in patients with acute respiratory failure. Anesthesiology 50:399–403, 1979
10. Jacobs HS, Craddock PR, Hammerschmidt DE, et al: Complement induced granulocyte aggregation. An unsuspected mechanism of disease. New Engl J Med 302:789–794, 1980
11. Lynch JP, Mhyre JG, Dantzker DR: The influence of cardiac output on intrapulmonary shunt. J Appl Physiol 46:315–321, 1979
12. Milley JR, Nugent SP, Rogers MC: Neurogenic pulmonary edema in childhood. J Pediatr 94:706–799, 1979
13. Popp AJ, Shah DM, Berman RA, et al: Delayed pulmonary dysfunction in head injured patients. J Neurosurg 57;784–790, 1982
14. Rackow EC, Fein IA, Leppo J: Colloid osmotic pressure as a prognostic indicator of pulmonary edema and mortality in the critically ill. Chest 72:709–713, 1977
15. Schumaker PT, Rhodes GR, Newell JC: Ventilation–perfusion imbalance after head trauma. Am Rev Resp Dis 119:37–43, 1979
16. Shapiro HM, Marshall LF: Intracranial pressure responses to PEEP in head-injured patients. J Trauma 18:254–256, 1978
17. Sibbald WJ, Anderson RR, Reid B, et al: Alveolar–capillary permeability in human septic ARDS: Effect of high dose corticosteroid therapy. Chest 79:132–142, 1981
18. Snow RL, Davies P, Pontoppidan H, et al: Pulmonary vascular remodeling in adult respiratory distress syndrome. Am Rev Resp Dis 126:887–892, 1982
19. Suter RL, Fairley HB, Isenberg MD: Optimum end-respiratory airway pressure in patients with acute pulmonary failure. New Engl J Med 292:284–289, 1975
20. Theodore J, Robin ED: Pathogenesis of neurogenic pulmonary edema. Lancet 2:749–741, 1975
21. West J: Pulmonary Pathophysiology: The Essentials. Baltimore, Williams & Williams, 1977
22. Wilson RS, Pontoppidan H, Rie MA: Acute respiratory failure, in Ropper AH, Kennedy SK, Zervas NT (Eds): Neurological and Neurosurgical Intensive Care. Baltimore, University Park Press 1983, pp 87–106
23. Zapol WM, Snider MT: Pulmonary hypertension in severe acute respiratory failure. New Engl J Med 296:476–480, 1977

*Doris A. Trauner*

# 22

# Acute Management of Seizures

## SEIZURES IN CHILDREN

The management of ongoing seizure activity constitutes a pediatric emergency. Prolonged generalized seizures may cause permanent brain damage or death, as found in both experimental and clinical situations. It is thus imperative that an orderly approach to seizures be maintained in order to avoid delay in treatment.

A seizure is a transient disturbance of electrical activity in the brain that results in alteration in consciousness and usually in abnormal motor activity. Status epilepticus is defined as a seizure that by persisting or by being repetitive produces an enduring epileptic condition. Continuous or recurrent seizure activity lasting 20 minutes or more is considered status epilepticus.

Prolonged seizures (more than 1 hour) are accompanied by metabolic disturbances both systemically and in the brain, including lactic acidosis and hypoglycemia. Increased intracranial pressure occurs, and a variety of autonomic disturbances may be present, including hyperthermia, hypertension followed by hypotension, and eventually shock. Cardiovascular and respiratory collapses may ensue. Excessive muscle activity results in rhabdomyolysis and myoglobinuria, which may impair renal function. In addition to hypotension, this problem may result in renal failure.

The incidence of seizures in children is 2–5 percent. Most of these are febrile seizures occurring between 6 months and 4 years of age. However, a significant number of children with seizures have metabolic causes, infections

BRAIN INSULTS IN INFANTS AND CHILDREN
0-8089-1723-4

of the brain or meninges, or underlying brain damage (e.g., anoxic encephalopathy). The cause of the seizure must be determined rapidly so that specific treatment may be instituted where appropriate.

## ACUTE MANAGEMENT OF SEIZURES

### General Considerations

Whatever the cause of the seizure activity may be, it is important to minimize potential complications from the seizure itself. Of utmost importance is maintenance of an adequate airway either with an oral airway or by endotracheal intubation if necessary. Likewise, blood pressure should be monitored and stabilized to prevent shock. The child must be protected from injury such as broken bones, head trauma, or asphyxiation from vomitus. If emergency medical equipment is not available, the child should be placed on the floor in a semiprone position with the face toward the floor, and away from any hard or sharp objects or furniture. If equipment is available, a nasogastric tube should be inserted and stomach contents aspirated. The child should not be tightly restrained because of the potential for bony fractures during intense tonic activity of the muscles but should, if possible, be placed in a bed with side rails up and padded as protection against bruises or other trauma.

### History

When a child is in active seizure, there is no time to take a detailed medical history prior to initiating therapy. A nurse or other assistant who is available can obtain the necessary information. Otherwise, the parents should be asked a few brief questions: Was there any history of recent trauma? Has the child been ill or febrile? Does the child have a previous history of seizures? Is there any known toxin exposure? Is there preexisting disease?

An equally brief physical examination should be performed at the outset, including checking blood pressure, adequacy of respirations, and temperature. External signs of trauma should be looked for especially to the head, as well as any evidence of focality such as unilateral tonic or clonic movements, eye deviation to one side, or hemiparesis. A more thorough examination should be deferred until treatment has been instituted and the seizure activity terminated.

### Laboratory Tests

An IV line should be inserted and blood drawn for complete blood count, electrolytes, glucose, calcium, magnesium, liver, and renal function tests and a toxicology screen. The IV line can then be used for administering anticonvulsant medications. Arterial blood gas determinations should also be obtained. Preparations should be made for performing a lumbar puncture after seizures have stopped.

### Treatment

General rules of treatment are to decide which medication to use and to follow a logical procedure in administering it. The choice of drug therapy will depend partly on the underlying cause of the seizure. For example, if the child has never before had seizures but has had recent head trauma or an unusual illness, one may choose not to use IV phenobarbital, which would be likely to sedate the child for several hours and preclude carrying out an adequate neurological examination. In these circumstances the slow IV administration of phenytoin (Dilantin; manufactured by Parke-Davis) might be the agent of choice (18 mg/kg in normal saline solution over 15–30 min).

A typical treatment approach in children over 1 year of age is the following: administer IV glucose, 25–50 percent, 1–2 ml/kg. If seizures continue, one of the following drugs may be used: (1) IV diazepam, 0.1–0.3 mg/kg at a rate of 1 mg/min (if seizures do not stop within 10 minutes, this dose should be repeated)—diazepam may cause respiratory depression, so intubation and mechanical respiration are essential; (2) IV phenobarbital, 5 mg/kg (this dose may be repeated if seizures do not stop after 10–15 minutes); or (3) rectal paraldehyde, 0.3 ml/kg mixed with an equal amount of mineral oil, up to a maximum of 6 ml. Paraldehyde should be injected through a glass syringe only. (Paraldehyde reacts with plastic materials.)

There is *no role* for the intramuscular (IM) administration of phenobarbital or diazepam in the acute treatment of status epilepticus. Absorption is slow and erratic and makes this route ineffective for rapid treatment. It can also complicate ongoing management since blood levels of the agent administered may rise a few hours later and cause sedation or interaction with other agents administered subsequently.

### Treatment Problems

Diazepam is short-acting and although seizures may be quickly stopped, the duration of action is only 15–20 minutes and the seizures may resume. If diazepam is used, therefore, it should be followed by a longer acting anticonvulsant, such as phenobarbital (3–5 mg/kg/day) or phenytoin (5 mg/kg/day). The combination of IV diazepam and phenobarbital may cause apnea, however, so one must be prepared to mechanically ventilate the patient if this combination is used.

If the child has a significant fever, this should be treated immediately in addition to administering anticonvulsant medication; a cooling blanket and cool wet sponges can be employed. Acetaminophen suppositories may also be used.

Most children with seizures will respond to one of these modes of therapy. If the seizure activity does not abate despite these attempts, several other means are available. Intravenous lorazepam at a dose of 0.1–0.2 mg/kg (maximum 6 mg) is very effective in stopping seizures. This agent has a longer duration of action than diazepam, and usually the anticonvulsant effect will last for 6 hours or more. Another alternative is IV diazepam by continuous drip at a rate of up to 5 mg/h or high-dose barbiturates to induce burst suppression on the EEG. This latter approach requires intensive care monitoring. When barbiturates are used, it is our experience that phenobarbital is more effective than the shorter-acting barbiturates, although the use of phenobarbital results in prolonged iatrogenic coma because of its long half-life. Finally, general anesthesia is recommended by some authorities when all else fails. This is discussed further in Chapter 17. Although this procedure will arrest motor activity associated with a seizure and may decrease the epileptiform discharges, it may not prevent the seizures from continuing or recurring when the anesthetic is discontinued.

### Treatment of Seizures in Infants

The approach to acute management of seizures in infants under 1 year of age is generally similar to that of older children with a few exceptions. Following administration of 25 percent glucose (1–2 ml) solution, IV calcium gluconate (30–90 mg/kg) or pyridoxine (50–100 mg IV) may be given as well. If the seizures do not abate, diazepam or paraldehyde may be used at the same doses as mentioned above; *or* IV phenobarbital 10 mg/kg (twice the dose used for older children) may be administered, repeated if seizures persist. If these measures are unsuccessful, phenobarbital may be repeated or lorazepam used. Intravenous phenytoin (18 mg/kg slowly) may be added. We have had a great deal of success in aborting recurrent seizures in infants using clonazepam by nasogastric tube, in doses of 0.125 mg every 6 hours. Although this will not be absorbed rapidly enough to be effective in status, it will prevent recurrent seizure activity in situations where it is likely to be a problem, such as anoxic encephalopathy and drowning.

### Further Evaluation of the Child with Seizures

Once seizures have been controlled, diagnostic procedures concluded, and specific treatment initiated for the underlying cause of the seizures where necessary, long-term seizure control should be considered. Phenobarbital is the usual drug of choice for chronic therapy.

## BIBLIOGRAPHY

Delgado-Escueta AV, Bajorek JG: Status epilepticus: mechanisms of brain damage and rational management. Epilepsia 23 (Suppl 1): S29–S41, 1982

Delgado-Escueta AV, Treiman DM, Walsh GO: The treatable epilepsies. Part II. New Engl J Med 308:1576–1584, 1983

Gastaut H: Clinical and electroencephalographic classification of epileptic seizures. Epilepsia 11:102–113, 1970

Meldrum BS, Vigoroux RA, Brierley JB: Systemic factors and epileptic brain damage: Prolonged seizures in paralyzed artificially ventilated baboons. Arch Neurol 29:82–87, 1973

Russman BS: Convulsive seizures in infancy and childhood. Pediat Ann, 5 5:304–312, 1976

Tharp BR: Recent progress in epilepsy—diagnostic procedures and treatment. Calif Med 119:19–48, 1973

# PART VI

# Management of Pediatric Head Injuries and Intracranial Pressure

*Hector E. James*

# 23

# Evaluation of Head Injury in Reference to Therapy

Of all pediatric hospitalizations due to trauma, 75 percent are attributable to trauma to the head. Approximately 70 percent of the deaths that occur following trauma occur within 48 hours of hospitalization.[8] Consequently, the health care personnel first coming into contact with a child with head trauma can determine the favorable or unfavorable outcome in each patient.

Mortality rates due to head injury in children differ in the literature. Reports of mortalities of 20–25 percent[9] and 35 percent[2] differ from others who have reported a 9 percent mortality rate.[1] The variation reported most likely reflects not only the outcome of decisions made in the early phases of management, but also the availability of the correct support systems for the management of the acutely ill child, such as ready accessibility to CT scanning and the presence of a pediatric intensive care team (Intensivists, pediatric nurses, pediatric neurosurgeons).[7]

## ASSESSMENT OF BRAIN INJURY

The actual clinical state of any child should be promptly assessed by the health care personnel first coming in contact with the child to determine the magnitude of brain insult. At that time, the brain insult can be estimated as being mild, moderate, or severe in nature. This assessment may be performed by applying the Glasgow Coma Score (GCS) in those instances in which it is

BRAIN INSULTS IN INFANTS AND CHILDREN
0-8089-1723-4

applicable. For that purpose, we will consider the following three categories:

1. Mild head injury. This is defined by a GCS of 13 or more or in an infant who, following a head injury, is stunned and cries but remains alert following a very brief period of unconsciousness.
2. Moderate head injury. This is defined in a child with a GCS of 9–12 or in an infant who, following a head injury, remains lethargic or has recurrent emesis. It also applies to patients who have posttraumatic convulsions.
3. Severe head injury. This is defined by a GSC of 8 or less or in infants with severe obtundation, with or without seizures, or with obtundation and multiple trauma.

### Mild Head Injury

Children who have been observed in the emergency room as long as considered necessary and have been found to show no evidence of child abuse or neglect may be discharged and reassessed as outpatients at a later date. If a skull injury, such as a subgaleal hematoma, is present, skull radiographs should be performed to determine the presence or absence of fracture. Linear fractures in infants are not of immediate therapeutic concern but should be followed up at a later date to rule out the occurrence of a growing skull fracture (leptomeningeal cyst).[7] Patients with depressed skull fracture should be admitted to the hospital and neurosurgical consultation placed (see section on skull injuries). If child neglect or abuse is suspected, the child should be promptly admitted, and the necessary referral to the medical social services should follow.[7]

### Moderately Severe Head Injury

These patients should be hospitalized for thorough assessment and follow-up. Skull radiographs and computed tomography (CT) scans are not mandatory unless a focal injury to the skull leads one to suspect that a depressed skull fracture is present. These patients usually are combative and uncooperative when studied; thus the yield from such studies is often inadequate and may lead to a false sense of security. On the other hand, sedation of these children may lead to airway embarrassment and intracranial decompensation (see Chapter 2). Intubation for studies in this category of patient is far too invasive since, for the most part, patients will improve rapidly over a period of a few hours.

Patients with moderately severe head injuries should be admitted to the pediatric intensive care unit and supported with maintenance intravenous (IV) fluids. The IV line not only serves for hydration, but should always be promptly instituted as an emergency access route for medications, such as anticonvulsants, should they become necessary. If deterioration of consciousness ensues or seizures occur, the patient should be promptly intubated, mechanically ventilated, paralyzed, and transported to the CT suite to determine the presence or absence of a mass lesion.[7] Diazepam (0.25 mg/kg) should be the anticonvulsant given immediately for seizure control if seizures have occurred, and phenobarbital (5 mg/kg/dose) or phenytoin (5 mg/kg/dose) should follow.

Children in the moderately severe head injury category who have not shown improvement (or deterioration) at 48 hours of their hospitalization should have a CT scan. This is because epidural hematomas in children may not be manifest in the first 24 hours following trauma, as they are in adults, but more commonly appear at 48 hours.[7] Likewise, hematomas that may have been small at the time of admission may enlarge following hospitalization[7]; consequently, a CT scan is needed to determine that epidural hematoma is not present in a child who is not improving in the 48 hours following admission.

## Severe Head Injury

### *Immediate Management*

Intubation should follow immediately for any patient determined to be in this category. Intubation will lead not only to adequate oxygenation, but will reduce the $Paco_2$ level and will improve pH. In turn, intracranial pressure (ICP) will be reduced and cerebral perfusion pressure (CPP) improved (see Chapter 8). Likewise, if posttraumatic seizures occur, the airway will have already been assured and the secondary brain insult due to the seizures impeded.[7] The intubation should be performed effectively and with minimal neck manipulation to prevent spinal damage from a potentially unstable cervical spine. As IV and arterial lines are placed, a lateral cervical x-ray should be obtained to determine the presence or absence of cervical injury.

The patient should be promptly transported for CT scanning to determine the presence or absence of an operative mass lesion. If a mass lesion such as a subdural or epidural hematoma is detected, the patient should promptly be taken to the operating room for its evacuation. If no operative lesion is detected, the patient is then transported to the pediatric intensive unit, where stabilization is continued and ICP monitoring systems instituted.

It cannot be overemphasized that there should be no delay in carrying out the steps mentioned above for a child who is severely head injured, since progressive mass lesions can lead to worsening of intracranial dynamics and decompensation; for these children there may be little time in which to prevent irreversible damage (see Chapter 2).

An indwelling bladder catheter is necessary to monitor urinary output and also may eliminate the combativeness that may accompany bladder retention in the comatose patient. Placement of a nasogastric tube will aid in preventing emesis and will serve as a pathway to administer antacids when the clinical course has been stabilized, thus preventing stress gastric ulcers.

### *Aspects of Medical Therapy*

*Anticonvulsant therapy.* The administration of anticonvulsants should always be performed in the acute phase of the management of the child with a severe head injury. The reason for this is that posttraumatic epilepsy occurs in 6–16 percent of head-injured children.[7] The seizures may not be detected in the patient who is paralyzed for mechanical ventilation, and uncontrolled electrical seizures may create further brain injury (see Chapter 22). Therapy may be performed with phenobarbital (5–10 mg/kg/dose), followed by a maintenance dose of 5 mg/kg/day; or phenytoin, in equivalent doses, may be administered. Blood samples should be measured at 24–48 hours of therapy to ascertain that the appropriate therapeutic blood levels have been attained.

*Steroid therapy.* It is now clear that steroids have multiple effects on neuronal and glial metabolism (see Chapter 1) and that the effect on the insulted brain is more than a purely antiedematous effect. The clinical effectiveness of steroids in conditions other than head injury is considerable.[4,10,11,12] The effectiveness of steroids in the outcome of head injuries remains controversial[5]; thus steroids are not routinely employed. Faupel et al.,[3] in a double-blind study in head-injured adults, noted that those receiving high-dose dexamethasone had a significantly better outcome and lower mortality rate than did those receiving placebo or low-dose dexamethasone therapy. A similar finding was noted in a preliminary study done in head-injured children,[6] and this study is currently being expanded. The concern for deleterious side effects, such as a high incidence of infections, pulmonary complications, and gastric hemorrhage, has not been documented.[3,6]

*Diuretic therapy.* The mainstay of diuretic therapy for the control of ICP is currently hypertonic mannitol. Its application in the child with head injury is outlined in Figure 23-1. Further discussion on diuretic therapy and dosages is given in Chapter 26.

*Barbiturate therapy.* Barbiturates are employed for sedation and control of intracranial hypertension as well as for the treatment of seizures in severe head injury. Their place in the treatment regimen of the severely head injured child is illustrated in Figure 23-1. Further analysis as to the role and dosage of barbiturates in such therapy is presented in Chapter 2.

*Mechanical ventilation therapy.* Mechanical ventilation therapy continues to be the mainstay of the management of the child with head injury. Its role in the child with a severe brain injury is illustrated in Figure 23-1. Further analysis of ventilation therapy is outlined in Chapter 25.

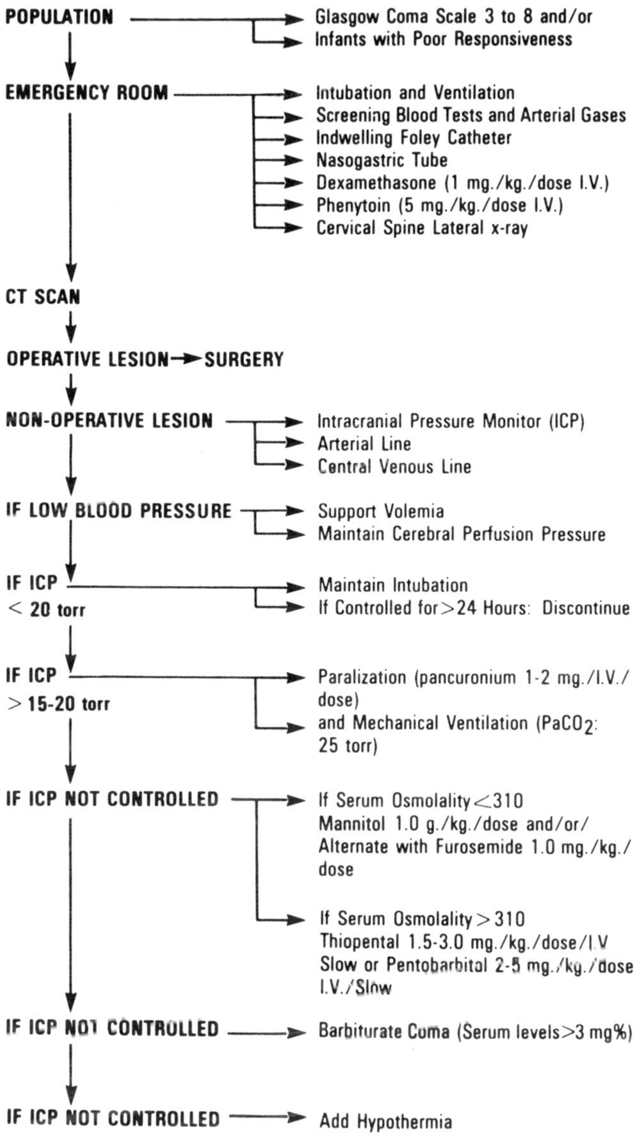


**Fig. 23-1.** Approach to the management of severe head injury.

## MANAGEMENT OF SKULL INJURIES

Contusions and abrasions do not require treatment other than topical therapy and assessment of tetanus prophylaxis. A subgaleal collection is commonly due to blood from a linear skull fracture. This requires no specific therapy, and management should be determined by the outcome of the assessment of the brain injury (see previous section). In follow up of an infant however, skull radiographs are needed to determine that a leptomeningeal cyst is not developing.[7] A comminuted skull fracture should be of no operative concern unless it is compound or depressed. In the compound skull fracture, immediate neurosurgical debridement and exploration is needed to prevent subsequent local and intracranial infections. A depressed skull fracture that is not compound should be assessed by the neurosurgical consultant as to whether surgical exploration and elevation is needed in each individual situation.[7] Periorbital ecchymosis or ecchymosis behind the ear in the mastoid region, or hemotympanum, indicate a basilar skull fracture. Bedrest will be needed, as well as careful monitoring of temperature. If febrile spikes occur, immediate blood and cerebrospinal fluid (CSF) cultures (lumbar puncture) should be obtained and the patient initiated on broad-spectrum antibiotic coverage, pending the results of the cultures. This phenomenon may occur when there is a CSF fistula at the base of the skull and organisms have entered the meninges.[7]

Following the initial evaluation of brain and skull injuries, the concomitant and subsequent systemic stabilization of the patient is mandatory. This is discussed in Chapter 24.

## REFERENCES

1. Bruce DA, Schut L: Recent advances in the treatment of head injuries. Pediatr Ann 5:643–656, 1976
2. Carlsson CA, Von Essen A, Lofgren A: Factors affecting the clinical course of patients with severe head injury. J Neurosurg 29:242–251, 1968
3. Faupel G, Reulen HJ, Schurmann K: Double-blind study on the effects of dexamethasone on severe closed head injuries, in Pappius H, Reulen HJ (Eds): Dynamics of Brain Edema. Berlin, Springer, 1976, pp 337–343
4. Gailich JH, French LA: Use of dexamethasone in the treatment of cerebral edema resulting from brain tumors and brain surgery. Am Practit 12:169–174, 1961
5. Gobiet W: The influence of various doses of dexamethasone on intracranial pressure in patients with severe head injuries, in Pappius H, Reulen HJ (Eds): Dynamics of Brain Edema. Berlin, Springer, 1976, pp 351–353
6. James HE, Madauss WC, Tibbs PA, et al: The effect of high dose dexamethasone therapy in children with severe head injury. Acta Neurochirurg 45:225–236, 1979
7. James HE: Head injuries in infants, children and adolescents, in Nussbaum E (Ed): Pediatric Intensive Care. Mount Kisco, New York, Futura Publishing Company, 1984, pp 55–77

8. Jamieson D, Kay HH: Accidental head injury in childhood. Arch Dis Childh 49:376–381, 1974
9. Jennet B, Teadsale G, Baakman R, et al: Predicting outcome in individual patients after head injury. Lancet 1:1031–1034, 1976
10. Long DM, Hartmann FJ, French LA: The response of human cerebral edema to glucosteroid administration. Neurology 16:521–528, 1966
11. Meinig G, Aulich A, Wende S, et al: The effect of dexamethasone and diuretics on peritumoral brain edema: Comparative study of tissue water content and computed tomography, in Pappius H, Reulen HJ (Eds): Dynamics of Brain Edema. Berlin, Springer, 1976, pp 301–305
12. Weinstein JD, Toy FJ, Jaffe ME, et al: The effects of dexamethasone on brain edema in patients with metastatic brain tumors. Neurology 23:121–129, 1973

*Robert C. Pascucci*

# 24

# Stabilization of the Patient with Head Injury and Multiple Trauma

Physical trauma is the principal cause of death among Americans between the ages of 1 and 38 years.[23] Since its victims are often those at or near the beginning of their most productive work years, its cost measured in terms of lost potential and productivity is high: the total annual cost of accidental trauma, including lost wages, medical expenses, and indirect work losses, amounts to about $58 billion. Children, because of incomplete physical and intellectual development, are especially vulnerable to trauma. Approximately 15,000 children under 15 years of age die from accidental injuries each year in the United States; most of these are motor vehicle injuries.[2,7]

Head injuries, either isolated or in combination with multiple-system injury, are extremely common in children. Various studies[5,10,13–15,17] have revealed head injury to be present in 70–80 percent of children with injuries severe enough to require admission to hospital; no other single body area was involved as frequently. Approximately half of seriously injured patients with head injury will be found to have injuries to another body system as well. Patients whose multiple injuries including head injury have a worsened prognosis, and the combination of head injury and other bodily injuries results in a poorer outcome than either injury alone.

The injured child is usually brought to the hospital emergency ward for initial treatment. Management of the patient may continue there; or, with a growing trend toward regionalization of health care, transfer of the severely injured child to a pediatric trauma center may be considered. We will consider here the provision of life support to the pediatric trauma victim, through

BRAIN INSULTS IN INFANTS AND CHILDREN
0-8089-1723-4

assessment of the injury and initial stabilization and transport of the child for definitive therapy.

## EMERGENCY RESUSCITATION

It is unusual for the child with isolated brain injury, unless that injury is devastating, to present in shock or with cardiopulmonary arrest. If multiple areas of injury are present or a hypoxic or ischemic event has intervened, however, such a presentation is more likely. In this circumstance, initial attention must be directed to global resuscitation of the child; more sophisticated efforts to protect and preserve brain function presume that adequate oxygenation and perfusion have been restored and are not indicated until that is the case.

### History

Although resuscitation of the child cannot be delayed while a detailed history is obtained, basic information should be obtained while it is fresh in the observers' and rescuers' minds. The specific circumstances of the head injury and the succeeding course should be sought. The mechanism of injury and the activity in which it was sustained may suggest the presence of associated injuries, as in the common occurrence of cervical spine injuries in diving accidents. Information regarding the patient's general medical health and preexisting medical conditions may be invaluable in directing further care. The circumstances of the trauma may raise suspicion of child abuse or neglect; although it may be inappropriate to pursue this possibility in the emergency room setting, it is useful to gather whatever information is available for later review.

### Rapid Physical Examination

The first few moments with the patient are spent in assessment of airway, breathing, and circulation and in immediate correction of abnormalities in these areas. A rapid examination of the entire child, with special attention to head and neck, chest, abdomen, and extremities, can proceed simultaneously with resuscitation. Active external hemorrhage is controlled, most often with direct pressure.

An initial neurological assessment is made as soon as practical. Such assessment includes examination of the head and neck for ecchymoses, obvious fractures or dislocations, and penetrating wounds. Bleeding or CSF drainage from the nose or ear is noted. Evaluation of the patient's global level of consciousness [as on the Glasgow Coma Scale (GSC)], cranial nerve and brainstem reflexes, or spinal cord function and examination for specific lateralizing signs are completed as quickly as possible and repeated at intervals throughout stabilization.

### Airway

An adequate airway must be established at once. Although simple positioning is the key to restoration of the airway in most children, in victims of head trauma it must be assumed that cervical spine injury is present until ruled out by examination and/or radiological study. Most unstable cervical spine injuries become worse with neck flexion and are generally improved by gentle axial traction or neck extension. The usual "sniffing" position, often best for airway maintenance and tracheal intubation, should not be used when cervical spine injuries are suspected.[19] A knowledgeable individual other than the one managing the airway should assume responsibility for maintaining the head in the "neutral" position with gentle but firm axial traction.[8] Sandbagging or splinting of the cervical spine early in the course of resuscitation may prevent inadvertent flexion or dislocation with consequent increase in pressure on the cervical cord.

Anterior displacement of the jaw and tongue by forceful dislocation of the mandible at its angles will relieve soft-tissue obstruction of the airway and can be employed even if cervical spine injury is present. Continuous gentle positive airway pressure may then "splint" the airway open and allow gas exchange; an oral airway (but not a nasal one, if fracture of the cribriform plate is suspected) may prove useful.

Oxygen is administered as soon as it can be made available, and bag–mask ventilation is begun if the patient's own efforts are inadequate. Both hypoxemia and hypercapnia are potent stimulants for the increase of cerebral blood flow (CBF); we recommend the use of 100 percent oxygen to ensure $Pa_{O_2}$ level of greater than 100 torr and sufficient alveolar ventilation and fresh-gas flow to reduce the $Pa_{CO_2}$ to the range of 28–32 torr. If adequate ventilation cannot be provided, the possibility of a foreign-body airway obstruction must be considered. Removal of such material may be accomplished with a finger sweep of the posterior pharynx or, preferably, with an instrument under direct vision. Direct trauma to the larynx and upper airway may also impede ventilation, and it may be appropriate to move directly to intubation or in more severe cases, to cricothyrotomy or tracheostomy. Adequacy of ventilation is confirmed by improvement of the patient's condition and by auscultation of bilaterally symmetrical breath sounds (see the following section).

### Endotracheal Intubation

Intubation of the trachea will provide a more secure airway and allow access for continued ventilatory assistance; if there is any doubt regarding the patient's ability to maintain an adequate airway, this procedure is indicated. It is better to err on the side of early intubation than to have serious airway difficulties develop a few hours later, requiring emergency intubation under less controlled circumstances. This procedure should not be the first priority of the physician, however; ventilation and oxygenation come first. When all necessary materials and personnel are available, intubation may be performed by the most experienced person present.

The pertinent differences in the anatomy and physiology of the pediatric airway have been discussed earlier and need not be repeated here. If cervical spine injury is not present, the conventional techniques of direct laryngoscopy and intubation may be performed as usual. It must be understood that these procedures are potent noxious stimuli, however, and have been shown to produce large rises in intracranial pressure in patients with decreased intracranial compliance.[21] Children recently subjected to head trauma are thought to have a relatively increased cerebral blood flow (CBF)[20,26] with possible decreased compliance and risk for developing increased ICP; therefore, it is essential to provide protection against further rises in intracranial pressure during laryngoscopy and intubation. The child in frank cardiopulmonary arrest must be intubated without use of depressant drugs. If cardiovascular performance is adequate, however, intubation should be performed swiftly and efficiently under anesthetic coverage.[22] Our practice is to anesthetize the patient with generous doses of thiopental and muscle relaxants (see Table 24-1); intravenous (IV) lidocaine has also been shown to modify the ICP response to laryngoscopy[3,9] and may be used in addition to the agents mentioned above. The anesthetic agents listed in Table 24-1 are useful in emergency intubation. Drugs other than atropine should be administered only by personnel experienced in their use and prepared to deal with possible adverse effects. Barbiturates should be employed with caution in patients with hypovolemia.

### Ventilation

Ventilation must be coordinated with chest compression if cardiopulmonary (CPR) is ongoing. The most reliable indicators of adequate ventilation are auscultation of the lungs, adequate chest wall movement, and clinical response. Chest wall and pulmonary compliance will vary from moment to moment during resuscitation, particularly if there has been chest or abdominal trauma; undue resistance to ventilation or newly assymmetric breath sounds may suggest a developing pneumothorax or hemothorax requiring

**Table 24-1** *Intravenous Anesthetic Agents for Children*

| Drug | Dose | Comments |
|---|---|---|
| Atropine | 0.02 mg/kg | Vagolytic |
| Thiopental | 2–6 mg/kg | Rapid induction; protection against increases in ICP; Avoid use in patients with hypotension or hypovolemia |
| Methohexital sodium | 1–2 mg/kg | Same as above; May induce seizures in susceptible patients |
| Succinylcholine | 1–2 mg/kg | Rapid-acting muscle relaxant. Bradycardia common in children and should be preceded by atropine; risk of hyperkalemia in susceptible patients |
| Pancuronium bromide | 0.1–0.15 mg/kg | Moderately rapid onset of muscle relaxation; protective of heart rate and blood pressure |
| Lidocaine | 1–1.5 mg/kg | Suppresses cardiovascular and ICP response to laryngoscopy and intubation |

prompt evacuation. Bleeding in the airway may lead to clotting and occlusion of the endotracheal tube; frequent irrigation and suctioning are essential.

### Circulation

External chest compression will provide subnormal but adequate circulatory support; it should be employed not only in the setting of complete cardiac arrest, but at any time that spontaneous cardiac output seems inadequate. The rate and technique are as recommended by the American Heart Association[16] and will vary with the child's age and size. Inadequate perfusion despite adequate heart rate and contractility implies hypovolemia and requires volume restoration as discussed in the following paragraphs.

### Venous Access

The techniques and landmarks for venous cannulation are identical in children and adults. Care should be taken to establish IV lines of sufficient caliber to allow rapid fluid resuscitation. It is often wise to establish two or more access points on opposite sides of the diaphragm, to ensure venous continuity between the IV site and the heart. Although central venous access may be helpful in later patient management, central venous pressure (CVP) measurements add little to the initial management of pediatric trauma, and prolonged efforts to insert a central line are unnecessary until the patient is more stable. If venous access is unavoidably delayed, certain resuscitation drugs (atropine, epinephrine, lidocaine) may be administered intratracheally with good effect.

### Volume

Hypovolemia is common in the pediatric trauma patient and must be corrected before adequate systemic and CNS perfusion can be restored. Tachycardia, rather than hypotension, is the hallmark of inadequate intravascular volume in the child. Volume replacement is begun early, guided by clinical history, physical and laboratory evidence of poor perfusion, degree of tachycardia, and response to volume challenge.

Volume replacement in the child is given in aliquots of 10–20 ml/kg, administered quickly by direct syringe infusion. Although isotonic crystalloid may be used at first, colloid may be preferable in the brain-injured child to avoid excessive leakage of fluid across the blood–brain barrier. Satisfactory response to volume infusion will be manifest by slowing of the heart rate, improved perfusion, and correction of metabolic acidosis. In the setting of brain injury, the goal should be sufficient but not overzealous volume administration, to ensure systemic and cerebral perfusion without occasioning fluid excesses and edema formation.

### Drug Administration and Other Support

The drugs used in pediatric resuscitation differ little from those used in adult practice; doses are noted in Table 24-2. All the drugs listed in Table 24-2 are intended for IV administration; atropine, lidocaine, and epinephrine may be diluted with sterile water and given intratracheally (IT). The intracardiac route (IC) is hazardous and should be avoided if possible. Special attention must be paid to correction of hypoglycemia (common in the stressed neonate) and hypocalcemia (with rapid infusion of citrated blood products).

Restoration and preservation of normal body temperature is essential; the cold infant will remain acidotic and poorly perfused, and resuscitation is frequently unsuccessful until core body temperature is greater than 34–35°. If defibrillation is necessary, an initial "dose" of 2–6 joules/kg is appropriate. Persistent arrythmias are unusual in children following successful correction of hypoxia, acidosis, and perfusion; if they are present, increased intracranial pressure or a posterior fossa lesion may be responsible, and further investigation is appropriate.

**Table 24-2** *Pediatric Resuscitation Drugs*

| Drug | Dose | Comments |
|---|---|---|
| Atropine | 0.02 mg/kg | Indications: Bradycardia<br>Cautions: Administer full dose; partial doses may paradoxically slow rate by central vagal stimulation |
| Epinephrine | 10 μg/kg (0.1 cc/kg of 1/10,000 solution) | Indications: Asystole, to stimulate cardiac activity; fine ventricular fibrillation, to coarsen before electroshock; to increase vascular tone and perfusion pressure<br>Cautions: Avoid in recurrent ventricular fibrillation |
| $NaHCO_3$ (Sodium) bicarbonate) | 1–2 mEq/kg (initial)<br>0.5–1 mEq/kg (repeat) | Indications: Metabolic acidosis<br>Cautions: Avoid excessive administration; dilute 1:1 with $D_5W$ for infants, infusing slowing<br>Repeat doses guided by measurements of arterial gases and pH |
| Naloxone (Narcan, Endo Pharmaceuticals) | 10 μg/kg; repeat as needed | Indications: Suspected narcotic overdose<br>Cautions: If effective, watch for renarcotization as effect of the drug wears off |
| Dopamine | 2–5 μg/kg/min<br>5–10 μg/kg/min<br>10–20 μg/kg/min | Renal–splanchnic effect<br>Some $beta_1$ action<br>Alpha effects begin |

**Table 24-2** *(continued)*

| Drug | Dose | Comments |
|---|---|---|
| | | Indications:<br>Low-output state; impaired renal or splanchnic perfusion<br>Cautions:<br>Tachydysrhythmias, excessive vasoconstriction |
| Isoproterenol | 0.05–2 μg/kg/min | Indications:<br>Bradycardia; refractory status asthmaticus<br>Cautions:<br>Vasodilator; may lower blood pressure; may precipitate tachyarrhythmias; increases myocardial oxygen requirement and may aggravate myocardial ischemia |
| Dobutamine | 2.5–20 μg/kg/min | Indications:<br>Low-output state<br>Cautions:<br>Tachycardia and dysrhythmias |
| Epinephrine | 0.05–1.0 μg/kg/min | Indications:<br>Refractory low-output state<br>Cautions:<br>May cause intense vasoconstriction |
| Calcium chloride | 10–30 mg/kg | Indications:<br>Hypotension; electromechanical dissociation; hyperkalemia<br>Cautions:<br>May aggravate digoxin toxicity; extravasation may yield tissue necrosis; rapid administration may produce bradycardia |

**Table 24-2** *(continued)*

| Drug | Dose | Comments |
|---|---|---|
| Calcium gluconate | 30–90 mg/kg | Indications:<br>Same as $CaCl_2$<br>Cautions:<br>Slightly less sclerotic; requires hepatic metabolism to release calcium ion |
| Lidocaine | 1 mg/kg (bolus); 15–50 μg/kg/min (infusion) | Indications:<br>Ventricular tachycardia or ectopy<br>Cautions:<br>Metabolism slowed in congestive failure; avoid in high degrees of AV block; rapid administration may cause seizures; infusion rarely needed in children |
| Bretylium tosylate | 5 mg/kg (initial)<br>10 mg/kg (repeat) to cumulative maximum of 30 mg/kg | Indications:<br>Ventricular tachycardia or fibrillation, especially if refractory to other antiarrhythmics<br>Cautions:<br>Orthostatic hypotension, especially if less than 5-mg/kg dosage is given; nausea, vomiting in the awake patient if given too fast |
| Dextrose | 0.5–1.0 g/kg<br>(2–4 cc/kg of 25% solution) | Indications:<br>Hypoglycemia (documented or suspected)<br>Cautions:<br>Hypertonic solution—administer slowly; do not overtreat |

## ASSESSMENT AND STABILIZATION OF THE INJURED CHILD

As the child improves, a more complete assessment of the extent of injury is made. The assessment process is a dynamic one, with the working diagnosis and plan being continuously updated by new information and by the child's response to therapy.[4] A complete, systematic physical examination is performed, with special attention to the areas most frequently injured: the chest, the abdomen, the extremities, and the head.

### Chest

Adequacy of oxygenation and ventilation should be assured and modest hyperventilation considered if increased ICP is suspected. Asymmetry of breath sounds, tracheal deviation, or displacement of the cardiac apex may suggest pneumothorax or hemothorax and the need for a tube thoracostomy. Open chest wounds and flail-chest segments will require attention; positive-pressure controlled ventilation is beneficial in these cases. A chest x-ray is of value in evaluating such conditions and may reveal clinically unsuspected areas of atelectasis or contusion.

Cardiac performance and peripheral perfusion are continuously reevaluated. Cardiac tamponade is rare in children but cannot be overlooked; muffled heart sounds, dyspnea, a weak and thready pulse, and distended neck veins all suggest the diagnosis. More commonly, poor cardiac output will be a result of residual hypovolemia and be manifest by tachycardia, peripheral vasoconstriction, and a persistent metabolic acidosis. If rapid volume infusion improves the child's condition but deterioration recurs after the volume load has been completed, ongoing losses are occurring.[18,25] It is unlikely that hypovolemic shock will ensue purely from closed head injury,[1,6,22] and other etiologies should be sought in these patients. Hypotension associated with warm and flushed skin, peripheral vasodilation, and flaccid limbs suggest a high spinal cord lesion with consequent functional sympathectomy.[11,20]

### Abdomen

Blunt rather than penetrating injury is seen in children, and perforation of a hollow viscus is rare. Conservative therapy is thus the rule, and surgery is avoided unless there is clinical evidence of deterioration. Abdominal distention from acute gastric dilation is common, and placement of an orogastric or nasogastric tube is recommended to ease ventilation and minimize the risk of vomiting and aspiration. Laboratory evaluation of the abdomen may include plain films, an IVP, a radionuclide liver–spleen scan, or an abdominal CT scan. Peritoneal lavage is seldom used to determine the need for operation in children unless serial abdominal examinations will be impossible or contraindicated because of other injuries or ongoing therapy.

### Extremities

Injuries to the extremities need little attention in initial therapy. Stabilization of injured areas and control of bleeding is necessary, and neurovascular integrity must be evaluated and appropriate measures taken to ensure peripheral perfusion.

## TRANSFER TO DEFINITIVE CARE

The greatest danger to critically ill patients is often during transfer from one hospital to another or from one area within a hospital to another. The injured child must receive continued close attention during such transfers to anticipate and resolve problems arising enroute. Ideally, the physician supervising the child's care from the onset will be able to stay with the child and provide ongoing care. If this is not possible, another physician should be asked to assume this responsibility. In areas with regional pediatric referral centers, a transport team (physician, nurse, and/or other personnel) and equipment may be available to move the child. The referring physician must provide adequate information on the child's condition and previous management to this team to ensure safe transfer.

Finally, care must be provided for the family of the injured child. Feelings of guilt are common in parents and siblings. Young children, particularly, do not understand the true causes for illness or injury. They often consider themselves at fault for injury of a brother or sister; the physician can provide reassurance that it was not. The prognosis for head-injured children is not always grim,[12,26] and parents will benefit from cautious optimism, if appropriate, and from the caring attention of the physician and other health care personnel.

## REFERENCES

1. Bartkowski HM, Pitts LH: Neurologic injury, in Trunkey DD, Lewis FR (Eds): Current therapy of trauma 1984–1985, Philadelphia, B C Decker, 1984
2. Christoffel KK, Tanz R: Motor vehicle injury in childhood. Pediatr Rev 4:247–254, 1983
3. Donegan MF, Bedford RF: Intravenously administered lidocaine prevents intracranial hypertension during endotracheal suctioning. Anesthesiology 52:516–518, 1980
4. Fallis JC: Initial assessment of the injured child, in care for the injured child, Toronto, The Surgical Staff, The Hospital for Sick Children; Baltimore, Williams & Wilkins, 1975
5. Fife D, Jagger J: The contribution of brain injury to the overall injury severity

of brain-injured patients. J Neurosurg 60:697–699, 1984

6. Fischer EG: Head injuries, in May HL (Ed): Emergency Medicine, New York, John Wiley & Sons, 1984
7. Gratz IR: Accidental injury in childhood: A literary review on pediatric trauma. J Trauma 19:551–555, 1979
8. Greifenstein FE, Gegg WS: Anesthesia in the presence of injuries to the cervical spine, in Zauder HL (Ed): Anesthesia for Orthopedic Surgery, Philadelphia, F A Davis, 1980
9. Hamill JF, Bedford RF, Weaver DC, et al: Lidocaine before endotracheal intubation: Intravenous or endotracheal? Anesthesiology 55:578–581, 1981
10. Holmes MJ, Reyes HM: A critical review of urban pediatric trauma. J Trauma 24:253–255, 1984
11. Hussey RW: Spinal cord injuries, in May HL (Ed): Emergency Medicine, New York, John Wiley & Sons, 1984
12. Mahoney WJ, D'Souza BJ, Haller JA, et al: Long-Term Outcome of Children with Severe Head Trauma and Prolonged Coma. Pediatrics 71:756–762, 1983
13. Mayer T, Walker ML, Clark P: Further experience with the modified abbreviated injury severity scale. J Trauma 24:31–34, 1984
14. Mayer T, Walker ML, Johnson DG: Causes of morbidity and mortality in severe pediatric trauma. JAMA 245:719–721, 1981
15. Mayer T, Walker ML, Shasha I, et al: Effect of multiple trauma on outcome of pediatric patients with neurologic injuries. Child's Brain 8:189–197, 1981
16. McIntyre KM, Lewis AJ (Eds): Textbook of Advanced Cardiac Life Support. American Heart Association, 1981
17. McKoy C, Bell MJ: Preventable traumatic deaths in children. J Pediatr Surg 18:505–508, 1983
18. Morse TS: The child with multiple injuries. Emerg Med Clin N Am 1:175–185, 1983
19. Pitts LH: The Management of Acute Cerebral and Spinal Cord Trauma, ASA Refresher Course Lectures, 1981
20. Raphaely RC, Swedlow DB, Downes JJ, et al: Management of severe pediatric head trauma. Pediatr Clin N Am 27:714–727, 1980
21. Shapiro HM, Wyte SR, Harris AB, et al: Acute Intraoperative Intracranial Hypertension in Neurosurgical Patients. Anesthesiology 37:399–405, 1972
22. Teasdale G, Galbraith S: Head trauma and intracranial hemorrhage, in Grenvik A, Safar P (Eds): Brain Failure and Resuscitation, New York, Churchill Livingstone, 1981
23. Templeton JJ, Broennie AM: Emergency department anesthetic management, in Fleisher G, Ludwig S (Eds): Textbook of Pediatric Emergency Medicine, Baltimore, Williams & Wilkins, 1983
24. Trunkey DD: Trauma. Sci Am 249:2,28–35, 1983
25. Zeigler MM: Major trauma, in: Fleisher G, Ludwig S (Eds): Textbook of Pediatric Emergency Medicine, Baltimore, Williams & Wilkins, 1983
26. Zimmerman RA, Bilaniuk LT, Bruce D, et al: Computed tomography of pediatric head trauma: Acute general cerebral swelling. Radiology 126:403–408, 1978

*Derek A. Bruce*

# 25

# Ventilation, Hyperventilation, Megaventilation, and Cerebral Blood Flow

Arterial $CO_2$ concentration has potent cerebrovascular effects. In the normal state, there is a 3–4 percent change in cerebral blood flow (CBF) for each 1-mm change in $Paco_2$ and a concomitant effect on cerebral blood volume (CBV). As described previously (Chapter 5), $CO_2$ response curves in adult human beings and experimental animals show that below a $Paco_2$ of approximately 20 torr no further decrease in CBF occurs despite continued hyperventilation. This suggests that a balance has been reached between the vasoconstrictor effects of decreasing $Paco_2$ in the vessel wall and the vasodilator effects produced by cerebral metabolic needs. The implication is that the cerebral metabolic control is dominant over the $Paco_2$ effect and thus adequate CBF for metabolism is preserved. Despite this finding there is a widespread belief that hyperventilation may induce brain ischemia. This is addressed later in this chapter. In normal volunteers, continued hyperventilation over 6 hours results in a gradual return of CBF toward normal.[6] This is the result of two mechanisms. The first mechanism involves gradual normalization of cerebrospinal fluid (CSF) alkalosis as bicarbonate increases. The other probable mechanism involves accumulation of metabolic end products resulting in a gradual reconstitution of the normal balance between blood flow and metabolism. In unconscious patients with decreased metabolism this reconstitution of blood flow despite continued hyperventilation does not appear to recur.

BRAIN INSULTS IN INFANTS AND CHILDREN
0-8089-1723-4

## VENTILATION

Mechanical ventilation alone will not produce any beneficial effects on children with head injury unless the child is hypoventilating as a result of pulmonary, medullary, or spinal cord injury. Preoperative tracheostomy has been shown to have a beneficial effect on the outcome of patients with head injury, as has the introduction of mechanical ventilation. There is increasing evidence to suggest that intermittent episodes of systemic hypoxemia occur spontaneously in head-injured patients, even in the intensive care unit (ICU) setting, and that mechanical ventilation may limit or minimize these. In small children there is evidence that spontaneous hyperventilation results in exhaustion of pulmonary musculature and a diminished ventilatory capacity[1]; thus another potential benefit from mechanical ventilation is present in children.[1] There are pitfalls, however, in the use of positive-pressure ventilation, particularly in patients with pneumothorax or reduced circulatory volume, and the ventilator settings must be adjusted appropriately to avoid prolonged elevated intrathoracic pressure. In small children the risk of pneumothorax is present and increases with greater degrees of positive end-expiratory pressure (PEEP).

## HYPERVENTILATION

An improved outcome has been obtained in head-injured patients with the use of mechanical ventilation. Further studies showed almost immediate improvement in EEG, particularly in young patients, following head trauma who were placed on mechanical hyperventilation. There are many potential benefits to be derived from hyperventilation. The obvious ones are decreases in cerebral blood flow and cerebral volume, resulting in lowered intracranial pressure (ICP). These may be the least important, however, especially in patients with already low ICP following trauma. A decrease in arteriolar pressure will result in decreased capillary pressure and decreased edema formation. This will also result in decreased venous capillary pressure and a tendency for removal of extracellular fluid from the brain down the hydrostatic gradient. Moreover, the reversal of brain tissue and CSF acidosis, which is a common accompaniment of severe head trauma, might be beneficial. There is also evidence that hyperventilation can improve the state of pressure autoregulation following trauma.[2] Finally, a decreased $Pa_{CO_2}$ may directly affect neuronal membranes, resulting in hyperpolarization and a decreased firing that would result in decreased energy utilization and might be a beneficial protective mechanism for the cell.[3]

Is hyperventilation dangerous? If done improperly, the answer is "yes." If the intrathoracic pressure is elevated, especially in a child with decreased blood volume, the decreased venous return can result in poor cardiac output, decreased arterial pressure and decreased cerebral blood flow.[5] The major concerns about hyperventilation, however, is the suggestion that primary brain ischemia can be produced. The evidence for this is poor. Slowing on the EEG is seen with voluntary hyperventilation and in at least one study could be abolished with hyperoxygenation. These changes, however, could be due to the direct effects on membrane potential of the decreased $CO_2$. Elevated lactate production in the brain at a $Paco_2$ around 20 torr has been reported. This, however, is probably a reflection of the pH sensitivity, of the phosphofructokinase enzyme with increased flux through this step in the glycolytic pathway as a result of the increased pH. If the energy needs are not changed, the excess pyruvate will go to lactate and dissipate from the brain.[3] Pyruvate crosses the blood–brain barrier poorly; thus an increase in lactate and lactate/pyruvate ratio cannot be equated with cerebral ischemia.[3] Studies in which cerebral high-energy phosphates have been measured have shown no change in adenosine triphosphate (ATP) or energy-charged potential despite $Paco_2$ levels around 10 torr in studies in mice, cats, and monkeys.[3] Increased lactate was found in all animal models, but as mentioned above cannot be taken as a hallmark for ischemia. Finally, a decrease in phosphocreatinine was seen in cats and monkeys.[3] This may demonstrate that as CBF falls to a critical level, the alteration in CBF triggers a response that results in local vasodilatation and thus no further decrease in CBF. As mentioned above, it appears that as CBF drops to a threshold level, metabolic autoregulation overcomes the effect of the $CO_2$-induced vasodilation and no further drop in CBF occurs. There is thus no reliable evidence that significant brain ischemia can be induced by hyperventilation.[1]

There is increasing evidence that the CBF responses to hypoxemia and hypotension are not altered by hyperventilation. One final concern is that the alkalosis will produce a shift in the hemoglobin dissociation curve that could result in inadequate tissue oxygenation. Although this is a theoretical problem, it does not appear to be of practical importance in children.[4,5]

## MEGAVENTILATION

The use of hyperventilation in clinical practice is directed mainly toward control of elevated ICP, but following head trauma in children, mild hyperventilation to $Paco_2$ levels of 25–30 torr may have other benefits as described previously: decreased edema formation, improved edema resolution, decreased energy utilization due to hyperpolarization, and improved pressure autoregulation. If ICP is elevated above 20 torr despite modest hyperventilation, how much further hyperventilation is desireable, and what monitoring may be helpful? Probably the single most useful measure is arteriojugular oxygen difference (AJD$O_2$). This will increase as CBF decreases and is a simple way to follow the oxygen level required by the brain. In hypoxemia normal brain bioenergetics can be demonstrated with jugular oxygen tensions below 10 torr, whereas a drop in energy change potential can occur during hemorrhagic hypotension with jugulovenous oxygens above 30 torr. We have taken a jugular venous $O_2$ of 20 torr as the lower limits of acceptable during clinical hyperventilation. The usual limiting factor to the use of hyperventilation in children is the response of the ICP. Our own unpublished data in children suggest that no further decrease in CBF occurs below a $Paco_2$ of approximately 15 torr; therefore, one would not expect any further ICP effect below this point. We frequently see a further decrease in ICP as $CO_2$ is lowered to the low teens. This may best be explained by some increase in red cell velocity that functions to maintain blood flow despite further decrease in vascular caliber, or that this further decrease in blood volume is produced at the venous end of the circulation and does not affect the resistance vessels and thus does not decrease CBF. In children in whom ICP cannot be controlled by combinations of hyperventilation to 20 torr, muscle paralysis, head-up position or administration of mannitol or barbiturates, we have no hesitation in decreasing the $Paco_2$ in a stepwise fashion to 15 torr or less as long as an effect of the ICP obtained.[1] We make no effort to treat the alkalosis. This degree of hyperventilation can, however, be a hazard when suctioning is performed. As the child's ICP is often very sensitive to minor increases in $Paco_2$, when suctioning is performed, manual hyperventilation should be done to control the ICP at the level that it was with mechanical ventilation. Suctioning must be done in short bursts to avoid significant ICP changes. After such hyperventilation for days, the $Paco_2$ response appears to be enhanced, and a slow return of $CO_2$ to normal over many days is necessary to avoid recurrence of elevated ICP.

In conclusion, hyperventilation lowers CBF with a plateau in the CBF–$CO_2$ curve in children somewhere between 15 and 20 torr.[1] There appears to be no evidence that brain ischemia can be produced by such therapy. There are risks involved, however, in maintenance of adequate systemic volume. Avoidance of increased intrathoracic pressure is necessary if such megaventilation is to be performed safely. Monitoring of jugular venous $O_2$ is recommended if prolonged hyperventilation below 20 torr is to be performed.

## REFERENCES


1. Bruce DA: Effects of hyperventilation on cerebral blood flow and metabolism. Clin Perinatol 11:673–680, 1984
2. Enevoldsen EM, Jens T: Autoregulation and $CO_2$ responses of cerebral blood flow in patients with acute severe head injury. J Neurosurg 48:689–703, 1978
3. McMillan V, Siesjo BK: The influence of hypocapnia upon intracellular pH and upon some carbohydrate substrates, amino acids and organic phosphates in the brain. J Neurochem 21:1283–1289, 1973

4. Okuda Y, McDowall DC, Ali MM, Lane JR: Changes in $CO_2$ responsiveness and in autoregulation of the cerebral circulation during and after halothane induced hypotension. J Neurol Neurosurg Psychiat 39:221–230, 1976
5. Raicle HE, Posner JB, Plum F: Cerebral blood flow during and after hyperventilation. Arch Neurol 23:394–397, 1970
6. Reivich M: Arterial $Pa_{CO_2}$ and cerebral hemodynamics. Am J Physiol 206:25–35, 1964

*Hector E. James*

# 26

# Diuretic Therapy for Intracranial Hypertension

Diuretics have been extensively employed in the management of intracranial hypertension. The basis for this approach has been the attempt to dehydrate the brain in the presence of brain edema through reducing intracranial volume and subsequently intracranial pressure.

In that context, the effects of many solutions of varying concentrations on CSF pressure in studies of animals and humans has been extensively reported.[2,8,10,18,39,57] We discuss here only those pertinent ones in reference to current use in clinical practice.

## HYPERTONIC DIURETICS

These diuretics reportedly act by extracting water from the brain through the osmotic gradient generated in the capillary lumen by the medication, across the blood–brain barrier.[44,47] It thus follows that these agents are effective only in the presence of an intact blood–brain barrier; they will then extract water from normal brain parenchyma, and not in the grossly edematous brain.[26,44,47]

The most commonly employed diuretic of this group is mannitol. Hypertonic urea is effective in reducing ICP,[3,20,23,35,43] but the concern for its rapid diffusion into the tissues, as well as the difficulty in its manipulation, lead to its clinical replacement by mannitol. Glycerol has been employed for the control of ICP[9] and for the management of acute stroke,[40,41] but concerns about hemolysis and hematuria have restricted its widespread use.

Hypertonic diuretics have been noted to reduce ICP within minutes of

BRAIN INSULTS IN INFANTS AND CHILDREN
0-8089-1723-4

their administration when given by intravenous (IV) bolus in experimental animals[4,11,20,24,46,48] and human patients.[25] Cerebral blood flow measurements following hypertonic diuretics have yielded contradictory results.[21,30,31] Cerebral blood flow changes may create an increase in cerebral blood volume and consequently will raise ICP; however, intracranial elastance improves following mannitol administration,[36] and consequent improvement in microcirculation can then lead to improved brain function.

There is no uniform agreement as to dosage in mannitol therapy. Some have recommended small, frequent doses (0.25 g/kg) to minimize pendulum swings in serum osmolality and sodium,[38] whereas other authors noted that a dosage of 0.5 g/kg reduced ICP in only one-third of the patients,[34] or that after the first administration of a similar dose, there was no further reduction of ICP in the subsequent ones.[30] Over 90 percent of patients receiving doses of 1.0 g/kg have a significant reduction in ICP.[28,58] In the acute setting, therefore, this should be the preferred dose for the control of ICP.[27,28]

The rapidity of the ICP return to its pretreatment value following mannitol administration is not dose-related but it is strongly influenced by the magnitude of fluid replacement following administration of the agent.[28] In a study with hypertonic diuretics in dogs, the authors[29] noted a persistent reduction of ICP for many hours in all subgroups of the study except for the animals that received continuous fluid replacement in equal amounts to the urine output. In this last subgroup, ICP not only returned to pretreatment values, but also increased over those values (the so-called rebound-effect). Shenkin et al.[50] noted a reduction of the requirements for mannitol when the adult patients where on restricted IV fluid replacement. The authors recommended maintaining the patients' serum osmolality in the 290-mOsm/l range.[50]

The hazards of hypertonic diuretics should be noted. The sudden overload of the circulatory system by the shift of water into it may be deleterious to the patient.[1] Serum osmolality over 340 mOsm/l causes renal failure because of interference of the renal counter current mechanisms.[53] Osmolalities over 375 mOsm/l lead to cellular disruption and systemic acidosis.[52] Values between 300 and 310 mOsm/l indicate that the threshold for the blood–brain barrier for mannitol may be exceeded.[51] It may then allow for mannitol to move into the CSF and brain, moving water into these compartments if the gradient is adequate, thus increasing ICP.[46] It is thus mandatory to closely monitor the patient's hydration, serum osmolality, electrolyte balance, and state of renal function, especially in the small child.

## LOOP DIURETICS

In this group of diuretics furosemide has been most commonly employed. It has been shown effective in subacute and chronic administration regimes in reducing experimentally induced[12,15,22,37] and clinical forms of cerebral edema and intracranial hypertension.[5,22,49,54] Its mechanism of action is possibly related to a direct reduction of sodium transport into the brain, thus decreasing brain size.[12,56] It could also reduce ICP by its mechanism of inhibiting CSF production when administered IV or intracisternally.[7]

Furosemide has a major advantage over hypertonic diuretics in that it creates far less of a change on serum sodium, potassium, and osmolality.[13] This, in situations where less acute shifts in intravascular volume and protection of the myocardium from sudden load and work are desired, can be advantageous.

The effect of furosemide on brain water content is controversial. Although some studies have revealed a reduction in brain water content in the cryogenic brain edema experimental model,[12,37,45] others have not.[22] This may be related to the timing of measurement of brain water content in reference to furosemide administration. In the former series the administration was subacute or chronic, and in the latter it was acute.

Some investigators believe that furosemide does not act as effectively as mannitol in reducing ICP; therefore, its application for the control of ICP has not been extensive.

## CARBONIC ANHYDRASE INHIBITORS

Acetazolamide is the protype of this group, and in the past multiple experimental and clinical experiences have been reported testifying to its effectiveness in cerebral edema and ICP.[6,14,22,33,37,59] Other reports have been made indicating its ineffectiveness in these aspects.[19,22] Acetazolamide has been shown to reduce carbonic anhydrase activity, thereby decreasing CSF production.[16,32,55] It has also been shown to reduce cellular sodium influx in vitro and hence reduce cellular permeability; it could then be a mechanism for reducing brain edema.

Because of its inhibitory effect on carbonic anhydrase activity, the increase in carbon dioxide in the tissues leads to cerebral vasodilation.[17,33] This sudden release following acute IV administration of acetazolamide can significantly rise ICP, prior to reducing it.[22] Thus acetazolamide should not be administered IV in patients with elevated ICP. Prolonged usage of acetazolamide may lead to systemic metabolic acidosis.

## COMBINATION DIURETIC THERAPY

Multiple therapies are commonly employed in the clinical setting to control brain edema and ICP. The combination of diuretics is not a common practice for the control of ICP. In previous work we demonstrated no

**Table 26-1** *Diuretics Employed in Control of Intracranial Pressure*

| Diuretic | Dosage | Method of Administration | Solutions |
|---|---|---|---|
| Mannitol | 0.5–1.0 g/kg/dose | Intravenous | 10% or 20% solution |
| Furosemide | 1–5 mg/kg/dose | Intravenous, intramuscular, or oral | Vials, tablets, suspension |
| Acetazolamide | 10–20 mg/kg/dose | Intramuscular or Oral | Vials, tablets, suspension |

reduction of ICP in the combination of two diuretics different from the reduction that occurred when each diuretic was given alone.[22,42] No prolongation (in the acute setting) of the ICP nadir was noted.[22] Furosemide did, however, block the natural rise in ICP when acetazolamide was given IV.[22] In the chronic setting there may be an advantage to alternating mannitol and furosemide administrations. The net result is a reduction of the total amount of mannitol since it is more effective in long-term administration. Furosemide administration results in decrease of the total body sodium, permitting a "resetting" of serum and tissue osmotic gradients. One must realize that measurements of urinary electrolytes and close monitoring of the patient's water and electrolyte balance are mandatory.

Table 26-1 demonstrates dosage and methods of administration of diuretics for the control of ICP.

## REFERENCES


1. Aviram A, Pfan A, Czaczkes JW, et al: Hyperosmolality with hyponatremia caused by inappropriate administration of mannitol. Am J Med 42:648–650, 1967
2. Bakay L, Crawford JD, White JC: The effects of intravenous fluids on cerebrospinal fluid pressure. Surg Gynec 99:48–52, 1954
3. Beks JWF, Groen A, Huizinga I, et al: Effects of intravenously administered hypertonic urea solution. Acta Neurochir (Wien) 13:1–10, 1965
4. Beks J, ter Weeme C: The influence of urea and mannitol on increased intraventricular pressure in cold-induced cerebral edema. Acta Neurochir (Wien) 16:97–107, 1967
5. Bergland RM, Page RB, Howland WS: Furosemide: A non-osmotic diuretic for neurosurgical use. Presented at the 43rd Annual Meeting of the American Association of Neurological Surgeons, Miami Beach, Florida, April 8, 1975
6. Buhan S: Effect of acetazolamide (Diamox) on the water content and distribution in various segments of the central nervous system. Acta Med Jugosl 14:341–352, 1960
7. Buhrley L, Reed DJ: The effect of furosemide on sodium-22 uptake into cerebrospinal fluid and brain. Exp Brain Res 14:503–510, 1972

8. Bullock LT, Gregersen, JI, Kinney R: The use of hypertonic sucrose solution intravenously to reduce cerebrospinal fluid pressure without a secondary rise. Am J Physiol 112:82–96, 1935
9. Cantone G, Guidetti B, Virno M: Oral glycerol for reduction of intracranial pressure. J Neurosurg 21:278–283, 1964
10. Clasen RA, Prouty RR, Bingham WG, et al: Treatment of experimental cerebral edema with intravenous hypertonic glucose, albumin, and dextran. Surg Gynecol Obstet 104:591–606, 1957
11. Clasen, R, Cooke P, Pandolfi S, et al: Hypertonic urea in experimental cerebral edema. Arch Neurol (Chicago) 12:424–434, 1965
12. Clasen RA, Pandolfi S, Casey D Jr: Furosemide and pentobarbital in cryogenic cerebral injury and edema. Neurology (Minneapolis), 24:642–648, 1974
13. Cottrell JE, Robustelli A, Post K, et al: Furosemide- and mannitol-induced changes in intracranial pressure and serum osmolality and electrolytes. Anesthesiology 47:28–30, 1977
14. Demailly P: Acetazolamide in intracranial hypertension. Gaz Med France 69:2123–2124, 1962
15. Di Rocco C, Gentilomo A, Maira G, et al: L'azione combinata dei corticosteroidie dei diruetici nella prevenzione e nel trahamento dell'edema cerebrale. Minerva Neurochir 15:121–124, 1971
16. Domer F: Effects of diuretics on cerebrospinal fluid formation and potassium movement. Exp Neurol 24:54–64, 1969
17. Ehrenrich DL, Burns RA, Alhman RW, et al: Influence of acetazolamide on cerebral blood flow. Arch Neurol 5:227–232, 1961
18. Fishman RA: Effects of isotonic intravenous solutions on normal and increased intracranial pressure. Arch Neurol Psychiatr 70:350–360, 1953
19. Fishman RA: Brain edema. New Engl J Med 293:706–711, 1975
20. Fremont-Smith F, Forbes HS: Intra-ocular and intracranial pressure: An experimental study. Arch Neurol Psychiatr 18:550–564, 1927
21. Goluboff B, Shenkin H, Hoft H: The effects of mannitol and urea on cerebral hemodynamics and cerebrospinal fluid pressure. Neurology (Minneapolis) 14:891–898, 1964
22. Harbaugh RD, James HE, Marshall LF, et al: Acute therapeutic modalities for experimental vasogenic edema. Neurosurgery 5:656–665, 1979
23. Irvine MD: Administration of urea for reduction of intracranial and intraocular pressure. Am J Ophthalmol 49:164–166, 1960
24. Jaird M, Andersen J: The effect of urea on cerebrospinal fluid pressure in monkeys before and after bilateral nephrectomy. J Lab Clin Med 53:484–489, 1959
25. James HE, Langfitt TW, Kumar VS, et al: Treatment of intracranial hypertension: Analysis of 105 consecutive, continuous recordings of intracranial pressure. Acta Neurochir (Wien) 36:189–200, 1977
26. James HE, Bruce DA, Welsh F: Cytotoxic edema produced by 6-aminonicotinamide and its response to therapy. Neurosurg 3:196–200, 1978
27. James HE: Analysis of therapeutic modalities for head injured children. Child's Brain 5:263–271, 1979
28. James HE: Methodology for control of intracranial pressure with hypertonic mannitol. Acta Neurochir 51:161–172, 1980
29. Javid M, Gilboe D, Cesario T: The rebound phenomenon and hypertonic solutions. J Neurosurg 21:1059–1066, 1964
30. Johnston IH, Paterson A, Harper AM, et al: The effect of mannitol on intracranial pressure and cerebral blood flow, in Brock M, Dietz H (Eds): ICP, Berlin, Springer, 1972, pp 176–180
31. Johnston IH, Harper AM: The effect of mannitol on cerebral blood flow: An experimental study. J Neurosurg 36:461–471, 1973
32. Kister SJ: Carbonic anhydrase inhibition: VI. The effect of acetazolamide on cerebrospinal fluid flow. J Pharmacol Exp Ther 117:402–405, 1956

33. Knopp LN, Atkinson JR, Ward AA Jr: Effect of diamox on cerebrospinal fluid pressure of cat and monkey. Neurology (Minneapolis) 7:119–123, 1957
34. Kullberg G, Sundbarg G: Reduction of raised intracranial pressure following infusion of mannitol, in Beks JWF, Bosch DA, Brock M (Eds): ICP III. Berlin, Springer, 1976, pp 224–227
35. Langfitt TW: Possible mechanisms of action of hypertonic urea in reducing intracranial pressure. Neurology 11:196–209, 1961
36. Leech P, Miller JD: Intracranial volume-pressure relationships during experimental brain compression in primates. 3. Effects of mannitol and hyperventilation. J Neurol Neurosurg Psychiatr 37:1105–1111, 1974
37. Long D, Maxwell R and Choi KS: A new therapy regimen for brain edema, in Pappius HM, Feindel W (Eds): Dynamics of Brain Edema, New York, Springer-Verlag, 1976, pp 293–300
38. Marshall LF, Smith RW, Rauscher LA, et al: Mannitol dose requirements in brain-injured patients. J Neurosurg 48:169–172, 1972
39. Masserman JH: Effects of intravenous administration of hypertonic solutions of dextrose. With special reference to the cerebrospinal fluid pressure. JAMA 102:2084–2086, 1934
40. Meyer JS, Channey JZ, Rivera VM, et al: Treatment of cerebral edema due to acute cerebral infarction with glycerol. Lancet 2:993–997, 1971
41. Meyer JS, Fukuuchi Y, Shimazu K, et al: Effects of intravenous infusion of glycerol on hemispheric blood flow in patients with acute cerebral infarction. Stroke 3:168–180, 1972
42. Millson CH, James HE, Shapiro HM, et al: Intracranial hypertension and brain edema in albino rabbits. Part 3. Effect of simultaneous diuretic and barbiturate therapy. Acta Neurochirurgica 61:271–280, 1982
43. McQueen JD, Jeanes LD: Dehydration and rehydration of the brain with hypertonic urea and mannitol. J Neursurg 21:118–128, 1964
44. Pappius HM, Dayes LA: Hypertonic urea: Its effect on the distribution of water and electrolytes in normal and edematous brain tissue. Arch Neurol 13:395–402, 1965
45. Pappius HM: Effects of steroids on cold injury edema, in Reulen HJ, Schurmann K (Eds): Steroids and Brain Edema. New York, Springer-Verlag, 1972, pp 57–63
46. Prill A, Volles E, Dahlman W: Stabilization and disturbance of osmoregulation in the cerebrospinal fluid, in Brock M, Dietz H (Eds): ICP. Berlin, Springer, 1972, pp 303–308
47. Reed DJ, Woodbury DM: Effect of hypertonic urea on cerebrospinal fluid pressure and brain volume. J Physiol 164:252–264, 1962
48. Reed D, Woodbury D: Effect of urea and acetazolamide on brain volume and cerebrospinal fluid pressure. J Physiol 164:265–273, 1962
49. Rose AL, Millac P: The treatment of benign intracranial hypertension with furosemide. J Neurol Sci 3:606–608, 1966
50. Shenkin HA, Beizier HS, Bouzarth WF: Restricted fluid intake. J Neurosurg 45:432–436, 1976
51. Silber SJ, Thompson N: Mannitol-induced central nervous system toxicity in renal failure. Invest Urol 9:310–312, 1972
52. Sotos JF, Dodge PR, Meara P, et al: Studies in experimental hypertonicity. Pediatrics 26:925–928, 1960
53. Stuart FP, Rorres E, Fletcher D, et al: Effects of repeated and massive mannitol infusion in the dog. Structural and functional changes in kidney and brain. Am Surg 172:190–204, 1970
54. Thilmann J, Zeumer H: Untersuchungen zur Behandlung des hirnodems mit hohen Dosen Furosemid. Deutsch Med Wochenschr 99:932–935, 1974
55. Tschirgi RD, Frost RW, Taylor JL: Inhibition of cerebrospinal fluid formation by a carbonic anhydrase inhibitor, 2-acetylamino-1,3,4-thiadiazole-5-sulfonamide (Diamox). Proc Soc Exp Biol Med 87:373–376, 1954

56. Tutt HP, Pappius HM: Studies on the mechanism of action of steroids in traumatized brain, in Reulen HJ, Schurmann K (Eds): Steroids and Brain Edema, New York, Springer-Verlag, 1972, pp 147–151
57. Weed LH, McKibben PS: Pressure changes in the cerebrospinal fluid following intravenous injection of solutions of various concentrations. Am J Physiol 48:512–530, 1919
58. Wise BL, Chater N: The value of hypertonic mannitol solution in decreasing brain mass and lowering cerebrospinal fluid pressure. J Neurosurg 19:1038–1043, 1963
59. Wistrand P, Nechay BR, Maren TH: Effects of carbonic anhydrase inhibition on cerebrospinal and intraocular fluids in the dog. Acta Pharacol (Kbh) 17:315–336, 1961

*Mark A. Rockoff*

# 27

# Barbiturate Therapy

Patients with severe head injury frequently develop intracranial hypertension. Occasionally, this is unresponsive to the most diligent use of conventional therapies. Brain death may result from herniation of brain tissue, but more subtle changes can occur as cerebral perfusion is compromised.[8] Since uncontrolled intracranial pressure (ICP) is invariably associated with death,[5,14,16,22] newer methods have been employed in those patients refractory to treatment. Although many agents have been utilized, barbiturates have received the most attention. The review presented in this chapter discusses the use of barbiturate therapy in these circumstances.

## HISTORY

Shortly after barbiturates were introduced into clinical practice, the ICP-lowering properties of these agents were described.[6] Even in these early studies, it was noted that doses sufficient to produce anesthesia were necessary to lower ICP; however, barbiturates were not used for this purpose until the 1970s. The first clinical reports involved the use of barbiturates as induction agents for anesthesia in patients undergoing craniotomy for tumor.[18] Although barbiturates were clearly useful, they did occasionally produce systemic arterial hypotension.

A natural extension of this experience was to use barbiturates outside the operating room in intensive care units (ICUs) to control ICP in patients refractory to conventional therapies. Thus the concept of "barbiturate coma" was developed. Actually, this term is a misnomer since patients were already comatose as a result of brain injury and barbiturates were utilized only in an attempt to treat intracranial hypertension. No patients were rendered coma-

BRAIN INSULTS IN INFANTS AND CHILDREN
0-8089-1723-4

tose by the administration of the barbiturates or any other drugs. Nevertheless, the concept of giving sedative or anesthetic agents to neurologically impaired patients provoked a great deal of controversy from its inception.

## RATIONALE

A multitude of explanations have been proposed to explain the central nervous system (CNS) protective effects of barbiturate anesthesia. Presumably ICP is lowered because barbiturates decrease cerebral metabolism and blood flow, resulting in a decrease in cerebral blood volume (CBV).[12,15] Since most inhalational anesthesia agents are cerebral vasodilators, barbiturates rapidly became the mainstay of neuroanesthesia practice.

In addition, the ability to decrease cerebral metabolism and induce an anesthetic state could be used to prevent adverse responses to noxious stimuli. Although a patient with severe head injury (or any other central nervous system insult) might be comatose, preservation of autonomic responses to painful stimulation persists unless the patient is brain dead. Many procedures necessary for the care of critically ill patients (including endotracheal intubation, tracheal suctioning, catheterizations, etc.) will produce hypertension, tachycardia, agitation and pain unless blunted by sufficient quantities of analgesics and sedatives. The ability of barbiturates to anesthetize patients is utilized daily in operating room anesthesia practice and may be beneficial in certain conditions in the ICU.

Barbiturates also are effective anticonvulsants and may be useful in prevention or treatment of clinical (or subclinical) seizure disorders. This may be particularly beneficial in patients who are given neuromuscular blocking agents to facilitate operative procedures and/or mechanical ventilation, in whom detection of seizures without continuous electroencephalographic monitoring is impossible. Other more speculative theories, including scavenging of free radicals, have been proposed but are unproven.

## CLINICAL APPLICATION

### Patient Selection

Those patients whose ICP remains refractory to conventional medical therapy may benefit from a trial of barbiturates. This implies that the patient already has:

1. Adequate oxygenation
2. Airway protection with endotracheal intubation

3. Mechanical hyperventilation
4. Hyperosmolality (osmotic agents and/or diuretics)
5. Normotension
6. Absence of hyperthermia
7. Control of abnormal motor function (use of muscle relaxants, if necessary)

Failure to respond to conventional therapy usually means that direct ICP monitoring reveals an abnormality. This includes a persistently elevated baseline ICP greater than 15 mmHg, a "normal" ICP (less than 15 mmHg) but with an abnormal intracranial compliance to formal compliance testing, or frequent pressure "waves" of ICP greater than 20 mmHg lasting more than a few minutes and occurring either spontaneously or with stimulation.

Occasionally, barbiturates can (and probably should) be utilized without ICP monitoring. In some emergency situations, ICP is likely to be elevated on presentation of the patient to the emergency room, and treatment is necessary before an ICP monitoring device can be inserted. For example, the child who arrives with decerebrate posturing, abnormal respirations, and systemic hypertension after an isolated head injury needs immediate airway control, and barbiturates (along with muscle relaxants) facilitate the smooth performance of this procedure. Furthermore, such a child will need an emergency computed tomography (CT) scanning, and the use of barbiturate anesthesia can help to produce a controlled immobile state. This is frequently preferable to administration of increasing amounts of intravenous (IV) sedative drugs to just "get by" during a brief radiological procedure. If scanning reveals an intracranial hematoma, anesthesia will be continued for the operative procedure. If no intracranial mass is appreciated, the patient will be transported to the ICU, where an ICP monitor can be inserted. This will assist in determining if further barbiturate therapy is necessary.

As with all medical therapies for patients with severe head injury, barbiturates are not a substitute for the rapid evacuation of intracranial hematomas.[3] It should be recalled that intracranial hematomas may occur late (after a normal CT scan) as a result of delayed bleeding or complications from ICP monitoring devices, and repeat CT scanning should be considered in patients not responding to treatment.

## Agents and Dosages

Many different barbiturates have been employed.[4,16,17] The amounts used would produce sleep in healthy patients and are sufficient to depress cortical electrical activity.[20] The ultra-short acting agents have the advantage of immediate onset and rapid redistribution. Thiopental (Pentothal, manufactured by Abbott; 2–5 mg/kg) works within seconds and has an effective duration of a few minutes to less than 1 hour. Although the half-life of this drug is quite prolonged, redistribution to tissue stores occurs rapidly and limits duration of action. Methohexital (Brevital, manufactured by Lilly; 1–2 mg/kg) has a similar effect but can promote seizures in some patients with complex seizure disorders. Pentobarbital (Nembutal, manufactured by Abbott; 3–30 mg/kg) may be used if a more prolonged effect is desired. Maintenance doses are on the order of 1–2 mg/kg/h. If pentobarbital is given by continuous IV infusion, marked fluctuations in blood pressure are less likely to occur. Similarly, thiopental may be given by constant infusion. When the drug is administered in this manner, redistribution becomes less important as body stores are saturated with drug, and a prolonged duration of action occurs as drug metabolism assumes the major responsibility for limiting drug effect. The starting dosage is then adjusted according to the values of ICP and blood pressure.

Phenobarbital (Luminal, manufactured by Winthrop) may also be administered in anesthetic quantities (50–150 mg/kg). It may have an advantage over the other barbiturates when anticonvulsant action is the major effect desired. However, it takes longer (minutes) to reach maximum brain concentrations and has a very prolonged recovery because it has a half-life of many days.

As with any anesthetic agents, drug doses are only a rough guideline to amounts necessary (or tolerated). Clearly, the minimal amount necessary to produce the desired effect should be utilized. If ICP control is of concern, the correct amount is that necessary to control ICP and no more. Likewise, if immobilization is desired (to facilitate CT scanning), these drugs should be titrated to effect. Generally, all administered drugs should be given slowly (over a few minutes).

#### Side Effects

It has already been mentioned that anesthetic quantities of barbiturates are usually necessary to lower ICP. On the other hand, sedative amounts of barbiturates may be helpful in preventing agitation, which can lead to intracranial hypertension. As increasing amounts of barbiturates are administered, respiratory depression will occur. This should not be a problem in patients already comatose and receiving mechanical ventilation. The most significant complication with anesthetic quantities of these drugs is arterial hypotension.[4,21] This will invariably occur in all patients if enough barbiturates are given. It is initially due to an increase in venous capacitance and will respond to IV volume infusions. Since free water is restricted in patients with cerebral edema, colloid solutions are probably best used. Central venous pressure monitoring is useful in estimation of fluid requirements, especially since urine output may be unreliable in patients receiving diuretic and/or osmotic agents. Hypotension is frequently exacerbated by high ventilatory pressures and dehydration secondary to fluid restriction and use of osmotic agents.

When systemic hypotension develops despite adequate intravascular volume, it is a reflection of myocardial depression. Sympathomimetic agents (such as dopamine) are useful in maintaining cardiac output, but this usually represents an unwanted effect of barbiturates. It is important to remember that attempts are made to lower ICP in order to improve cerebral perfusion pressure (the difference between blood pressure and ICP). The adverse effects of hypotension may outweigh any ICP-lowering effect of the drug at these levels. Although sympathomimetic agents may be helpful to counterbalance this response transiently, hypotension is usually a sign that an excessive amount of barbiturates is being administered. There is little evidence to support the use of even more barbiturates during simultaneous administration of more sympathomimetic agents. Blood levels can be followed but usually add little to the clinical management of patients beyond that provided by carefully titrating the drug. Assays for specific barbiturates must be performed if multiple different barbiturates have been administered.

### Patient Monitoring

When sufficient quantities of barbiturates are given to produce an anesthetic state, the clinical neurological examination is lost and it is difficult to follow the patient's clinical course to look for signs of improvement or deterioration. The only neurological reflex that persists with high-dose barbiturate anesthesia is pupillary function. Barbiturates usually cause pupillary constriction, and dilated pupils are indicative of light anesthesia, hypoxia and ischemia, seizures, or uncontrolled ICP. Dilated pupils may also develop in patients receiving dopamine.

However, additional monitoring can be used to provide information about the brain in the absence of the clinical examination.[7] Most important is direct ICP monitoring. Certainly problems are encountered with all currently available techniques; however, only through knowledge of the ICP can barbiturates be titrated to produce the best effect with the least complications. Except for the brief emergency use of barbiturates, all patients who are receiving high-dose barbiturate therapy for intracranial hypertension should have continuous ICP monitoring.

Electrophysiological monitoring may be helpful. Although high-dose barbiturate anesthesia invariably suppresses the electroencephalogram,[1] it permits a direct assessment of the presence or absence of seizures. Auditory, visual, and somatosensory evoked potentials may be followed and maintain their integrity to a high degree despite administration of barbiturates. Severely impaired responses are usually indicative of significant neurological damage.

Computed tomographic scanning is performed to assure that no surgically correctible lesion is present. Repeat scans are helpful to assess progress and to detect lesions that may subsequently develop.

### Cessation of Therapy

When a stable clinical state has been maintained for approximately 24 hours, withdrawal of therapy is usually considered. The most potentially problematic treatment is the first to go. If induced hypothermia has been employed, for example, body temperature is gradually returned to normal. Barbiturate dosage should be tapered to avoid sudden changes; the dose is conveniently reduced approximately 25 percent every 6–12 hours. If ICP elevation develops, barbiturates can be augmented if more conventional methods fail to produce a response. If a therapeutic phenytoin level is obtained before barbiturates are withdrawn, prophylaxis against seizures may be provided and will not obscure the neurological examination. Patients who receive high-dose barbiturates for many days may have a slow recovery despite a fall in their measured blood levels.

### Results

When ICP is monitored, there is no doubt that high doses of barbiturates can lower ICP when conventional methods fail.[9–11,16,19] What is controversial is whether this decrease in ICP improves outcome.[13] Nevertheless, it appears reasonable that since intractable intracranial hypertension following an acute brain insult is almost invariably fatal, methods that reduce ICP should be utilized as long as ICP is being monitored to guide drug administration to minimize adverse effects.

Patients whose ICPs do not respond (at least transiently) to barbiturates almost invariably have an unfavorable prognosis (death or vegetative survival).[14,16] These patients rarely respond to other methods of ICP control either, and probably have sustained a sufficient amount of neurological damage to impair cerebral vascular responsiveness.

Some patients will respond only transiently to barbiturates and then "breakthrough." Hopefully, the time gained will have been used to treat surgically correctible lesions or maximize other medical therapy. Barbiturate anesthesia may also be helpful in simplifying medical management. For example, mannitol requirements may be reduced in head-injured patients treated with barbiturates, and this may help to prevent the development of fluid and electrolyte problems.[10]

Certainly, nursing procedures are easier and more effectively performed in patients who are well anesthetized and, therefore, not struggling, coughing, and so on. This "nonspecific" effect of barbiturate anesthesia may contribute to some reports of improvement in outcome following barbiturate anesthesia in animal models of acute neurological injury.[2]

## REFERENCES


1. Bird TD, Plum F: Recovery from barbiturate overdose coma with a prolonged isoelectric electroencephalogram. Neurology 18:456–460, 1968
2. Bleyaert AL, Safar P, Stezoski SW, et al: Amelioration of postischemic brain damage in the monkey by immobilization and controlled ventilation. Crit Care Med 6:112–113, 1978
3. Bruce DA, Schut L, Bruno LA, et al: Outcome following severe head injuries in children. J Neurosurg 48:679–688, 1978
4. Carlon GC, Kahn RC, Goldiner PL, et al: Long-term infusion of sodium thiopental: Hemodynamic and respiratory effects. Crit Care Med 6:311–316, 1978
5. Dean JM, McComb JG: Intracranial pressure monitoring in severe pediatric near-drowning. Neurosurgery 9:627–630, 1981
6. Horsley JG: Intracranial pressure during barbital narcosis. Lancet 1:141–143, 1937
7. Lundar T, Ganes T, Lindegaard KF: Induced barbiturate coma: Methods for evaluation of patients. Crit Care Med 11:559–562, 1983
8. Marsh ML, Marshall LF, Shapiro HM: Neurosurgical intensive care. Anesthesiology 47:149–163, 1977
9. Marshall LF, Hoi Sang U: Treatment of massive intraoperative brain swelling. Neurosurgery 13:412–414, 1983
10. Marshall LF, Shapiro HM, Rauscher A, et al: Pentobarbital therapy for intracranial hypertension in metabolic coma (Reye's syndrome). Crit Care Med 6:1–5, 1978
11. Marshall LF, Smith RW, Shapiro HM: The outcome with aggressive treatment in severe head injuries: I. The significance of intracranial pressure monitoring; II. Acute and chronic barbiturate administration in the management of head injury. J Neurosurg 50:20–30, 1979
12. Michenfelder JD. The interdependency of cerebral function and metabolic effects following massive doses of thiopental in the dog. Anesthesiology 41:231–236, 1974
13. Miller JD: Barbiturate and raised intracranial pressure. Ann Neurol 6:189–193, 1979
14. Miller JD, Becker DP, Ward JD, et al: Significance of intracranial hypertension in severe head injury. J Neurosurg 47:503–516, 1977
15. Pierce EC, Lambertsen CT, Deutsch S, et al: Cerebral circulation and metabolism during thiopental anesthesia and hyperventilation in man. J Clin Invest 41,1664–1671, 1962
16. Rockoff MA, Marshall LF, Shapiro HM: High-dose barbiturate therapy in humans: A clinical review of sixty patients. Ann Neurol 6:194–199, 1979
17. Sawada Y, Sugimoto H, Kobayashi H, et al. Acute tolerance to high-dose barbiturate treatment in patients with severe head injuries. Anesthesiology 56:53–54, 1982

18. Shapiro HM, Galindo A, Wyte SR, et al: Rapid intraoperative reduction of ICP with thiopentone. Br J Anaesth 45:1057–1061, 1973
19. Shapiro HM, Wyte SR, Loeser J: Barbiturate-augmented hypothermia for reduction of persistent intracranial hypertension. J Neurosurg 40:90–100, 1974
20. Steen PA, Michenfelder JD: Cerebral protection with barbiturates. Relation to anesthetic effect. Stroke 9:140–142, 1978
21. Traeger SM, Henning RJ, Dobkin W, et al: Hemodynamic effects of pentobarbital therapy for intracranial pressure. Crit Care Med 11:697–701, 1983
22. Woodcock J, Ropper AH, Kennedy SK: High dose barbiturates in non-traumatic brain swelling: ICP reduction and effect on outcome. Stroke 13:785–787, 1982

# Index

## B



## C

## I



## K



## L

## M



## N